ADVANCE PRAISE FOR
WHEN HEALING BECOMES A CRIME

"This book needs to be read by every health care professional and legislator, as well as every citizen, since we are all potential patients during our lifetime. I hope it will allow people to open their minds and explore true healing. True healing should never be a crime, nor healers criminals."
Bernie Siegel, M.D., author of *Love, Medicine, and Miracles*

"This book is indispensable to anyone interested in botanical medicine, but it is also of urgent importance to everyone concerned about health and cancer and government regulation. In fact, this masterful telling of a fascinating story should appeal to everybody who likes a great yarn. Not just good information, good reading. Enjoy."
James Duke, author of *The Green Pharmacy*

"The saga of Harry Hoxsey has long been enshrouded in myths promoted by zealous promoters and detractors. At long last, Kenny Ausubel has cut through this thick fog of legend to bring us a detailed, factual, and exciting account of Hoxsey's treatment for cancer. He has dug up obscure sources with incredible energy and ingenuity. Every reader who is interested in medical history and in the question of what really works in cancer therapy will want to read and re-read this incredible true story."
Ralph Moss, author of *The Cancer Industry* and *Cancer Therapy: The Independent Consumer's Guide to Non-Toxic Treatment and Prevention*

"Ausubel's book is a triumph of elegant prose and scholarly understatement. It is the last word on the history of the decades-old 'Quackbuster' conspiracy by the cancer establishment—the National Cancer Institute, the American Cancer Society, and the AMA—to protect the monopolistic drug industry against competition from promising alternative therapies."
Samuel Epstein, M.D., author of *The Politics of Cancer* and *The Safe Shopper's Bible*

When Healing Becomes a Crime

When Healing Becomes a Crime

The Amazing Story of the Hoxsey Cancer Clinics and the Return of Alternative Therapies

KENNY AUSUBEL

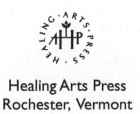

Healing Arts Press
Rochester, Vermont

Healing Arts Press
One Park Street
Rochester, Vermont 05767
www.InnerTraditions.com

Healing Arts Press is a division of Inner Traditions International

Note to the reader: This book is intended as an informational guide. The remedies, approaches, and techniques described herein are meant to supplement, and not to be a substitute for, professional medical care or treatment. They should not be used to treat a serious ailment without prior consultation with a qualified health care professional.

Library of Congress Cataloging-in-Publication Data

Ausubel, Kenny.
    When healing becomes a crime : the amazing story of the Hoxsey cancer clinics and the return of alternative therapies / Kenny Ausubel.
        p.   cm.
    Includes bibliographical references.
    ISBN 978-0-89281-925-6 (alk. paper)
    1. Cancer—Alternative treatment. 2. Herbs—Therapeutic use. 3. Hoxsey, Harry M. I. Title.

RC271.H47 A975 2000
616.99'406—dc21   99-461975

Printed and bound in the United States

20 19 18 17 16 15 14 13 12 11

Text design and layout by Priscilla Baker
This book was typeset in Janson, with Tiepolo as the display typeface.

Contents

PART THREE

Money, Power, and Cancer: Healing the Politics of Medicine

Foreword

by Bernie Siegel, M.D.

Dr. Bernie Siegel is a cancer surgeon, bestselling author, and pioneer in the field of mind-body healing. He founded the Exceptional Cancer Patient Program, a support group system enabling cancer patients to mobilize their full human resources for healing.

When Healing Becomes a Crime needs to be read by every health care professional and legislator, as well as every citizen, since we are all potential patients during our lifetime. Its importance lies not in convincing anyone of the efficacy of Hoxsey's treatment, but in demonstrating the closed-mindedness of the medical profession. We must not keep repeating the scenario and making criminals out of well-intentioned people.

Twenty-five years ago I was chastised for suggesting that personality, life events, and state of mind had an effect on the course of one's cancer. Although this was something others had seen fifty years prior to my awareness, I am still on some Web site quack lists. Years ago I was on all the talk shows and was exposed to criticism for causing guilt and blaming people for their illness. None of this was true, but no one wanted to support my research or listen to what I had to say—except the people who had the illness. Today many doctors have come around to my view because they or their loved ones developed cancer and they experienced first-hand the power of the human spirit under desperate circumstances.

We need to change the system so that future doctors do not receive just medical information but are given a true education. They need to learn how to treat *people*, not diagnoses. They need to be trained to be willing to accept that which is experienced. We have to remember there is more to healing a person than there is to curing a disease.

The system needs to open up so that the pages of medical journals are not 50 percent pharmaceutical ads, thus closing minds and doors to alternative and integrative treatments. In the future, companies need to be rewarded for researching alternative treatments that cannot be patented.

Our government could easily remedy that with tax breaks and deductions for the cost of the research, while allowing the company doing the research to profit from its work in a similar manner to any other commercial venture.

I hope this book will awaken people to the possibilities of true healing. Yes, I am against quackery—taking advantage of sick people—even though believing in a quack may cure someone whom a doctor has declared hopeless. What I seek is an open system to assure that we do the research and give people the information, enabling them to make rational choices that are appropriate for them. Life is a labor pain and we each have the right to decide what pains we are willing to experience to give birth to ourselves.

When my father was dying of cancer, I ordered medication from overseas to give him hope. One day I received a phone call from the post office. They told me the FDA wouldn't allow the package to be delivered unless it was labeled botanical products rather than medication, so the change was made and we received the medication. Someone in the post office treated us like human beings and cared. We are all entitled to make decisions about our lives and health. Let us hope that some day our medical and health care systems include freedom of choice, communication, appropriate research, and the *desire* to help the patient experiencing the disease.

I've had it easier than Harry Hoxsey because I was a doctor, and when people saw that what I did worked, it became policy. Today the things I was criticized for are a part of quality treatment. No one is against success, so let us approach health care with an open mind and acceptance of what works. And as healers, let us not forget the Hippocratic Oath, whose central message is, "First do no harm." True healing should never be a crime, or healers criminals. May *When Healing Becomes a Crime* herald the beginning of a new era of medical care that is inquisitive, compassionate, and devoted to making people well.

Acknowledgments

Because my work with Hoxsey began in 1983, there are many to thank: My special thanks and admiration to Peter Barry Chowka, whose inquisitive reporting and tireless activism first alerted many of us to the Hoxsey story and the clinic's survival in Mexico.

To Mildred Nelson, who gave of herself generously in the creation of both this book and the film, though these were some of her least favorite things to do. It is hard to know what more to say about Mildred than what I have portrayed in these pages. And to her sister Liz Jonas, who also cooperated freely.

To Catherine Salveson, an ally in this work since we undertook it together in 1983, whose dedication to a more humane, patient-centered medicine continues admirably.

Special gratitude to the Hoxsey patients who gave so openly and courageously in the telling of their personal stories, including Margaret Griffin, Stephen Crutcher, Martha Bond, Rex Major, and most especially to Gwen Scott, who assisted in many other ways. Also to Mike Oller, although his story did not make it into the book. To Raul, who amazingly still drives that van and brings hope, comfort, and help to cancer patients.

To J. P. Harpignies, who doggedly read draft after draft and offered uniquely insightful criticism, perspective, and fortitude.

To Nina Simons, my partner and wife, who did the same, while tolerating my intermittent obsession throughout a twelve-year cycle.

To my agent and friend Nina Reznick, who provided astute editorial guidance and worked far beyond the call of duty to bring it to publication.

To Susannah Schroll, the perennial angel who kept me on the Hoxsey path and repeatedly facilitated my ability to pursue this book.

To Ehud Sperling, Jon Graham, and Rowan Jacobsen of Inner Traditions for sharing the vision and bringing it to fruition.

To Ralph Moss, Francis Brinker, Gar and Christeene Hildenbrand, Dr. Samuel Epstein, Mary Ann Richardson, Dennis McKenna, Dr. Bernie Siegel, Catherine Salveson, and Mark Blumenthal for their participation as well as their generosity in checking relevant portions for accuracy. To

Uzondu Jinuike for his assistance with surfing the medical Web and making sense of it for me. To Nancy Carleton for her keen editorial eye and encouragement at a crucial transition. To my brother Jesse Ausubel and mother, Anne, for critiquing the manuscript honestly.

To: Dr. Larry Dossey and Dr. Andrew Weil for their encouragement and assistance; Steve Cary, who shared the original vision of the book and helped make it happen; Alice Martell for her early belief and efforts; Micalea Sullivan, who began and ended the project with incalculable assistance in research and citations; and Karen Farrell and Debbie Doyle of Wordswork, my transcription angels.

To all those who helped the documentary film happen: Researcher extraordinaire Ray Hemenez, who picked up the scent and has still not stopped pursuing it with me, and whose contribution has been inestimable; Josh Mailman and John Ross, who bravely anted up the first adventure capital; the late Ernie Shinagawa, the exceptional editor who found the movie when I got lost in the weeds; and Nina Simons, who helped decisively in securing the film's distribution and sales and never lost faith even against unlikely odds. The crew, whose dedication proved that "it all shows on screen": David Brownlow, Alton Walpole, Murray Van Dyke, Ernie Shinagawa, Suzanne Jamison, and Sarah Gartner. Max Gail, who brought his heart and soul to the screen. Peter Rowan and Jeff Nelson, who gave elegant music to the story, and Baird Banner, who captured it. Dr. Hugh Riordan, who checked all medical records and verified the new reality we all entered. The associate producers: David Brownlow, Laurel Hargarten, Ray Hemenez, Diana Sottler Lee, Andrea Nasher, Murray Van Dyke. Production associates: Luke Gatto, Alan Marks, Carolyn Bruce Rose, John Ross, Josh Mailman. To Carroll Williams and the Anthropology Film Center. And to: Gilbert Asher, Ann Farr Bartol, Ravi Batra, Julie Berman, Cheri Briggs, Jeffrey Bronfman, Gene Cameron, Barbara Chamberlain, William Cunningham, John Garvey, Neal Goodwin, Jerald Juhnke, Robert Klavetter, Patrick and Tina Lancione, Michael Lattimore, Ann Marks, Jan Marks, Rick Moss, Greg Pardes, Jenane Patterson, Vernal and Vita Salveson, Elvie and Melvin Sites, Milton and Pamela Sites, Jan Sultan, Andrea Swift, Christine Westfeldt, and Maguerite Wainio.

To Moctesuma Esparza and Robert Katz, who also assisted greatly in the film's distribution, and who have kept the faith along with Jan Wieringa toward producing its next expression as a dramatic feature film. Special thanks in this regard also to Susannah Schroll, Robert Barnhart, Edward Naumes, Dr. Robert Dozer, Dr. Alex Cadoux, Susanna Dakin, Tara Sterling, and Nina Reznick.

Introduction

"**M**y fight against cancer includes chemotherapy, Swedish massage, and relaxing to the muffled rhythms of Tibetan drums." This advertising tag line, floating above the close-up of a smiling middle-aged woman wearing a cheerful bandanna to hide her hair loss, looks at first glance like a feel-good promotion for a holistic California clinic. Expensively placed in the *New York Times*, instead the ad heralds the opening of the new Integrative Medicine Center at Memorial Sloan-Kettering Cancer Center, the bulwark of the cancer establishment that has historically abhorred such alternative influences—until 1999, that is.

Although this shift appears sudden, it actually marks the surprising reversal in a centuries-long power struggle, a bitter medical civil war between conventional and alternative approaches. After a long exile, these alternative therapies are now ascendant, riding a crest of popular demand, scientific validation, and commercial promise. Actually the tide is just starting to turn, and the face of cancer treatment may soon become almost unrecognizable as valuable alternative therapies permeate mainstream practice.

If Harry Hoxsey had lived to witness this apparent sea change in medicine, he would likely feel very mixed emotions. He would heartily cheer the grassroots surge propelling the movement, the same kind that once carried his Hoxsey Cancer Clinics to unmatched heights of popularity and validation. He would be exhilarated by the philosophical conversion of his enemies. But he would also be cynical, suspicious that a clinging monopoly was fighting to save face and above all keep its corner on the cancer market. But then, Hoxsey survived decades of being "hunted like a wild beast" only to see his clinics padlocked without a scientific test. He died a broken man, anguished over the future he felt was robbed from himself and from humanity. The Hoxsey treatment did live on, thriving as an underground legend still attracting more patients today than any of the other banished therapies, irrepressible after all.

The astonishing saga of the rise and fall and rebirth of the Hoxsey Cancer Clinics provides a classic case history of the corrosive medical politics that have long prevented the fair investigation of promising alternative cancer therapies, the kinds of practices whose ultimate acceptance now seems inevitable. When the government's Office of Alternative Medicine, part of the National Institutes of Health, recently commissioned a preliminary scientific review of Hoxsey, it signaled a radical departure, a seeming cease-fire in organized medicine's nearly seventy-five-year crusade against this reputed "cancer quackery." The government was finally giving a state nod to what is arguably the most notorious alternative cancer therapy in American history.

Hoxsey's powerful archenemy, the American Medical Association, had previously crystallized the medical establishment's sentiments in its supremely influential *Journal of the American Medical Association (JAMA)*. "It is fair to observe that the American Medical Association or any other association or individual has no need to go beyond the Hoxsey label to be convinced. Any such person who would seriously contend that scientific medicine is under any obligation to investigate such a mixture or its promoter is either stupid or dishonest."[1]

Paradoxically, this long-standing denunciation has not been based on the objective scientific evidence that is supposed to determine the acceptance or rejection of medical therapies. Rather, the dismissal typifies the kind of prefactual conclusion that has characterized "scientific" medicine's century-long pattern of condemnation without investigation.

Today substantial laboratory data indicates that the Hoxsey herbal tonic could have genuine value against cancer. Thousands of patients believe it saved their lives. There is no dispute that the Hoxsey remedies for *external* cancer are effective. Over the course of this century, numerous prominent figures including senators, congressmen, judges, and even doctors have affirmed Hoxsey's reputed cures and repeatedly called for an investigation. Why, then, has it taken so long?

The answer is buried in medical politics. It revolves around a fierce trade war fought over money as well as a fundamental conflict of medical opinion. Its consequence has been the exclusion and outright suppression of Hoxsey as well as numerous other unorthodox cancer therapies.

In fact, that war is subsiding at the precise moment when yesterday's "quackery" is repeatedly emerging as tomorrow's medicine. As the preeminent herbal cancer therapy, Hoxsey is now revisiting a therapeutic terrain dramatically expanding to embrace botanical and natural medicine. Its return symbolizes a much larger social transformation.

This book is a kind of investigative biography of this granddaddy of alternative cancer therapies. By exploring the unorthodox careers of renegade healers Harry Hoxsey and Mildred Nelson, we hold a mirror to the turbulent social and economic forces shaping medicine across the rich arc of the twentieth century. The story provides a perfect miniature of modern cancer politics while unearthing its ancient roots. It helps decode the arcane legacy of retrograde public policies still haunting us today, illuminating the emerging path to a future that is meaningfully inclusive of natural medicine.

This journey through the shadow side of medicine does raise very disturbing questions. If there were unorthodox treatments for cancer that were effective, would doctors even know about them? By refusing to investigate, has organized medicine denied countless people access to potentially life-saving therapies? And who has the ultimate right to determine the health-care choices of patients, especially people facing life-threatening illnesses for which conventional medicine has little to offer?

I began my odyssey into the Hoxsey story as a filmmaker and journalist in 1983, launching my own investigation into the treatment and its amazing history. Collaborating with public health nurse Catherine Salveson, I produced a documentary film on Hoxsey, and we both subsequently stepped through the lens to become players. The book also tells the personal story of how we slipped through the looking glass into the upside-down world of cancer politics during this era of dramatic flux.

Catherine and I bore witness to the creation of the Office of Alternative Medicine (OAM) in 1991, which grew directly from years of extreme public pressure mobilized by the large, highly organized alternative medicine community. In particular, the ardent constituency demanding the fair evaluation of unconventional cancer treatments led the effort. Congress firmly set the OAM's mission: to "investigate and validate" alternative therapies, with a priority on cancer. As early as 1987, national polls showed Congress that over half the American public favored the complete legalization of alternative cancer treatments.[2]

The tacit reason for such widespread and passionate popular interest in alternatives is sadly obvious: The medical establishment has largely lost its celebrated "War on Cancer" using surgery, radiation, and chemotherapy. But what has remained hidden from most people is the existence of another cancer war: the zealous campaign against unconventional cancer treatments and their practitioners. Over the course of the twentieth century, innovators such as Harry Hoxsey advanced more than one hundred alternative approaches, several of which seem to show significant promise. Yet rather than inviting interest and investigation from mainstream medicine, their champions have been ridiculed, threatened with the loss of professional licenses, harassed, prosecuted, or driven out of the country.

The facts clearly reveal that a consortium of interests has repeatedly condemned these treatments without investigation: the American Medical

Association (AMA), Food and Drug Administration (FDA), National Cancer Institute (NCI), and American Cancer Society (ACS), as well as certain large corporations that profit from the cancer industry. It is important to emphasize that this confederation of interests known as *organized medicine* consists principally of medical politicians and business interests, not practicing doctors. Physicians themselves have often objected to the unscientific rejection of alternative therapies and to restrictions on their own freedom to research or administer them.

The news blackout muffling this scandal has been so effective that most people do not happen into the underground of "disappeared" therapies until the fateful moment when they or their friends or relations are diagnosed with the dread disease. It is usually while fighting for their lives that patients discover the plethora of alternative cancer therapies claiming to offer hope and benefit, though with little if any scientific evidence to support their assertions.

Depending on whom you believe, Harry Hoxsey was either a fabulist of epic proportions who led credulous cancer sufferers to a certain death, or an effective healer persecuted by a medical trust. Often called the wildest story in medical history, Hoxsey is worth the telling sheerly as a great yarn. Beginning with the treatment's reputed discovery by a horse, it is a chestnut of Americana that might have sprung from the pen of Mark Twain. Were it presented as fiction, no one would believe it possible.

For over thirty-five years, Harry Hoxsey doggedly sought a scientific test of his herbal cancer remedies while organized medicine systematically blocked him. Though largely forgotten today, Hoxsey's quest ignited a cancer war that blazed across the national stage from the 1920s through the 1950s. Against all odds, he won a formidable series of victories, especially against his medical nemesis: AMA chief Dr. Morris Fishbein, the "Voice of American Medicine" for twenty-five years. These two figures came to personify the acrimonious schism dividing medicine.

In the McCarthyite wake of the 1950s, Hoxsey ultimately lost the war when the treatment was forced out of the country to Tijuana, Mexico. It was the first alternative clinic to set up shop south of the border. Hoxsey's successor, nurse Mildred Nelson, has quietly treated patients there ever since. Like Hoxsey, she claims a success rate as high as 80 percent, but her contention is unverifiable since the treatment has yet to be rigorously tested.

The campaign against unconventional cancer therapies has continued to boil, and the story of Hoxsey remains acutely relevant because it vividly illustrates how this struggle is nothing new. Where just a hundred years ago medicine was a rich grove teeming with diverse practices, it has been supplanted over the course of the twentieth century by a medical monoculture. How did this happen?

What radically tipped the balance of power was the arranged marriage between organized medicine and big business. Only since 1900 has medicine transformed itself into a vastly lucrative industry. Intent on eliminating economic competition, this medical-industrial complex has ballooned into today's $1 trillion medical-corporate state, within which cancer treatment is *very* big business. It has often been profitability that has driven the adoption of official therapeutics, and, as we shall see, organized medicine has been far more successful at controlling the cancer industry than at controlling cancer itself.

Along with economic competition, at the heart of the conflict is also a pronounced polarity of medical philosophies. In truth, both traditions, known as the *allopathic* and *empiric* schools, have made important contributions. Yet patients facing a life-threatening illness often poorly treated by conventional means have been denied access to all but the allopathic brand of cancer treatment.

Medical politics aside, Hoxsey may well represent a valuable cancer therapy. In these pages, you will travel through the underground of cancer patients who appear to have recovered using Hoxsey's "snake oil." Their positive experience bespeaks the contemporary renewal and validation of herbal and folk medicine. It marks the return to a rich materia medica empirically gleaned by keen clinical observers and intuitive healers throughout the ages.

Ironically, actual snake oil, the favorite archetype of medical charlatanism, seems to have gotten a bad rap after all. Contemporary research has found it to have important therapeutic value, possibly even against cancer. It contains the same omega-3 essential fatty acids that have elevated fish oil to a highly prized therapeutic agent. Recent studies demonstrate that natural compounds in these same fish oils increase immune response and prolong survival among cancer patients. Snake oil itself has a long history of medical usage that continues today in China, where it is successfully employed to treat arthritis and skin disorders.[3]

When researcher Dr. Richard Kunin bought snake oil from a Chinatown herbal shop in San Francisco and subjected it to laboratory analysis, it proved to have even higher levels of key therapeutic fatty acids than does fish oil. Intrigued by the results, Dr. Kunin went on to test two U.S. species of rattlesnakes against the principal variety used in China. He found that the Chinese species has at least five times the active constituents of the others. How did Chinese healers know? How is it that traditional and folk-medicine systems have consistently prefigured and predated innumerable scientific "discoveries?"

Empiricism is a way of knowing based on direct observation and experience. Outcomes are its first measure of success, emphasizing pragmatic results over theory or understanding. To the contrary, *allopathic rationalism* has asserted that practice must be the application of preexisting theory, not of therapeutic experience. The heritage of this conflict between allopathic and empiric philosophy is sharply expressed in *Webster's* definition of *empiric*: "One who enters a practice without a professional education and the proper experience; a quack."

In 1927 Dr. Morris Fishbein, whose overarching influence would guide orthodox medicine for the rest of the century, wrote, "Obviously a system of therapeutics that depends on ancient empiricism in its use of drugs cannot hope to be permanent in the present system of scientific medicine."[4] Clearly he never got to Chinatown, much less to China.

When all the tangled politics are cut away, Hoxsey is really about plant medicine. Herbs are today enjoying a renaissance and the Hoxsey tonic epitomizes the bountiful botanical legacy that is the cornerstone of modern pharmacy. The very word *drug* derives from the Dutch term *droog*, which means "to dry," since people have historically dried plants to make medicinal preparations. Whether the Hoxsey herbal tonic does successfully treat cancer remains an open question, but it is well proved that many botanicals possess powerful anticancer properties. Several major chemotherapy drugs derive from plants, as do numerous primary pharmaceuticals.

The tragedy framing this story is that cancer has reached epidemic proportions. Cancer incidence in the United States has risen by 60 percent just since 1950, and by twenty-seven times since 1900.[5] Each year, a staggering 1.2 million Americans—one in two men and one in three women—develop some form of internal cancer.[6]

The cancer death rate has also climbed precipitously. Where in 1899 the disease killed 30,000 people, in 1999 over 560,000 died.[7] Cancer is poised to become the top killer in the United States, making cancer treatment the "dominant specialty" of American medicine.[8] This most feared affliction has become the very emblem of modern civilization.

Yet outside a small handful of success stories, the cure rate using conventional cancer treatments has hardly improved since the 1950s. Then as now, despite $30 billion spent on the "War on Cancer" since 1971, over half of cancer patients die, every year more than twice as many Americans as were killed in all of World War II.[9] As we shall see, credible critics say that even these disappointing success rates may be doctored to appear more favorable than they really are.

Although organized medicine has summarily rejected unconventional therapies as unproven, we shall see that conventional cancer treatments are themselves largely unproven according to standard scientific protocols.

There are few major breakthroughs on the horizon, and even respected mainstream oncologists are calling for new directions. As we will also discover, a very large proportion of cancer is preventable, which is not a medical problem but a political one.

The bottom line is that ever-growing numbers of patients are turning to unconventional therapies, with or without the approval of their physicians. Varying estimates suggest that as many as 64 percent of cancer patients are now using alternatives, a startling figure suggesting the depth of desperation.[10] Their footprints are easily tracked to places like Tijuana, the Bahamas, and Europe. Patients are seeking alternative options despite organized medicine's opposition, the lack of insurance coverage, and the fact that most doctors can provide little or no information about them.

This runaway popular demand is triggering tectonic shifts in the orientations of medical practice, government policy, insurance coverage, and the mass media. Alternative cancer therapies are gaining dramatically heightened prominence and some are already starting to enter the repertoire of mainstream medicine.

Yet even now terminally ill cancer patients whose doctors have given them up to die are compelled to cross international borders in search of potentially life-saving therapies. These basic human-rights issues are echoing loudly through the halls of Congress, where a relentless movement of cancer patients and activists seeking medical civil rights is steadily influencing public policy to allow more options for both patients and doctors.

What we may be witnessing at last is a rapprochement between these polarized camps, a long-overdue truce in the cancer wars. Conventional medicine is approaching alternatives with a tentative handshake, though only time will tell whether the gesture is sincere or just a temporary concession in the winner-take-all game that has dominated U.S. medical politics for so long.

But what we are unequivocally witnessing is a marked increase in formal research on alternative cancer therapies. The government's creation of the Office of Alternative Medicine inaugurated a new openness, giving society permission to probe these taboo treatments through unbiased research and discussion. The OAM has recently been elevated to the National Center for Complementary and Alternative Medicine with increased funding, and other federal agencies including the National Cancer Institute are expanding their research into alternatives. Among the participants are top mainstream medical institutions, universities including Harvard, Columbia, and Stanford, as well as elite cancer centers such as Memorial Sloan-Kettering and M. D. Anderson.

Because some of these alternative therapies could represent the cutting edge of cancer treatment, a profit motive is kicking in. Corporate medicine sees a sizable market and large companies are staking a claim. Ironically, the underlying commercial agenda that has long worked against the acceptance of alternative medicine is now spurring its rapid growth. This economic imperative is accelerating its legitimization and relaxing the political polarization.

Using Hoxsey as a compass, these pages navigate this extraordinary transformation. The book is divided into three main parts. Part 1 begins with the story of how I got involved with Hoxsey through making the film and describes my first life-changing visit with Catherine to the Bio Medical (Hoxsey) Center in Mexico. It goes on to explore the dramatic recoveries of Hoxsey patients "who got well when they weren't supposed to." Subsequent chapters paint the colorful tableau of the rise and fall of the Hoxsey Cancer Clinics until shortly after the government drove the treatment from the United States in the 1960s.

Part 2 delves into the fascinating and long-standing conflict of medical opinion around the Hoxsey medicines. It probes both the science and folklore behind Hoxsey's herbal tonic and external salves, and reveals surprising evidence of both their possible worth and proven efficacy. It also examines the nutritional and attitudinal elements of the treatment, general practices that are being scientifically validated today. The therapeutic investigation moves into a critique revealing the severe limitations of conventional cancer treatments. Threaded throughout is the hidden history of how these two schools of medicine have been at odds for centuries, culminating with the Hoxsey dispute as the quintessential modern expression of this conflict.

Part 3 cuts to the pitched cancer wars of the 1980s, when the antagonism between conventional and alternative cancer camps heated to a flash point, with Hoxsey sharing center stage. This clash unexpectedly catalyzed a historic shift and precipitated a shaky resolution that included the start of the first-ever government investigation into Hoxsey. Several chapters look inside the profit-driven corporatization of the cancer industry and the commercial entry of alternative therapies. Subsequent chapters examine emerging solutions and "policy cures," including basic human-rights questions of freedom of choice, now gaining political momentum.

Finally, the book points to the signs of a hopeful healing now under way, of both cancer and the wounds of medical politics. Courageous visionaries from all bands of the spectrum are leading a powerful movement to forge a new medical model. Buoyed by widespread popular support, they are reinventing a therapeutics centered on positive outcomes.

They are forming a healing partnership between doctor and patient and cultivating a medicine alive with the restorative forces of nature and the spirit.

Since releasing the Hoxsey movie over a decade ago, I've witnessed changes in attitudes toward alternative cancer treatments that were once unthinkable. There is a profound healing taking place within medicine. This mending embodies a reintegration of the tragic split that has cleaved it in two, separating allopath from empiric, doctor from patient, technology from nature, mind from body, body from spirit. That healing is beginning to knit together the fractures of what in the end is one body that would do well to have all its parts joined.

There are many questions and challenges ahead, and the sorry history of the cancer wars gives ample pause to remain circumspect. The chilling tale of injustice the Hoxsey story portrays may make you angry, but above all it offers hope. We are balanced on the cusp of a transformation in medicine, a tenuous bridge to what could be one of the most vibrant and fertile eras in the history of medical discovery.

Ending the medical civil war is bound to result in a greater menu of choices for patients, and what is best for the patient surely ought to be the first consideration. We have the unique opportunity to create an authentically collaborative medicine embracing the best from all worlds.

PART ONE

The Wildest Story in Medical History

The Ballad of Harry and Mildred

"Harry fought 'em longer and harder than anyone, but politics is bigger than one man any day."
Mildred Nelson

I

Riding the Cancer Underground

In 1840 Illinois horse farmer John Hoxsey found his prize stallion with a malignant tumor on its right hock. As a Quaker, he couldn't bear shooting the animal, so he put it out to pasture to die peacefully. Three weeks later, he noticed the tumor stabilizing, and observed the animal browsing knee-deep in a corner of the pasture with a profusion of weeds, eating plants not part of its normal diet.

Within three months the tumor dried up and began to separate from the healthy tissue. The farmer retreated to the barn, where he began to experiment with these herbs revealed to him by "horse sense." He added other popular ingredients from home remedies of the day and devised three formulas: an internal tonic and two external preparations. He soon became known for treating animals with cancer and tumors. Folks said he had "the healing tetch."

The empiricist handed the secret formulas down through the generations. His grandson John C. Hoxsey, a veterinarian in southern Illinois, was the first to try the cancer remedies on people, and claimed positive results. His son Harry showed an early interest and began working with him. After his father's death, Harry founded the first Hoxsey Cancer Clinic in 1924, heralded by the local chamber of commerce and high school marching bands on Main Street.[1]

So begins the Hoxsey legend, and with it the thirty-five-year cancer war between organized medicine and the folk healer. Orthodox medicine branded Hoxsey the worst cancer quack of the century. He would be arrested more times than any other person in medical history.

Yet by the 1950s Hoxsey's stronghold in Dallas, Texas, grew to be the world's largest privately owned cancer center, with branches spreading to seventeen states.[2] Two federal courts upheld the therapeutic value of the treatment.[3] Even his archenemies the American Medical Association and the Food and Drug Administration admitted that the therapy does cure certain forms of cancer.[4]

Nevertheless, medical authorities denied Hoxsey's insistent plea for a fair scientific test. Instead they worked to ban the treatment, outlawing it entirely in the United States in 1960.[5] Hoxsey's chief nurse, Mildred Nelson, took the treatment to Tijuana in 1963, abandoning any hope of offering it in the United States.[6]

When I first stumbled upon Hoxsey in 1980, I saw it as a sleeping giant of a story that somehow submerged from view after the clinic's demise. I had a far more personal motive, however, for taking a serious interest. One evening in 1976, over dinner at the small farm where I was living north of Santa Fe, New Mexico, I got a phone call from my mother. My father had cancer. Six months later, at age fifty-five, he was dead.

About two weeks after my father's death, I received a newsletter in the mail unbidden. It contained testimonials of cancer patients who swore that a complex nutritional program developed by dentist Donald Kelley cured them after their doctors gave them up to die. I read with shock, amazement, and disbelief.

Like many people in 1977, I believed what the doctors told me: Cancer was largely incurable. I certainly knew nothing of alternative treatments. I was skeptical, even hostile, to the idea, but with my father freshly buried and my heart broken, I was open. If there was anything at all to this, I had to know.

I started reading everything I could get my hands on and spoke to anyone I could find who had a direct personal experience. I quickly discovered a subterranean netherworld of purported cures using a variety of therapies—from nutrition and mental imaging to herbs and immunology. It was only when I came across an obscure article about the Hoxsey Cancer Clinics that a lightbulb flashed in my head, illuminating the warp I found myself in. The article by Peter Barry Chowka detailed the astonishing social history of Hoxsey.[7] I began to realize that, like most human affairs, medicine is political. Had ideology buried science without an obituary? Were "unorthodox" treatments being politically railroaded instead of scientifically tested?

Chowka's piece mentioned Hoxsey's autobiography, and I set out to find a copy. I located it by mail order, and when the self-published book, *You Don't Have to Die*, finally arrived, I sat down to scan it. For the next four hours, I read transfixed.

Hoxsey revealed a hidden history of the AMA and U.S. medical politics. He described a venal culture of tyranny and corruption, a medical dictatorship supported by avaricious vested interests. He accused an AMA official of unsuccessfully trying to buy his formulas before subsequently blackballing him.

Would spurned medical politicians suppress a cure for cancer? The seemingly outrageous charge represented nothing less than a crime against humanity. Was it to be believed?

I was a budding filmmaker at the time, and decided to channel my interest in alternative medicine into movies. After my wife illustrated a book about southwestern herbs, I became friendly with the herbalist author and ended up producing my first documentary, *Los Remedios: The Healing Herbs*, about the rich legacy of plant medicine in the Southwest. A friend showed the program to Catherine Salveson, a registered nurse with a background in cancer care, herbs, and media. Over lunch, I shared with her the story of Hoxsey. Catherine, who even in her nursing uniform bore an uncanny resemblance to singer Joni Mitchell, turned out to be extremely bright, articulate, and open. We connected strongly, and by the end of the meal, we resolved to make a trip to the Tijuana clinic to see for ourselves. Perhaps we would find a film there.

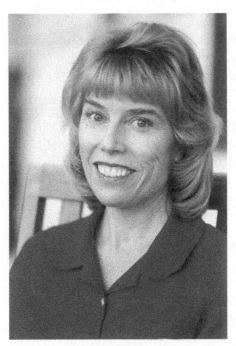

Catherine Salveson

I carried a great deal of trepidation as we set out for San Diego. My only direct experience with cancer had been the horror of my father's death. Visiting him in Memorial Sloan-Kettering Cancer Center in New York, the flagship of conventional cancer treatment, branded my psyche with the indelible imprint of a medical concentration camp. Hopeless patients in blue smocks hovered like phantoms, their emaciated bodies ravaged by radiation and chemotherapy. A skeletal cluster of bald-headed children looking strangely like old men and women formed a macabre audience around a color TV spewing out violent cartoons and commercials for sugar-coated cereal. The place smelled of death and despair. The doctors, aloof and cold, seemed to have hardened themselves against the incredible pain and their own helplessness.

Flying into San Diego, Catherine and I stayed at the "cancer motel" at the edge of the U.S. border. In the morning we boarded the van taking patients to the various Mexican cancer clinics. The mood was somber and anxious. Raul, the Mexican driver, kept up a steady stream of cheerful patter, trying to ease the grim disquietude. As a hospice nurse, Catherine had more equanimity than I did. The van cruised easily through Mexican customs and we entered another country. The only images in my mind of Tijuana were bare lightbulbs and dirty needles.

Climbing steep hills overlooking the city, we arrived early at the Bio Medical Center, as the Hoxsey clinic was now known. Raul pushed back giant wrought-iron gates and shepherded us into the tiny cafeteria to wait for the clinic to open. The huge white building was an elegant Greco-Roman anomaly with large pillars at its carved wooden front doors. Cheerful yellow-and-white-striped canopies shaded the fancifully curving walkways. Brilliant tropical birds sang noisily in a big cage in the welcoming courtyard. An empty swimming pool displayed an enigmatic tiled emblem: a painted horse's head. I had always loved Mexico, and the place felt good.

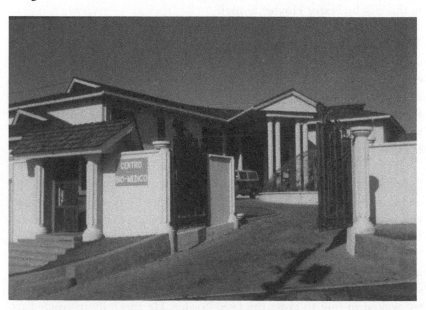

The Bio-Medical (Hoxsey) Center moved to Tijuana in 1963

The huge front doors swung open and I caught the eye of an older woman. Spontaneously, we smiled broadly at one another. I realized it was Mildred Nelson, with whom I had spoken briefly by phone before arranging to come to the clinic. When Catherine and I introduced ourselves,

Mildred became brusque. She was very busy. If we wanted to know the real story of Hoxsey, she said, go talk with the patients. Trailed by an entourage of clinic staff, Mildred moved so swiftly that she seemed to walk through walls, vanishing down a long hallway before we could open our mouths to respond. It was certainly not the reception we planned after months of anticipation and preparation.

We wandered into the waiting room, which was filling with yet another vanload of patients. We were on our own. The spacious room looked out grandly through large plate-glass windows across the sprawl of bustling Tijuana. Sunlight ignited the buzz of early-morning activity as medical orderlies started taking blood and performing other tests. The mood was definitely not what we expected. People laughed, joked, and circulated freely. As the day wore on, we came to recognize the new patients. They were the ones looking distressed and depressed. As the hours passed, they shared the same experience we did, listening to countless older Hoxsey patients cheerfully tell how Mildred had cured them three, five, and twenty years ago. And healed their mothers, their neighbors, and their best friends. Even their dogs. A few said they'd been cured in Dallas in the '50s by Harry Hoxsey himself.

We were stupefied. The stories were miraculous and they were legion. They involved almost every type of cancer, including the most deadly forms such as pancreatic, lung, and melanoma. Many people complained bitterly of prior abuse by doctors in the States, such as one lady who told how the doctor had removed one-and-a-half lungs, charged $100,000, and then informed her he hadn't expected it to work anyway. We also heard several accounts of relatives who had died while trying Hoxsey, but who experienced a relief of pain pronounced enough to stop taking painkillers.

The treatment was inexpensive, too. Mildred then charged a one-time fee of $1,500. Many patients paid in installments as low as $5 a month, and those who were destitute paid nothing. In his book, Hoxsey said that this tradition came from his father's deathbed charge that no patient be turned away for lack of funds.

Riding the van back to the cancer motel that afternoon, we found the mood decidedly upbeat. The passengers laughed uproariously at the idea of writing a cancer patients' joke book. Raul became serious, however, as we waited in line to cross the U.S. border. He carefully instructed us exactly how to answer the question of what we were bringing back from Mexico. "Just say 'herbs and vitamins,'" he cautioned with sudden sobriety. "Do not say 'drugs.' Just herbs and vitamins." The blocky border guard scowled inside the van. He asked a couple of people to open their little brown bags carrying the Hoxsey tonic and vitamins. Grudgingly, he let the van through. The effervescence went flat. We all knew we had crossed not just a political boundary, but a philosophical border as well.

After a couple of more days at the clinic, Catherine and I passed the better part of Memorial Day weekend holed up with Mildred in her small trailer next door where she had lived since coming to Tijuana. A once mobile home, it was now stationary atop the tiny pharmacy that originally served as the first Bio Medical Center. According to rumors, the beautiful new clinic next door was a former house of ill repute whose *señora* got busted on narcotics charges. Mildred put in an improbably low bid on the repossessed estate and, to her amazement and delight, she got it.

Imbibing a steady stream of coffee and smoking her trademark long brown cigarettes, Mildred regaled us in her thick Texas twang with countless anecdotes of Hoxsey's war with the AMA and FDA, stories regularly seasoned with rambling recollections of remarkable remissions. After a while, it became clear to us that Mildred was utterly sincere. She got involved with Hoxsey when her mother was successfully treated in Dallas in 1946 after being given up on by her doctors. Initially hostile, Mildred became a believer.

The phone interrupted constantly, day and night, with the frantic calls of cancer patients from all over the United States, Canada, and the world. Mildred answered every call, no matter what day of the week or time of day. "How would you as a cancer patient like to get an answering machine?" she challenged us sharply. As nurses on the front lines of caring for the sick, Mildred and Catherine understood each other perfectly.

In the course of conversation, we learned chillingly that Mildred had no successor. Sixty-five years old with two strokes behind her, she was searching. Interested doctors had come and gone, but none had the devotion and moxie it would take to preserve the contentious legacy. Because the Mexican government exacted a prohibitive fee of $50,000 a year for working papers for U.S. physicians, Mildred employed solely Mexican doctors, none of whom had the political savvy, in her opinion, to keep the Hoxsey clinic alive. Either the right person will show up, she told us, or it will be lost. She seemed to have more serenity about the prospect than we did. We had seen enough to convince us that this treatment needed to be explored.

At the end of the weekend, Catherine and I looked at each other nervously, and finally I popped the question. Could we make a film about Hoxsey? Perhaps a film would help spur an investigation. Mildred took one of her characteristically endless pauses, blowing smoke softly into the air. "I've turned down everybody that's ever asked, you know," she said evenly, and smoked it over some more. "But I like you kids." She was saying yes.

Back in Santa Fe, we swiftly made plans. I had primary responsibility for producing the film, since Catherine kept her day job, but we worked closely as coproducers. We started by holding a series of receptions for funders. As an independent filmmaker, you are actually very *dependent*— on funding. Raising money for a movie is just slightly easier than raising the dead. The film additionally started out with three strikes against it in 1984. It was the "D" word, documentary; the "C" word, cancer; and the "P" word, political. Filmmaking is often perceived as a somewhat glamorous occupation, but we quickly learned that the surest way to deflate a conversation at a party was to say we were making a film—about cancer. Yet we believed passionately in its importance, and if anything could make cancer entertaining, it would be the larger-than-life story of Hoxsey.

Over the next few months we raised enough money from good-hearted angels and people interested in natural medicine to do the first shoot in Tijuana and start the research. The film would take a harrowing four years to complete and launch us on an irrevocable journey into the mind-bending realm of cancer politics. With only one hiatus after the initial filming, I managed to keep it funded continuously to completion, although it was white knuckles every step of the way, never knowing from week to week where the money would come from.

Working with film researcher Ray Hemenez, I began to grope my way into the vaporous mists of Hoxsey. Using *You Don't Have to Die* as a road map, we sought to confirm or deny its many seemingly preposterous claims and allegations. Ray started in Dallas, exhausting all public records including newspapers and court transcripts. He also began to try to track down any living survivors of the struggle. If there was a needle in a haystack, Ray invariably found the thread with it, too.

One reason it took four years to produce the movie was that the documentation had to be impeccable. I am a journalist, not a doctor or scientist, and especially in matters of life and death like this, we all felt the acute responsibility to be fastidious in our factual accuracy. We gained access to the private files of the AMA, where we found a King Solomon's Mines of materials. The AMA's Bureau of Investigation gathered and kept virtually every scrap of information on Hoxsey and generated a vast output of its own. I sifted through original newspaper clippings dating back to 1924 that were so brittle I feared they would disintegrate in my hands. I carefully examined everything there, making voluminous notes and copies.

We had to file twice through the Freedom of Information Act to get Hoxsey records from the FDA, which apparently still considered these

documents a threat to national security. We also tracked down obscure
private collections across the country and searched all public and court
records. At the completion of the film, the National Library of Medicine
requested our research as a donation to its archives.[8]

We did manage to find a surprising number of individual players from
the Hoxsey drama still alive. The terrain was as polarized as Bosnia or the
Middle East, and both sides were deeply suspicious of us. The pro-Hoxsey
people were often reluctant to talk, fearing reprisals comparable to the
quack attack of the 1950s when federal and private health authorities instigated a broad prosecutorial assault on unorthodox practitioners. The
anti-Hoxsey forces were equally hesitant, loath to risk letting the genie
back out of the tonic bottle.[9]

Finally we managed to piece together most of the puzzle. Some parts
remained elusive. "Facts" swayed like seaweed in a shifting current. A
neptunian haze clouded key events, while time and memory lapses made
verification of certain incidents impossible. Fraught with charges and countercharges, the story was riddled with irreconcilable dispute and unprov-
able mystery. Overall, though, a distinctive picture did finally emerge, which
led me to call the movie *Hoxsey: How Healing Becomes a Crime*.

But to grasp the slippery story of Hoxsey, it's necessary to ask the
central question: Do people get well using the treatment? As Mildred
Nelson first told us, go talk to the patients.

"People Who Got Well When They Weren't Supposed To"

Catherine and I flew into Pittsburgh in 1986 with the film crew, where we had to rent two gleaming oversized American luxury cars to accommodate the cumbersome equipment. Having left our Subarus and pickup trucks at home, we felt strangely like movie mogul impersonators driving flashy Lincoln Continentals into the city suburbs. There we met Mrs. Margaret Griffin, the Hoxsey patient whom we came to film.[1]

Mrs. Griffin was graciously attired for her screen debut in a powder blue dress and pearl necklace. She had waited a long time to tell her story and was eager to start. Speaking with a distinctive Pennsylvania lilt, she related her encounter with cancer.

"Around November of 1966, I kept blacking out, and repeated X-rays in three different hospitals showed that I had two tumors around my aorta leading into my heart. The diagnosis was lymphosarcoma [cancer of the lymph system]. When my friend said to get another opinion, I went to two other doctors, and it was the same verdict: two tumors around the aorta. I didn't want to accept that, but in time I had to. So I finally went into one of the hospitals. A doctor did exploratory surgery, and he didn't remove anything, but he scooped back a large area under my right breast from the front to the back. What he saw was two tumors blocking the superior vena cava (the vein leading into the heart), lesions in the right lung, and cancer in all my lymph glands.

"I did take thirty treatments of cobalt radiation," Mrs. Griffin continued, "but I was rapidly going downhill. They gave me a year to live. That's the verdict that the doctor gave my family.

"In the meantime I was reading the *Enquirer* magazine and there was an article where various psychics were giving predictions. Jeane Dixon was one of the them. She said, 'This is the year for a cure for cancer.' So I immediately wrote to her through the *Enquirer*, and fortunately somebody forwarded it to Jeanne. It went through her secretary, and one day I got a phone call from Lee Alexander, a wonderful guardian angel, as I call him. He had been a pilot with American Airlines, which flew into Dallas, and so he knew about the Hoxsey therapy. He proceeded to talk about Hoxsey, and I knew that it was something controversial because Harry Hoxsey went to court against the FDA and, of course, he lost.

"So Lee had befriended the secretary and asked her, if anybody inquired about cancer, to turn their name over to him. That's how he contacted me to tell me about the Hoxsey. I was receptive because I knew my time was short. I had no other choice. If I die, I die, and all I'd lost was a few thousand dollars, and I don't even consider that a great loss. I decided I'm going. By that time the clinic had been closed, but Dr. Durkee had been part of the Hoxsey clinic and he had the formula. So underground, he would furnish a supply of the tonic." (Dr. Joseph Durkee was Hoxsey's leading doctor at the Dallas clinic from 1946 to 1952 before a falling out with his employer. He continued to treat cancer patients illegally underground with the Hoxsey formulas into the 1960s.)

"I had this premonition when I went out onto the tarmac that October morning. It was a gorgeous morning, and the sun was shining on this great big silver plane that I called the silver bird. I had never flown. I was always afraid to fly, but I was determined that I had to go. So I walked out onto that tarmac and looked at that beautiful bird and I thought, 'You're taking me to life.' And it did."

When she started her cancer odyssey, Margaret Griffin recalled that she was in very bad shape. "I had just taken a leave of absence from work. My face was puffy and red, and my breathing was terribly impaired." Then her trip to Dallas began to show results. "I was on the tonic for ten months when I started to notice a decided improvement in how I felt. So I knew then that it was working. All of a sudden everything got better. By the tenth month, everything turned around. The X-rays of my chest where the two tumors were around my aorta showed that there were no longer tumors. I went back to work and I worked many years after that. From time to time I'd fly down to Dallas, get a supply of the tonic, bring it home. Here I am today to talk about it. It truly worked."

Eager to share her great good fortune with her physician, Mrs. Griffin was shocked by his response. "When I went back to my regular doctor who had originally diagnosed it, I was all thrilled. I made the appointment and his nurse said, 'I'm sorry, Mrs. Griffin, but Dr. So-and-So doesn't want you as his patient anymore because you didn't believe in him.' So that was the end of that. I thought, 'Well, forget you.' I'm going my way and I'm not going to be looking for trouble going to this doctor and that doctor. If I drop in my tracks, so be it. I figured this worked and that's how I live. I haven't bothered to do any follow-up, and the Hoxsey works beautifully."

Mrs. Griffin told us she later paid the fee at the Bio Medical Center to receive a lifetime supply of tonic, which she used continuously for eight years and intermittently since. She followed the Hoxsey program of the tonic and a prescribed diet. "It's very simple. It doesn't make you ill. Your hair doesn't fall out like chemo, and it's almost too good to be true, you might think. But it does work."

In preparing this book, I decided to try calling Mrs. Griffin over ten years later to see if she was still alive. She answered the phone and happily told me that she is cancer-free at the age of seventy-nine, thirty-four years after starting Hoxsey. She does have heart trouble and other ailments, but her greatest anguish lies elsewhere.

"My friends look askance at me," Mrs. Griffin said with exasperation. "I've been able to convince a few people to go to Hoxsey and they too have benefited by it. But the majority of people don't believe me, and they don't want to believe me. What can I do? I write letters to the editor and I loan that [Hoxsey] film out, but nobody ever calls. We lost a daughter at the age of four to a brain tumor, and I was very supportive at that time of the American Cancer Society, but I lost confidence and faith in them. That was another reason why I thought I have to go this route. I think really we need anarchy in the streets. Then maybe we'll get something done."

Surprising sentiments emanating from a staid Pittsburgh suburban neighborhood, though not uncommon ones. As we bounced around the country tracking down Hoxsey patients, we slipped into a kind of parallel universe of "people who got well when they weren't supposed to," as cancer surgeon and author Dr. Bernie Siegel terms these remarkable recoveries. Like Mrs. Griffin, their stories have been stricken from the record. Orthodox medicine, rather than studying such cases, dismisses them as "anecdotal evidence" lacking credibility since they were not part of a controlled scientific study. Was Mrs. Griffin indeed cured by Hoxsey? Or possibly by the radiation she received? By other influences? By standard measures, we do not know.

For the film, we worked closely with Dr. Hugh Riordan to document the validity of patient histories such as Mrs. Griffin's. Dr. Riordan is the head of a large Kansas clinic and former president of the American Holistic Medical Association. In documenting new cases for this book as well as rechecking the others, I consulted with Gar Hildenbrand, whom you will meet again later in these pages. Former director of research for the Gerson Institute, a nutritional cancer therapy with its own beleaguered history, the cancer activist went on to become an epidemiologist, working for the OAM and other respected groups verifying medical data. I asked him and his partner Christeene Hildenbrand to assess all of the cases discussed here, for both the validity of the medical records and the prognosis for their disease with the treatment they had.

The Hildenbrands confirmed Mrs. Griffin's cancer diagnosis and commented, "This tumor was originally believed to have a particularly adverse prognosis. Today she would have been treated aggressively with chemotherapy and radiotherapy. The outcomes of these combined treatments show approximately a 50 percent five-year survival rate. But when she was originally treated, the expectation would be for her cancer to recur after radiation therapy, even if the doctors had achieved complete remission, which we doubt they did. Her memory of the event was that the cobalt therapy did nothing and her physician told her she had about a year to live. Without Hoxsey, that prognosis would have been pretty accurate."[2]

In writing this book, I searched for more case histories of cancer patients who seem to have benefited from the Hoxsey treatment. While visiting Mildred, I noticed her reading a letter from New Zealand and inquired whom it was from. It turned out to be Gwen Scott, a breast cancer patient who started the *Hoxsey Connection* newsletter in her region.[3] New Zealand and Australia are home to an unusual cluster of Hoxsey patients because a local medical doctor there, Dr. Eva Hill, journeyed to Dallas in the 1950s and received successful treatment for a severe skin cancer on her face.[4] Upon returning home, she began offering the Hoxsey treatment against considerable legal difficulties. Although a protracted and high-profile court clash with medical authorities was ultimately resolved in her favor, she continued offering Hoxsey for the rest of her many days under constant pressure from medical authorities. Dr. Hill cultivated a large and thriving Hoxsey practice there, but after her death at the age of ninety-two, patients like Gwen had to resume the trek to Tijuana.

Speaking in a sing-song down-under dialect, Gwen Scott described to me her encounter with cancer. "It started late in 1993. I had a lump on my breast for eight months. It was testing negative in the needle biopsy [a method for diagnosing cancer] in January 1994, so I wasn't really worried about it, although I have a family history—I lost a sister with breast cancer. I didn't actually understand that these biopsies are not always accurate. It tested four times as being a benign cyst, but it was growing all that time, and I wasn't happy about it."

Gwen's general practitioner wasn't able to get her an appointment at the hospital because her biopsies showed up negative for cancer. "In that eight-month period," Gwen recalled with a deep sigh, "it grew huge, and when I was finally seen, it was almost ulcerating. It was about four inches long and about two inches around. It was certainly very cancerous and was described as 'Grade III, infiltrating carcinoma with vascular permeation and axillary lymph node metastases.'" Gwen's condition is considered a very advanced and usually deadly breast cancer with involvement of the lymph system. "Vascular permeation" implies malignant seed cells in the circulating cells, which would be very bad news. The additional circumstance that her case was initially misdiagnosed could easily have cost Gwen her life.

When the biopsy showed potentially fatal cancer, she opted for surgery. "I had a lumpectomy and then a mastectomy in the hospital here in August 1994, and the advice of the surgeon was that there's no [further] treatment that would be any good because I was going to die anyway. There was no chemo or radiation—they were not offered to me. The doctor expected for it to be in the brain or lung within a month's time— that was August, September, 1994—and that October they expected me to be in a bad way." Gwen was also given Tamoxifen, a pharmaceutical drug used to treat breast cancer.

"What the surgeon actually said to me was, 'No treatment will do you any good because you are going to die anyway.' I asked, 'Well, when?' because I didn't know whether to spend what little inheritance money I'd thought was coming, get the bathroom fixed, or blow it all on a trip overseas. I really wanted to know when this demise was going to take place. He said, 'Within a month's time you will be in a bad way, and then we will be able to tell more accurately when that demise will be.' There was nothing more, in their opinion, that would help me."

Gwen decided to take action on her own, a pattern typical of many cancer survivors. She saw it as the crucial moment to take personal responsibility for her situation by doing some homework. "At that time I didn't feel like dying and I also had a problem. I got partially paralyzed for some reason, whether it was a reaction to their drugs or whatever it was. No medical doctor could actually give me a reason of what it was, and that started me searching in libraries. I did start straightaway on a course of antioxidants [vitamins, minerals, and other natural substances believed to have anticancer activity and other health benefits] and things like that.

"Visiting the libraries and looking at things on breast cancer medically as well as on alternatives was so confusing, because every time I found something, I would go back to the doctors, and they either didn't know what I was talking about or didn't have an answer for it. I gradually lost respect for them, but I did gain a knowledge that they actually didn't know a hell of a lot about. In that time, I was searching for something that would suit me.

"I could not plow myself through all the different confusing and conflicting reports, medically as well as alternative. I didn't have the faith in either to provide me with any answers because there were so many conflicting reports. The more you read, the more confusing it became. I really had to go by the cost, for one thing, and the easiest to follow, because I'm basically a lazy person. And the highest success rate. That was pretty obvious: It was the Hoxsey treatment."

Gwen was still not sure what to do. The clinic lay thousands of expensive miles away. Like most cancer patients, she was starkly confronting her looming mortality and still had little solid information to go on. "I couldn't say that I was actually praying for help—I suppose, meditating and asking for guidance to find something. I went into a secondhand book shop. A book fell off the shelf at my feet. I picked it up and put it back. It fell off again. So I actually bought it for $3, and it was a book called *Cancer and Cure*. It told the story of Dr. Eva Hill. The same day I also bought a magazine from a health food store which told the story of the [Hoxsey] clinic in Tijuana. I got in touch with the writer and the editor of the magazine and got the phone number. I rang the clinic.

"I started immediately on the Hoxsey treatment through the generosity of Mrs. Nelson, on a trial basis. Another patient was able to put me on it until I was financially able to make the trip over to Tijuana. The clinic told me that if I could stay cancer-free for two years, I *may* have a chance."

Gwen began to feel a portentous effect immediately. "The first night I took it, I had a wonderful sleep. The feeling of well-being was almost immediate. I had an incredible dream."

Gwen soon noticed palpable physical progress. "I did have other lumps, which may or may not have been cancer [on the other breast and under the arm] that disappeared. I didn't actually know that I had them until the oncologist here said, 'Oh, those lumps have gone.'

"One of the things I found quite surprising was the oncologist here told me I was wasting my money, which I thought was funny, because I didn't have any money. It wasn't a problem. Hoxsey seemed the right thing to me all the way through. I'm cancer-free. All around, the whole thing has been immensely successful for me."

Gwen Scott has now passed the five-year survival mark since her diagnosis, the medical standard to deem a cancer patient cured. After starting Hoxsey, she is completely free of cancer with a stage of disease that her doctors expected would kill her in a matter of months. Her medical records confirm her original cancer as well as malignancy remaining after her surgery.

After confirming Gwen's documentation, the Hildenbrands also validated her grave prospects. It included an "invasive neoplasm [cancer tumor] with the poorest prognosis of all ductal cancers" at a stage considered the worst. The fact that it infiltrated ten different lymph nodes again put her in the worst category for recovery. "Even using Tamoxifen," they went on, "she would have been expected to have a recurrence within the first couple of years, and the staying power of the drug is under two years [after it is discontinued]."

However, because Gwen did receive Tamoxifen, her case is not entirely clear-cut. She did stop the drug after two years and has not taken it for over three. Because most Hoxsey patients have previously received various forms of conventional treatment, her case is representative of the ambiguity characterizing many such cases. What seems certain is that she was not supposed to get well.

Through Gwen, I came in contact with Rex Major, a retired policeman from New Zealand who shared with me his struggle against both the disease and his doctors. His personal drama exemplified the tug-of-war that has plagued Hoxsey patients since the 1920s.

Rex checked into the emergency room in 1993 feeling "terrible." He ascribed his condition to his diabetes and a severe flu. Following a blood test and colonoscopy (internal examination of the colon) in September, he was diagnosed by an Australian doctor with Duke's C cancer of the colon, a very serious form of the disease. He had major surgery to remove the tennis-ball-sized tumor. Convalescing at home, he got a call a week later from the doctor, who told him that a biopsy revealed four lymph nodes invaded by carcinoma that was *metastasizing*, spreading elsewhere. Rex asked what his options were, and the doctor gave only two: chemotherapy or face death in three to six months.

"I was fortunate in having a cancer researcher as a friend and associate here in New Zealand," Rex related passionately to me, "and this guy gave me information and showed me documentation and an admission by the oncology department at Auckland Hospital on the subject of chemotherapy. That article indicated that, of every two hundred people that went through the oncology department at Auckland Hospital, one hundred and forty are dead in two years. Now my question was, 'What happened to the other sixty?' The answer was they went through all the traumas of the adverse reaction to the chemotherapy. I said, 'No, I'm not going to do that.'" Because chemotherapy drugs are powerful and debilitating poisons, many patients such as Rex Major consider the treatment as devastating as the disease. (For a full discussion of chemotherapy and conventional cancer treatments, see chapter 15.)

Rex Major recalled his confrontation with the oncologist over his rejection of chemotherapy. "He rang me up, and he and I had a real set-to over the telephone. I told him, 'I am going to discontinue this conversation. I'm going to put the phone down because I will not have you planting any seeds of doubt in my mind. I have made my decision. Thank you for your advice and I appreciate what you've done. This is my existence we're talking about. I'm going to be in control of it from here on.'"

Rex started shopping around for other choices. "I didn't just settle on Hoxsey straightaway. I actually looked at eight different options. I eliminated the ones that I didn't like, particularly chemotherapy once I'd investigated it. Being a policeman all those years, I always investigate anything that I got involved in, and when my life was at stake I had the utmost motivation to be sure that I was doing exactly the right thing. So it was a case for me of checking these out, ticking them off as they fell by the wayside, and ending up with one. Not that there's anything wrong with a lot of the others. There was quite a lot of merit with some of them, but they didn't fit the bill for me."

Part of Rex's latter working career was with the Dale Carnegie Organization, famous for its utilization of the "Power of Positive Thinking." Through the group, he knew a former Hoxsey patient and decided to hear her story. Yvonne Chamberlain recounted to him her brush with melanoma, a deadly form of skin cancer. She had no other treatment and credited Hoxsey with saving her life.

"I was blessed with the information on what to do when my turn came to be diagnosed with cancer," Major related to me. "Yvonne's recommendation and the conversations I had over the telephone with Mildred in those early days convinced me that that's what I needed to do. So, three weeks to the day, I was on an airplane. I went through the airports in a wheelchair. My wife had to be alongside me because I was still pretty weak after the operation, but I got myself over there as quickly as I possibly could. My experience was one of amazement, particularly at the facility. I was really taken with this beautiful big building that looks like something out of *Gone With the Wind*. A big bird aviary in front and a beautiful view looking back toward San Diego—it's a marvelous place."

Rex Major started treatment immediately with the Hoxsey tonic and diet. "The thing that I was intrigued about was the attitude of most of the people in the waiting room. There's an awful lot of very sick people there, usually the first-timers. But the laughing and the jokes and the friendly camaraderie that are created in that place are something to behold. I was very, very taken with the place, and very taken with Mildred."

Rex quickly began to feel positive effects from the treatment. He located a new doctor in New Zealand who worked closely with him to test and monitor his ongoing condition, including regular examinations of his colon. "I've got some beautiful, clear Technicolor photographs of the inside of my colon, which is in perfect condition today." Six years later, Rex Major is cancer-free.

Did Rex Major in fact have cancer in the first place? The official biopsy reports confirm that he did. Was he cured by prior surgery? He still had the disease in his lymph nodes when he went to Hoxsey, as a biopsy showed.

Was Rex Major really cured by Hoxsey? The Hildenbrands assessed Rex's case. "He refused chemotherapy from a physician who was very concerned about recurrence. The staging of the cancer had a very poor prognosis. The five-year survival rate for Duke's C is only 15 percent with state-of-the-art contemporary treatment, including chemotherapy. The fact that he did not receive this makes him a rarity indeed. Although one would not want to argue that surgery alone might not result in the occasional random cure, it would be foolish to argue that the Hoxsey management might not have contributed." Colon cancer, the second leading cause of cancer deaths in the United States, is considered one of the most curable only if it is found in the early stages.[5]

Could Rex Major be the rare one in 100,000 case of spontaneous remission? Could there be other factors besides the Hoxsey tonic responsible for his recovery, such as his faith and positive attitude?

These kinds of questions can be answered definitively only by an objective scientific test. The recoveries of Rex Major, Gwen Scott, and Margaret Griffin would all be discounted by the orthodox medical profession as unscientific anomalies whose causes cannot be known outside carefully controlled studies. Doctors have often contended that patients such as these were actually cured by prior conventional treatments of surgery, radiation, or chemotherapy. Their cases fit the classically intriguing but inconclusive profile of Hoxsey patients caught in a medical hall of mirrors amid a confusing volley of claims and counterclaims.

The case of Mrs. Martha Bond was more clear-cut, however. In 1986 our film crew traveled to Colorado to visit with this soft-spoken woman of about sixty years of age. She sat shyly behind tinted glasses in a perfectly pressed white dress as she told us her remarkable story from the heart of middle America.

"I first noticed it in about 1974—a mark on my cheek—but we didn't pay any attention to it because it was flat and there was no pain. We never thought it was cancer. Then in 1979 I got a dark mark on my leg, and that started to grow faster and it raised up high. So I told my husband about it. He's blind, so he didn't see it, but he felt it. He said, 'Oh, that's cancer. We'd better go down to Tijuana to the Bio Medical Center.'

"We went down there and they looked at it. They gave me the tonic and vitamins, and told me to keep taking it and to call them back and let them know how I was doing. That was in April. Around August, a friend of ours thought we ought to get a second opinion, so we went to our local doctor, a skin doctor, and he said that it was melanoma cancer. So he suggested I see Doctor X, a surgeon, and have it surgically removed. We asked Dr. X if there was any way we could take it off just locally by putting any salve or taking any tonic. He said, 'No way. There's no way but surgery. If you don't go into surgery, you're not going to live long.' I said to him, 'I've been taking something, a tonic, and it is getting flatter.' He says, 'No, it just can't.' He wanted to put me in the hospital that next week."

Melanoma is an especially deadly form of cancer. Usually manifesting as a black mole on the skin, it is not considered solely a skin cancer readily treatable by surgery because it also can spread internally to form tumors elsewhere with frightening speed. Surgery can be effective if the tumor is entirely removed before it has spread, but the knife can be a chancy proposition because cutting can spread it rapidly through the body. Doctors generally advise immediate and radical surgery for early-stage melanoma. Advanced melanoma is almost always fatal, with an expected survival time of only about seven months. Mrs. Bond's surgeon clearly saw her condition as very urgent and dangerous.

Mrs. Bond held up her hands to show our camera the size of the tumors. "The large one on my face was about a silver-dollar size, and the one on my leg was not quite as large, but it was thicker and deeper. The second one on my leg would be about a dime size or maybe quarter size. They just kept forming pus and blood around them."

After several months on the tonic, Mrs. Bond contacted the clinic again. "We talked to Mildred Nelson," she remembered, "and she looked up my records and said I must come down there and they would remove it, and not to let anyone cut it at all. So we went down to the clinic. It took three weeks." This time, Mildred applied the external salves.

"While I was taking the tonic, the one on my leg was going down and getting flatter after three and a half months. Mildred said that was a big help that it was going down. Then she put on a salve right directly on the two lesions. I could feel the feelers going to the roots of the cancer. She said not to touch it, and all we did was leave this cotton on it. When enough pus and blood seemed to form around them, they just fell out automatically. As soon as they fell out, there was no more pain. It was only painful while they were eating their way out. That's all Mildred did. In three weeks, they just fell out by themselves.

"When the second one was removed from my leg, there was one dot left, just like a pinhead, very small. She said, 'If we don't remove this, you're going to be sorry because it's going to spread, and then we've got to start over again.' So, we started over again with the salve, and that took about ten days, and then that one came out. Then she just put another salve on my face, and that closed up the opening on my cheek and that's all we did."

We asked Mrs. Bond what the conventional procedure proposed to her would have been. "The original surgeon wanted to scrape my face. If he had, he'd have left all these roots in my face. He told me that the hole he would cut on the one on my leg would be about the size of a fist. Now I only have just a slight indentation there. But if he had done the same for my face—because it was just as large on my face, if not larger, than on my leg—he'd have taken half of my face off. This way I have just a very slight scar.

"This was seven years ago and I am still here," Mrs. Bond said proudly, holding up a mason jar of pickled tumors. "I asked Mildred to let me have these cancers because I wanted them in a jar so I could show other people to prove that it really works. I would go around in the clinic and show all the people this cancer in the jar. I said, 'Look, I'm walking around carrying my cancer in the jar instead of inside of me, which is much better.' It made them happy to think it really works. I've kept it, wondering what I should do with it, but I thought I should keep it in case I meet someone else that needs the encouragement of seeing this."

Mrs. Bond provided us not only with the biopsy from her original doctor, but also with an alarming letter from the surgeon she consulted. It read, "Mrs. Bond, the skin tumors that you have are a very serious problem and I would urge you to reconsider this decision. I would strongly urge you to have these lesions surgically removed. Local therapy is not effective in treating a malignant melanoma, and these tumors will spread and ultimately result in your death, if not surgically removed."

The Hildenbrands confirmed her records. They indicated that the prognosis for leaving melanoma untreated is extremely poor, and the likelihood of surviving for seven years is very small, as her doctor stated in his fatalistic letter. The sole treatment she had was Hoxsey. (After this time, I lost track of Mrs. Bond and could not ascertain her status.)

Only after first putting Mrs. Bond on the tonic for several months did Mildred Nelson apply both a caustic red paste and a yellow powder directly to the tumors. The salves "ate" and removed the tumors, and Mildred then kept Mrs. Bond on the tonic for five years. Like Harry Hoxsey before her, she views melanoma as both an internal and external phenomenon.

What are these external remedies? The red paste and yellow powder, whose formulas have been published and are discussed in depth later along with all the Hoxsey remedies, are *escharotics*, caustic substances that burn tissue and kill cells. Escharotics are an old form of folk medicine with a long history of popular usage in both human and veterinary medicine. Surprisingly, organized medicine has not disputed the efficacy of these treatments since around 1950 and classifies them as a "standard" treatment, though one that is seldom if ever used.

The red paste is a "true" escharotic that will "eat" anything it touches. It is intensely painful. Mildred uses it mainly on large tumors. "You apply it daily over a period of time," she described. "You start at the top and go to the bottom of the tumor. When it comes out, when this dies, it separates just like you cut it out with a knife." The red paste contains several chemical and mineral ingredients, as well as bloodroot, a plant used on external cancers by Native Americans for centuries.

The yellow powder is a modified escharotic, unusual because it is claimed to be selective, killing only malignant cells. Normally it is applied topically on the surface. "The tissue where you put it that is malignant dies," Mildred explained. "Only the malignant part dies. Then it separates itself from the normal tissue by an accumulation of white cells underneath, which pushes it off. It separates cleanly. I have put the yellow powder in the eye." To emphasize its safety, Mildred dipped her fingers in a small jar of the powder, ate a pinch, and arched her eyebrows provocatively. It can also be injected internally, as the case of Stephen Crutcher, presented in chapter 13, demonstrates.

While filming, we observed Mildred treating several external cases. One man had a cavity in his upper back and shoulder at least three inches deep, a hideous, foul-smelling cancer. She peered intently over her bifocals and extended long agile fingers that looked like those of a young woman. To clean the festering mass, she dipped a cloth into a large bowl containing Pine Sol, which she uses as a disinfectant. Pine Sol is an off-the-shelf house-cleaning fluid she favors as the most effective agent not only for disinfecting these masses, but also for eradicating their unbearable stench.

Several patients told us that this treatment marked the first time they were relieved of the horrific odor that intensified their discomfort and made it hard to be around other people.

Mildred sprinkled some of the yellow powder into the gaping wound with a large Q-tip, and dressed it with bandages. The patient seemed none the worse for wear, put his shirt back on, and went off to the waiting room.

Mildred retreated across the room to her desk. Expansive picture windows looked out over Tijuana across to the U.S. border in the distance. She started another cigarette and settled comfortably into her spacious chair, framed by a photograph of natty Harry Hoxsey hanging on the wall behind her. The streaming sunlight highlighted deep lines on her weathered face as she ruffled through a folder and readied herself for the next case. Patients walking to consult other clinic doctors necessarily traversed the hallway at the open end of her office, and she nodded knowingly to each of them.

We found the Bio Medical Center a modern, competently run facility. Employing six Mexican physicians, the clinic had a laboratory, X-ray quarters, and a professional staff. It has always been an outpatient clinic, and except for external cases that may take several weeks or months to treat, most people spend about two days going through tests and then meeting with Mildred and the doctors. If they have cancer, they get a bottle of Hoxsey tonic that lasts about six months, along with other supportive treatments and instructions for the special diet.

The clinic today charges a one-time fee of $3,500, plus the costs of tests. If necessary, patients are permitted to pay on an honor-system installment plan. The clinic has never sent out a bill, and does not even have the administrative apparatus for mailing invoices. Poor people are treated free, contingent on verification of their need from a minister, doctor, or another reputable party.

Organized medicine has long accused the Hoxsey clinic of financially exploiting cancer patients. We found no evidence to support the charge. "My surgeon got so mad," chimed in Stella Gladis, a patient in for a checkup. "When he found out I wouldn't take chemotherapy and radiation from his friends, then he really screamed and hollered at me. He said, 'Why are you going down there? They'll only take all your money.' I said, 'Uh-uh—'cause you already did!" Stella Gladis paid $900 for her Hoxsey treatment. She estimated her bills from her cancer operations in the tens of thousands of dollars.

The famous Hoxsey tonic, which comes in a large old-fashioned glass bottle, is a dark brown liquid tasting a bit like flat root beer. It contains potassium iodide and herbs. (For people with stomach sensitivities or ulcers, there is another form called the "pink tonic" in a base of lactate of pepsin without a couple of the laxative herbs.)

A strict diet emphasizing fruits and vegetables is recommended in tandem with the tonic. According to Mildred, it evolved mainly from empirical observation that certain foods appear to negate the tonic's activity. Compared with many natural foods dietary programs for cancer, it is a relatively simple program.

The clinic also offers a multitude of supportive treatments, including vitamins, yeast, garlic, and a host of other natural medicines. The list changes as Mildred learns about new developments, and she is perpetually experimenting with new treatments that she hopes may help.

There is another ingredient to the treatment that Mildred considers essential. Sitting back in her reclining office chair, she squinted with a fierce gaze, exhibiting the no-nonsense gravity of someone who sees a lot of serious illness, "Probably the greatest success comes with the patient's attitude. When they come in the front door saying, 'I'm here to get some medicine because I'm going to get well,' then I'm just as happy as they are. But when they come through the door saying, 'Well, I don't think anything's going to help, but they wanted me to do this' "—Mildred grimaced—"you can't make 'em get well. They have to want to do it themselves."

There is a term in Spanish flamenco called *duende*. The best dancers are said to carry it with them always. *Duende* signifies the awareness that death is always on our shoulder, ready to take us in the wink of an eye. Its gift is the heightened awareness of the precariousness and preciousness of life. Cancer patients dance with *duende*, bringing a palpable immediacy to life. To face cancer fully demands a choice, Mildred suggests, at the inescapable moment of truth when the results of the tests come back. Whatever the outlook may be, people must first want to live. Only then can healing happen. Many patients we met had made this choice to live. According to Mildred, getting well at the Bio Medical Center is a healing partnership that takes two to work.

After spending considerable time at the clinic and filming repeatedly, we became convinced that Mildred Nelson's dedication as a nurse and her belief in the Hoxsey treatment are genuine. A cross between Mother Teresa and Calamity Jane, she certainly never expected the life she has led. A compassionate caregiver, she despises politics almost as much as sitting in front of a camera. Unlike Harry Hoxsey, she has long shunned both controversy and publicity.

"The first question the press may ask," Mildred sharply told our camera, "is, 'What's your fight with the AMA?' I have no fight with anybody.

I try to do the things that I know are right for the people, take care of 'em, help 'em. But I'm not here to fight." She long ago gave up any hope of a scientific investigation and is content to treat her patients in a setting far removed from U.S. medical politics.

When Mildred told us to go talk with the patients, she knew exactly the kinds of stories we'd find. They were like the ones she herself first heard when she came to the Hoxsey clinic in 1946, like the cases she would share with researchers from the Office of Alternative Medicine arriving in 1997 with Catherine to pore over records. They were what Harry Hoxsey built his career on and what won him an unlikely series of court trials all the way to the federal bench. But they were not sufficient to get the investigation he pleaded for.

The cases documented here are but a modest sampling, tantalizing leads tracked down by an independent journalist and a public health nurse. Although they are in no way definitive, one might expect such seeming successes to provoke interest from the medical community. Why did it take the government seventy-five years to investigate?

It is hard to believe that such a seemingly harmless program of a non-toxic herbal tonic, folk salves, a nutritional program, and an attitudinal approach to healing ignited one of the most bitter controversies in medical history, a spectacular cancer war between organized medicine and one man: Harry M. Hoxsey.

Since the Hoxsey treatment has never been rigorously investigated, the question remains: Was Harry Hoxsey a hoax, or was he "the quack who cured cancer"?

We set off to find out for ourselves.

3

A Formula for Conflict

One afternoon in Mildred's trailer, Catherine and I were relaxing after a strenuous day of filming. Mildred arose abruptly from her Lazy-Boy recliner and whisked to the closet. She emerged mysteriously with a large film can and handed it to us. It contained Harry Hoxsey's own movie, a promotional film we had not known about made at the Dallas clinic in 1957.[1] Incredulous at our great good fortune, we raced back to San Diego, rented a 16 millimeter projector, and gazed at the black-and-white images flickering on the motel wall.

The film opened with a title card displaying the antique cameo of a horse grazing by a steepled church, above the words: "This is a film based on a story of intolerance, in the best American tradition. Our fathers left us with a heritage of Freedom of Speech, Freedom of Religion, and Freedom of Choice. If you have the right to choose your own church, your own minister or priest, why not your own doctor?"

Then there was Harry Hoxsey, larger than life. A big man wearing a snappy suit and diamond ring, he cut an embattled figure. He was haggard, with deep black bags under his eyes, but fire burned through his fatigue. "We now have in our files and our records many, many thousands of case histories, pathological proofs, and X-ray photographic studies showing that we do *positively* cure cancer, both internal and external. We now have records proving the cure stands up for many, many years, as far back as over twenty years here in Texas."

Later in the film, holding up a copy of his newly published book, which he had just sent to every senator and representative in Washington, he thumped on his big desk and thundered, "This book, entitled *You Don't Have to Die*, is filled with dynamite. In fact, it should have been printed on asbestos paper. I give you names, dates, times, names of doctors, names of institutions. But they have never proven this treatment *don't* cure cancer."

It was easy for the medical profession to paint Hoxsey as a quack: He

35

fit the image perfectly. Brandishing his famed tonic bottle, he arrived straight from central casting as the stereotype of the snake-oil salesman. His fast-talking, carnival-barker manner pegged him as the huckster of the ages. Throughout his career, he was buffeted by a tempestuous conflict of medical opinion. The surviving players from the Hoxsey melodrama reflected these wildly divergent views.

"He knew the treatment worked," commented Mildred Nelson matter-of-factly. "He had no doubt in his mind that he was going to get all of them well if he could get a chance to get them."

The AMA could not have disagreed more vehemently. "He did persuade people that he had something of merit, and that he was being treated unfairly," said Oliver Field, who zealously pursued Hoxsey while heading the AMA's anti-quackery Bureau of Investigation in the 1950s. "The idea of being for the underdog is one of the things that most people have in their way of thinking—they favor them. He wasn't an underdog at all, as far as the medical profession was concerned. He was doing his thing and he had no business doing it. In fact, Hoxsey met the legal and dictionary definition of a *quack:* one who pretends to medical skill he does not possess."

"Some people say that if you walk like a duck and look like a duck and quack like a duck, you must be a duck," observed James Wakefield Burke, an accomplished journalist who wrote about Hoxsey and briefly worked for him. "Many people judged Harry at first impression like that, which didn't always bide good with strangers and certain officials in the AMA and in Washington. But those who got to know him, you didn't think that. He had a great deal of basic nobility about him, and any person with any intelligence would see that."

"I think everybody agrees that he was a great con man, a great salesman," countered William Grigg, public affairs director of the Food and Drug Administration, which battled Hoxsey for over a decade. "He was the kind of person who understood the value of publicity. Even though he was a very poorly educated man, he was very good at playing all the angles and wrapping up state governments, the AMA, and the FDA itself. Clearly, however, he had no belief that this treatment was useful. He was a great liar."

"As a crime reporter for ten years," remembered Jimmy Kerr, a Dallas TV newsman who covered Hoxsey for many years, "I was pretty good at recognizing a con man a mile off. Hoxsey was a bit of a used-car salesman, but I really don't believe he was a con man. He certainly believed in what he was doing. And I have to say, personally, that I believe he truly helped some people with cancer."

"For internal cancer he had absolutely nothing to offer," charged Dr. Harry M. Spence, a professor emeritus at the University of Texas whose

Dallas practice grew up alongside Hoxsey's in the 1930s, and who testified in court against him. "Hoxsey was certainly a bad man. He was bad in so many ways that are obvious, but I think perhaps the main way he was a force for evil was that he prevented so many people from getting treatment at an appropriate time."

"Hoxsey was honest," ruminated Jimmy "Trombone" Martin, his attorney in the 1940s and 1950s. "He really and truly believed in it. It takes lots of nerve to put up a big nice place in a big city like Dallas and hold yourself out as being able to furnish medicines that'll cure cancer. It takes nerve to do that. I don't believe a man that knew he was lying could do it. Be hard to do."

"Mr. Hoxsey was a rainmaker," offered Robert Heath, the director of the Dallas County Medical Society and son of its past director, Millard Heath, whom Hoxsey sued in the 1950s. "There were people who desperately needed an answer to the problem they had. Whether he had the answer or not, he was able to persuade them that he had the answer. The interesting thing about it is that, even with the rainmaker who used to travel the country during the late 1800s and early 1900s, occasionally it would rain. There were enough people who felt they were benefited that caused Mr. Hoxsey to be successful."

"Dad was always what I would call eighty/twenty," added Hoxsey's son. "Eighty percent of what he said was true, but he couldn't resist embellishing things that extra 20 percent. He didn't have to do it, but that's the way he was. He was a bit of a showman."

These living players helped me construct a unique oral history of Hoxsey never recorded elsewhere. Several died not long after we filmed them, including James Burke and Jimmy Martin. When I located Hoxsey's son and daughter, they spoke to me only on the condition of anonymity because they had once been so severely stigmatized as the children of a "quack." I have respected their privacy, just as I have omitted details of Hoxsey's personal life because I do not find it germane to the central meaning of the story: his quest for an investigation. He was a ladies' man, married four or possibly five times. Otherwise, he was a man obsessed with his mission, and that is what this book explores.

Through exhaustive research, I was able to document much of Hoxsey's story. Where accounts are at odds, I have tried to present the disparity of views and allegations. For Hoxsey's youth and very early years, there is primarily his own account. By the founding of his first clinic in 1924, I was able to find substantial documentation against which to measure his own rendering of events. In subsequent periods, I found a great deal of other material to confirm, deny, or color his depiction of the story.[2]

Harry Hoxsey was an American original. "I come of pioneer stock," he attested in *You Don't Have to Die*, a self-aggrandizing chronicle amply colorized with the Hoxsey legend. He traced the original "Hoxie" lineage from Scottish, English, Welsh, and Dutch stock back to Plymouth Colony in 1650.

According to Hoxsey, early colonial records indicate that the family became Quakers and ran into trouble with hostile local authorities. "The Friends are a religious fellowship without formal creed or priestly hierarchy," he wrote, "hence the Hoxseys were inclined to reject all religious, political or scientific dogma, to deny the authority of witch-doctors of any kind to impose their theories upon the community as divine doctrine. The Friends are opposed to violence, regard human life as sacred; hence the Hoxsey conviction that the preservation of human life is the sacred duty of all men, not merely those entitled to add 'M.D.' to their names." Throughout his career, Hoxsey cultivated the persona of a populist folk healer and working-class hero.

The family migrated to Rhode Island and later to West Virginia, Kentucky, and finally Illinois, where Harry Mathias Hoxsey was born on October 23, 1901, in the small burg of Auburn near Springfield, the state capital. His father was John C. Hoxsey, a veterinarian who had inherited his own grandfather's cancer formulas. John C. became known in the region for treating animals with cancer and tumors, and boarded sick horses during winters for the Ringling Brothers circus.

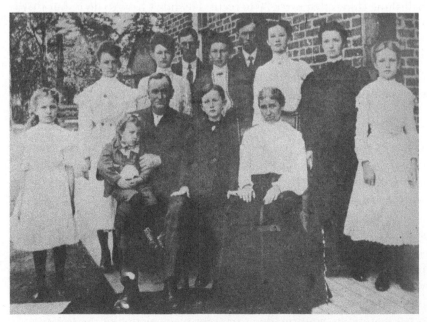

Young Harry Hoxsey (sitting on his father's knee) with family, c. 1905.

By the turn of the century the fertile farmlands of southern Illinois were giving way to coal mines, smokestacks, and waves of poor European immigrants. Flush wages for miners spawned a boomtown rush of raucous saloons, gambling joints, and brothels. Industrialism was ascendant, and so was cancer.

Vacating the small Auburn farm, John C. Hoxsey set up shop in a modest home office in small-town Girard, where he quietly began treating cancer patients under the auspices of two local doctors. In a cramped livery stable next to the town square, he kept a stock of the three medicines in locked cabinets along with bandages and surgical dressings. Each summer the veterinarian returned to the family farm to brew a year's supply of the cancer remedies. Harry, the baby of twelve children, was the only one to show an interest in the cancer work, and started apprenticing with his father at the age of eight.

Harry Hoxsey's defining moment shone during the first healing he witnessed as a young boy assisting his father. Cancer sufferer John Frommie, a prominent local citizen, came for treatment of two tumors including one on his nose the size of a walnut. For each session, Harry was permitted to cut bandages and tie elaborate strings reaching around the man's nose and behind his ears. After six months, Frommie reputedly recovered. Placing his hand on the child's head, he exclaimed, "Doc, it was Harry and his halters got me well!" As Harry recalled, "Right there and then I resolved that when I grew up I would cure people like my dad did." He said it was presumed from then on that he would go to medical school.[3]

Harry spent all his spare time helping out in his father's office. As the cancer practice grew, John C. gave over his veterinary business to an assistant in order to devote himself to it full time. The move entailed financial sacrifice in an impoverished community that seldom had more than a sheep or goat for payment. Yet he never turned people away for lack of funds, instructing Harry, "Son, cancer don't pick and choose. It hits rich and poor, black and white, Catholic, Protestant and Jew. All of them have a right to be treated, whether they can pay for it or not. Healing the sick and saving lives isn't a business; it's a duty and a privilege."[4]

Then tragedy befell the family. John C. tripped over a loose board, breaking his nose. Complications set in, his health declined precipitously, and the family had to sell the farm. At the age of fifteen, Harry quit school and went to work in the coal mines to support the family. Because of his expertise in handling animals, he soon graduated to muleskinner, driving ornery teams two and a half miles into the dark pits. During summers, he drove a taxi, shuttling miners to brothels and saloons. He built silos and chauffeured salesmen around the county in a horse and buggy. On the side, he sold insurance.

As Hoxsey's son told me, it was Harry's athletic period. The tall, robust farm boy played semiprofessional baseball for three teams under different names. He boxed and wrestled for cash, and sported a scar from a bout with a seven-foot Indian who flipped him out of the ring. He worked as a human fly carrying Coca-Cola signs up seven-story buildings. He picked up a bullet during a wave of bloody labor strikes in a region locked in violent class war between labor and capital, rocked from half a world away by Bolsheviks seizing power to establish a workers' state.

By 1919 John C. Hoxsey was bedridden. According to Harry, the diagnosis was erysipelas, an acute bacterial infection of the skin that resembles cancer. Before antibiotics, such conditions were often fatal. Deteriorating rapidly, the invalid father directed the boy to go to the People's Bank to retrieve his safe deposit box and then stop at the drugstore to buy three Big Chief writing tablets.

John C. propped himself up in bed and riffled through the metal box, withdrawing a small white envelope. "These are the cancer formulas I got from my father and he got from his. Now it's my turn to pass them on. When you were just a little shaver, asking questions about my work and watching me treat patients, I knew you had the call to be a doctor. That's why I picked you to inherit the family formulas."[5]

John C. gravely removed the contents of the envelope and handed Harry the first of the Big Chief tablets, illustrated on the fire-red cover with an Indian chief in full headdress. Slowly he read aloud the formula for the internal tonic. Harry copied it down word for word. The father instructed him to go in the dining room and write the formula on each of the 250 blank pages. Around midnight, young Harry fell asleep at the table half done. Roused by his mother in the dawn light, he refused breakfast and wrote all morning to finish.

The lad brought the tablet to his father, who asked sternly, "Do you have it by heart?" Harry recited the formula flawlessly, and his father tore the original and copies into little pieces, put them in a wastebasket, and motioned him to incinerate them in the woodstove. John C. then dictated the formula for the external red salve, and Harry went to work inscribing the second Big Chief tablet. He finished the next night, and brought the work back. Again he parroted the formula and burned the papers. His writing hand aching and stiff, he took down the last recipe for the yellow powder.[6]

When Harry completed the task the next day, he returned to find his father enfeebled and dying. Taking the boy's hand, the patriarch solemnly passed on the family legacy. "Now you have the power to heal the sick and save lives. What I've managed to do in a tiny part of this state, you can do all over the country, all over the world. I've cured hundreds of people; you can cure thousands, tens of thousands.

"But it's not only a gift, son; it's a trust and a great responsibility. Abe Lincoln once said God must have loved the common people because He made so many of them. We're common, ordinary people. No matter how high you go, you must never lose touch with the common people. You must never refuse to treat anybody because he can't pay. Promise me that!"[7] This counsel would inform the rest of Harry's unorthodox career.

"I wish I could have done more for you," lamented the elder as he summoned his last reserve of strength. "Sent you to college, helped you become a doctor. Now you'll have to go it alone. You've got a long hard battle ahead, and you're going to make yourself a lot of enemies. Many doctors won't like what you're doing because it will take money out of their pockets. They'll organize against you, fight you tooth and nail, persecute you, slander you, try to drive you off the face of the earth. Don't underrate them, they're powerful, they're the *High Priests of Medicine*. But in the end, you'll win. Because there's one thing they can't do, and that's put back the cancers you removed."[8]

With the transmission of the family legacy complete, John C. Hoxsey shut his eyes and sank into the bed. Several days later he was dead. According to Hoxsey, a local doctor came and signed the death certificate, citing the cause as erysipelas.

Charged with a daunting deathbed patrimony, Harry Hoxsey dedicated himself to curing cancer. To accomplish the mission, he recognized he had to become a doctor. With no money and a widowed mother and sick sister to support, he focused on making a living at his medley of jobs. He returned home late every night to study for a high school diploma, which he gained by correspondence course. He deposited his earnings each week in a cigar box marked COLLEGE. Tellingly, he also took a mail-order course in forensic medicine, the legal aspects of medical practice. He was apparently girding himself for the rules of the road as an unconventional healer.

Locals in the community knew that Hoxsey had a supply of the medicines locked in the cabinet, and over the next two years several came pleading for treatment. He rebuffed them for fear of jeopardizing his medical school plans. After the death of his mother and sister, he moved to nearby Taylorville to save on expenses by living with another sister. Toiling in the mines with his premium mule Shorty, he was now stashing over half of each paycheck in his cigar-box college fund.

But Hoxsey soon saw his plans subverted. Coming home from the mines one evening, he found a visitor waiting in the kitchen. A retired insurance broker and Civil War veteran, S. T. Larkin was a local citizen of wealth and standing whose lower lip and chin were disfigured with a running sore diagnosed as cancer. He knew Harry's father well and demanded treatment. Harry declined because he had no license to practice medicine. "Nobody needs a license to save lives," Larkin objected stubbornly. "If I was drowning, would you stand by and watch me go down because a sign on yonder tree says 'no swimming?'"

Hoxsey still resisted, refusing to break the law, but the Civil War veteran raised the ethical stakes. "The first thing they teach doctors is that human life is sacred. You have the power to save mine, if you treat me now. If you don't, I'll surely die, and you'll be guilty of murder."[9]

Torn by the life-and-death decision, Hoxsey reluctantly relented, agreeing to treat Larkin only if he swore to secrecy. Larkin consented, but when he returned for his next session, he brought a friend, E. C. McVicker, a director of the Farmer's Bank who had a black sore on his temple diagnosed as cancer. Hoxsey protested angrily, but McVicker promised he would give him a big check for college if Hoxsey cured him. "Might as well treat two as one," the banker quipped, and Hoxsey suddenly acquired a second patient and the financial means to a higher education.[10]

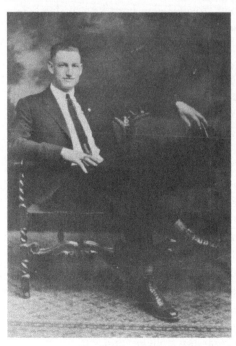

Hoxsey founds his first clinic in 1924.

When the two men returned for their next treatment, they brought along yet another cancer sufferer. After a heated argument, Hoxsey realized that—ready or not—he was in business. His patients became his patrons, and he quit his job in the mines and began discreetly treating cancer. Over the next two years, he claimed numerous cures. McVicker and Larkin appeared for years afterward as convincing Hoxsey testimonials at rallies and revivals.[11] (There are no medical records of these cases, and in that era, diagnosis was dicey. There is no way of knowing whether they actually had cancer.)

Having at last acquired enough money for college and

medical school, Hoxsey said he planned to halt his illicit practice and lay the tracks for his medical training. Seeking guidance, he consulted Dr. Maxamillian Meinhardt, a physician with a Chicago sanitorium. Dr. Meinhardt proved to be far more interested in Hoxsey's cancer remedies than in his prospective education. "You don't need to go to medical school if you have a cure for cancer," Meinhardt lobbied him. "If this thing will work, your troubles are over." He invited the credulous young man to treat some test cases at his Chicago facility.[12]

There Hoxsey met Dr. Bruce Miller, who would figure prominently in his future. The physician came down to Taylorville to check out some of Hoxsey's alleged successes. Impressed with the cases, Dr. Miller explained to Hoxsey that the medical profession was largely helpless against cancer using surgery, radium, and X-ray once the disease had spread. But, he warned, organized medicine would nevertheless oppose him as an outsider to the medical fraternity. When Hoxsey explained that he was going to become a doctor and bring the remedies in through the profession, Dr. Miller broke the news that various doctors were already complaining to the State Medical Board against the outlaw healer. Hoxsey was blackballed and stood no chance of admission to medical school.

Hoxsey listened numbly as Dr. Miller went on to propose that they go into business together. They could use the fifty-seven-year-old physician's medical license to comply with legal requirements, with Hoxsey legitimately serving as a medical technician. This structure became his modus operandi for the rest of his career. His course in forensic medicine may well have prepared him for this eventuality.

Hoxsey and Dr. Miller formed a legal partnership predicated on the condition that Hoxsey not be required to divulge his secret formulas. On March 1, 1924, they opened the first Hoxsey clinic in Taylorville. "I tried it out after long and careful investigation," Dr. Miller was

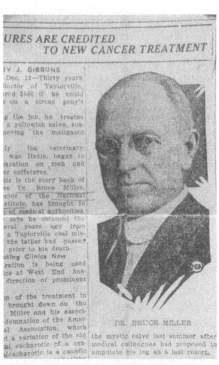

Dr. Bruce Miller heralds Hoxsey's therapy, c. 1925.

quoted in a 1924 newspaper, "and saved the life of my first patient. Since then it has never failed to remove any cancer except the sarcoma variety [arising from connective tissue]."[13] Miller said he was treating only external cancers at that time. The physician would continue working with Hoxsey or his treatment for decades to come.

The clinic was soon deluged with patients, and within two months the partners had to find bigger quarters. Hoxsey had his eye on a spacious building on Main Street owned by the Loyal Order of the Moose, and held a meeting with the Lodge board where he presented a dozen cured cases including McVicker and Larkin, as well as a secretary of the Lodge. The sensational testimonials did the trick. His dramatic cures were already emerging as his stock-in-trade.

Though never one to think small, Hoxsey could hardly have imagined the synchronous connections awaiting him at the Loyal Order of the Moose. Lucius O. Everhard, a Chicago insurance broker and Moose Lodge member, attended the fateful gathering. "This is the biggest thing on earth," Everhard reportedly told Hoxsey, boasting that he had recently written a large insurance policy for Dr. Malcolm L. Harris, chief surgeon of the Alexian Brothers Hospital in Chicago and secretary of the American Medical Association. Everhard proposed contacting Dr. Harris to arrange a demonstration.[14]

Hoxsey was elated when Dr. Harris agreed. Hoxsey, Dr. Miller, and Everhard drove the two hundred miles to Chicago the very same night, landing at the swanky Sherman Hotel. The following morning at 8:30, they waited eagerly outside the hospital until a chauffeured car delivered the distinguished Dr. Harris. The small, dapper physician stood in awkward contrast to Hoxsey in his ill-fitting Sunday best, and uncomfortably shook the ex-miner's rough, pawlike hand.

Dr. Harris led the trio to the funereal hospital room of Thomas Mannix, a sixty-six-year-old former police desk sergeant. A terminal cancer patient, the ghostly Mannix had a severe epithelioma, a grotesque mass of diseased flesh festering four inches across his shoulder. His distraught daughter Kate kept vigil, clasping his limp hand. The cancerous area had been treated with surgery and badly burned by intensive radiation. As Mannix later described in court testimony, "The surgeon done everything but cut my arm off. He advised me to take some [radiation] treatments. It was a red, raw sore, and there was a lump there. It covered pretty nearly my whole shoulder. When he sent for my wife and told her to take me home, he said that I had about four weeks to live. I had the good fortune to meet Dr. Miller. He said, 'My, that is a whopper.'"[15]

Dr. Miller reportedly objected to treating such an advanced case, but

Hoxsey insisted on proceeding. Leaning in to Mannix, he whispered words of encouragement and thought he detected a flicker of hope in the veteran's dim eyes. He applied a generous portion of the yellow powder and left a supply of the internal tonic with instructions, promising to return in a week. Hoxsey said Dr. Harris guardedly told him, "We are giving it to him for the sole purpose of seeing whether this treatment is toxic. We want it understood that I do not expect any results from it."[16]

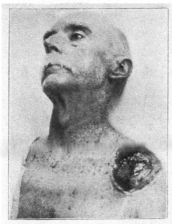

SERGEANT THOMAS MANNIX
Desk Sergeant
Sheffield Avenue Police Station
Chicago, Ill.
(1)

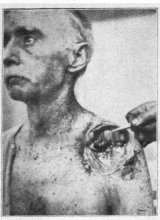

SERGEANT THOMAS MANNIX
Desk Sergeant
Sheffield Avenue Police Station
Chicago, Ill.
(2)

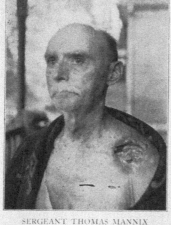

SERGEANT THOMAS MANNIX
Desk Sergeant
Sheffield Avenue Police Station
Chicago, Ill.
(3)

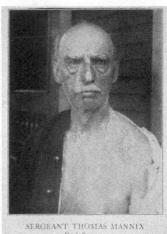

SERGEANT THOMAS MANNIX
Desk Sergeant
Sheffield Avenue Police Station
Chicago, Ill.
(4)

Graphic proof shows the success of Hoxsey's reputed demonstration to the AMA.

Within two weeks Mannix began to improve. Four weeks later, the cancer hardened and turned black, and started separating from the healthy tissue. His general health improved as well. Hoxsey told Dr. Harris that within a few days it would be possible to remove the dried, hardened tumor entirely. Dr. Harris suggested that the procedure take place in the hospital amphitheater in front of the entire staff.[17]

The amphitheater swelled with ten doctors and another fifty interns and students. Hoxsey said Dr. Harris introduced him to several physicians, among them Dr. Morris Fishbein, editor of the influential *Journal of the American Medical Association (JAMA)*. Dr. Miller and Hoxsey successfully removed the necrosed tumor, slipping off the stony mass cleanly with a knife. Hoxsey said the electric crowd descended around them and fired agitated questions for hours.

Here the accounts diverge radically. According to Hoxsey, the next morning he was invited for a meeting with Dr. Harris, who effusively dubbed the treatment "the eighth wonder of the world." The AMA official then made him an offer. "Do you remember Dr. Fishbein? He is the biggest man in medicine. He is the man that dictates the policy of medicine in this country. With this treatment, or this put in the proper hands, we will take it over and it will be the greatest boon to humanity on earth. Now, I drew up a contract for you to sign."[18]

The alleged contract proposed an extensive five-year testing period and stipulated that Hoxsey turn over his formulas with a large supply of the medicines. It further specified that Hoxsey would have no further involvement with the treatment and must immediately cease his own operations. The formulas were to become the property of a consortium of doctors including Dr. Harris and Dr. Fishbein, with Hoxsey allotted 10 percent of profits after ten years, if the treatment panned out.

Taken aback, Hoxsey suggested that he would have to show the document to his lawyer to review possible changes. "I promised my father," Hoxsey recalled objecting, "I would never give these formulas to anybody without an agreement they would carry his name, and they would agree to treat poor people, whether they had money or not."[19] Dr. Harris sidestepped the query and pressured him that no reputable doctor would have anything to do with him unless he signed the document.

Hoxsey stood his ground, prompting Dr. Harris to reach for the phone to call the hospital to deny Hoxsey access to Mannix until he inked the agreement. "I waited until he hung up the receiver," Hoxsey related, "and called the Mannix home. Before I could be connected, Dr. Harris reached over the desk and tried to take the telephone away from me. My left elbow flipped up, caught him squarely in the chest and sent him flying into his chair. It promptly toppled over, depositing him in a most undignified position on the floor." Hoxsey urgently warned Kate to get her father out of the hospital.[20]

Hoxsey said Dr. Harris put the contract back in the drawer and retorted, "Hoxsey, you are the biggest damn fool on earth. You are either going to sign that contract, or you will never treat any more cases of cancer, and you will rot in jail." "That is your opinion," Hoxsey replied evenly. "Miller and I can go back to Taylorville." Dr. Harris threatened, "If you go back to Taylorville and start working there, Fishbein and I will hound you as long as you live." "That is your opinion," Hoxsey repeated coldly, exiting under a shower of recriminations from the AMA official.[21]

Whatever actually transpired between Hoxsey and Dr. Harris, that's when the battle started. Hoxsey's charges became shrouded in inscrutable mystery. Did AMA doctors try to suppress a cancer cure they couldn't control? After extensive research, I was able to verify the medical case but not the allegations. Dr. Harris did later admit in a court deposition that Hoxsey held a demonstration in the hospital. In the AMA archives, I found grisly before-and-after pictures of Mannix, whose corrosive cancer visibly vanished following Hoxsey's treatment. He later lost his collarbone after an accident shoveling coal, though the AMA contended that it was the destructive result of Hoxsey's powder. As Mannix testified on behalf of Hoxsey in a later court trial, "If anybody got closer to hell than I did, I would like to see them. Bruce Miller today is the best friend that I have got. He saved my life." Mannix died in 1934 of heart disease and high blood pressure, twelve years after receiving the Hoxsey treatment. The AMA did finally acknowledge Mannix's recovery but maintained that he had actually been cured by the prior surgery and radiation.[22]

Dr. Harris and Dr. Fishbein subsequently contended that they had instantly flagged Hoxsey as a quack, and they flatly denied offering him a contract for his formulas. Yet one thing was certain: Hoxsey had made a very powerful enemy. By crossing swords with Dr. Morris Fishbein, he alienated the most powerful figure in medicine. Dr. Fishbein held a unique position. As *Journal* editor, he controlled the main income-producing organ of the AMA, and thus the organization. The *Journal* also set the accepted standards of medical practice, and without its blessing the medical gates were soundly shut. For the next twenty-five years, Hoxsey would battle Dr. Fishbein and the AMA for an investigation in a spectacle of national dimensions.

In 1924, however, the AMA had but recently gained the centralized power that Hoxsey suddenly found opposing him. Founded in 1847 in Philadelphia, the AMA had remained an insignificant trade organization until the turn of the century when it claimed only 9,000 members among the nation's 100,000 doctors. At the time, medicine was diverse, pluralistic, and financially unrewarding.[23]

When Dr. George Henry Simmons secured a job as editor of the inconsequential *Journal* in 1898, he moved to the AMA's sole rented room in Chicago and quickly dispatched the only other employee. The *Journal* was somnambulant, a dull instrument peddling an assortment of proprietary remedies and patent medicines. Organizationally, the AMA was a flimsy guild presiding over a loose collection of state medical societies that paid scant attention to their titular national representative, and over which the AMA exerted marginal influence. Dr. Simmons designated himself secretary and general manager of the AMA, as well as editor of the *Journal*. He set about designing an ambitious strategy to control national medical politics and secure a prosperous future for doctors.[24]

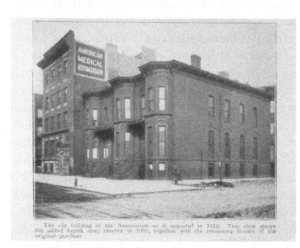

The modest 1910 headquarters of the AMA just before its dramatic rise to prosperity.

The old building of the Association as it appeared in 1910. This view shows the added fourth story erected in 1905, together with the remaining houses of the original purchase.

Dr. Simmons's AMA happened into a synchronous convergence of forces that would permanently alter the landscape of medicine. During this era of the great trusts of John D. Rockefeller, J. P. Morgan, John Jacob Astor, and Andrew Carnegie, the enterprising Dr. Simmons recognized medicine as an unexcavated gold mine and aligned the AMA with these interests. To do so, he started touting a political plan to restructure the AMA and endow it with authority to set national medical policy. With two compatriots, he quietly commenced revamping the AMA into a rigid hierarchy of county, state, and national medical societies, with power residing exclusively in him at the apex of the pyramid. The sole source of AMA income was the *Journal*, of which Dr. Simmons was in complete control. He signed all checks and approved all expenditures.

Dr. Simmons instituted a marketing drive to enlist all doctors to join the AMA, rapidly gaining 30,000 members by 1903. Doctors could belong to the AMA only by simultaneously holding membership in their local and state medical societies in a vertical consolidation. Within twenty years, the vast majority of doctors were members, and it became professional suicide not to belong to the AMA.

This process marked a crucial turning point in what Pulitzer Prize–winning medical sociologist Paul Starr has characterized as the unique "rise of a sovereign profession" within the "social transformation of American medicine." As Starr notes, the profession was soon able to convert its authority into "social privilege, economic power, and political influence."[25]

Dr. Simmons also launched a crusade against "irregulars" and "quacks," which encompassed all schools of medicine other than allopathic M.D.'s. He vigorously targeted homeopaths, herbalists, osteopaths, chiropractors, and the diverse array of "irregular" practitioners who populated medicine at the time. Some were coopted through admission to the AMA, and the many who were excluded found themselves increasingly restricted from most medical practice.

Simmons set up the Department of Propaganda for Reform, later to become the Bureau of Investigation, to catalog all irregular practitioners. The thrust of the bureau was "the collection and dissemination of information on 'patent medicines,' quacks, medical fads, and various other phases of pseudomedicine."[26] Heading the Propaganda Department was Dr. Arthur J. Cramp, who was inspired to become a doctor after his daughter reputedly died at the hands of a quack. His voluminous steel-cased card files kept fastidious track of every "irregular," and already numbered over 10,000 names. The Dickensian Dr. Cramp lifted a fiery sword in the AMA *Journal* to smite the

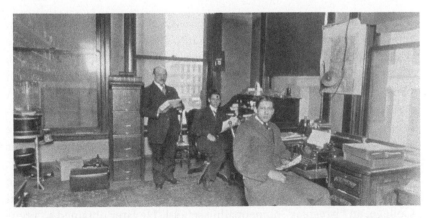

The AMA's newly centralized authority angered even the medical profession, c. 1920.

"nostrum evil or quackery" with smoldering editorials and columns.[27] Tellingly, the press room was the biggest at AMA headquarters.

The AMA team instigated aggressive legislative action against the irregulars in most states around the country to curtail or eliminate their practice. The organization also consolidated its dominion over the regular medical profession. By 1922, resistance to Simmons's controversial actions was fermenting across the land even within the orthodox community. The Illinois Medical Society in the *Illinois Medical Journal* openly attacked the AMA.

> Few of the members of the AMA realize the centralizing changes that have taken place in their organization within the last twenty-five years. So adroitly and insidiously have these changes been brought about that the majority of the members, dazzled by the material prosperity of the AMA, have entirely overlooked the fact that the Association has been converted from a democratic and self-governed body of professional men into a highly centralized machine with absolute control concentrated in a single individual.
>
> In the twenty-five years of expansion of the Association and the *Journal*, the anomalous condition has developed whereby the *Journal*, which is the property of the Association, now absolutely controls the Association to which it belongs. The editor of the *Journal* has developed into an absolute Dictator of the Association and its affairs through his control of the finances of the Association. The AMA is not a business enterprise.[28]

The Illinois Medical Society was deeply mistaken on the last count. Dr. Simmons had already built the *Journal* into a formidable financial engine while he deployed its revenues to acquire stocks, bonds, and the valuable real estate that now housed the AMA's grand new headquarters on Chicago's high-toned Dearborn Avenue.[29] Yet the new direction the AMA was charting appeared to be in direct conflict with its own Code of Ethics. Adopted at the organization's founding, the code specified that the AMA would always represent the ethical values of the profession over business interests.

Dr. Simmons, who emigrated to the U.S. from England in 1870 at the age of eighteen, ironically gained his M.D. from Hahnemann Medical College, an "irregular" homeopathic school. He later obtained a "regular" M.D. diploma from Rush Medical College in 1892. However, private

investigators subsequently discovered that Dr. Simmons had never graduated from college and had no medical degree when he commenced his
practice. After starting out as a homeopath, only ten years later did he
obtain a medical diploma by attending at most a day or two of classes a
month in Chicago. Simmons also advertised his services extensively, a
direct violation of the AMA's stern Code of Ethics. His ads promoted his
services as a "specialist in diseases of women," a common code of the day
for abortionists. He also adver-
tised his tenure for a year and a
half in the largest hospitals of
London and Vienna, where it was
not clear he had ever practiced.[30]

Confronting the charges, Dr.
Simmons claimed to have re-
nounced his "sectarian" origin,
and said he was afforded academic credit for his past practice
by agreement with the medical
school, which exempted him
from the "rigid requirements" of
undergraduate attendance.[31] He
insisted that his advertising activities were not regarded as "unethical" where he practiced at the
time.

Dr. Simmons survived the
insurgency, but was deposed two
years later in a lurid personal
scandal. His wife charged in
court that he had forced her to

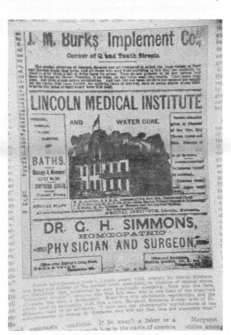

*Dr. Simmons's controversial
ad in which he still calls
himself a homeopath.*

undergo multiple abortions by drugging her into submission, and then
coerced her into a mental hospital.[32] Under fire, Dr. Simmons resigned
his post at the AMA for "reasons of health" and landed in luxurious retirement in Hollywood, Florida.

Dr. Simmons's chosen successor was his assistant and attentive under-
study of eleven years, Dr. Morris Fishbein. By the time the thirty-five-
year-old Dr. Fishbein succeeded his mentor at the *Journal* in 1924, the
apt pupil had learned his lessons well. He would go on to anchor the
AMA in a golden harbor of prosperity and emerge as the undisputed "Voice
of American Medicine." His organ was the *Journal*, and he played it
masterfully. Following Dr. Simmons's lead, he methodically set about

consolidating medical power and perfecting a medical plutocracy that punished any who dared diverge from the narrow AMA line, especially the irregulars. Among his most cherished refrains was a chorus against quacks that now rose regularly in his signature arpeggios in the *Journal*.

When Dr. Fishbein walked upstairs to the Bureau of Investigation on the fifth floor of AMA headquarters, he found Dr. Cramp already had a working file on Harry Hoxsey. Even prior to the ill-starred confrontation at the Alexian Brothers Hospital, Hoxsey had gotten on the wrong side of the AMA's bedside manner. Hoxsey and Dr. Fishbein were now fated to play out a highly personal contest that would come to personify the deep rift dividing medicine.

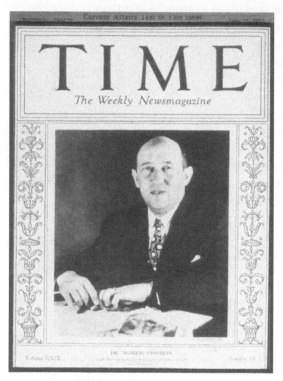

Dr. Morris Fishbein rises to national prominence.

Quacking Around

A deflated Harry Hoxsey returned to Taylorville to reconfigure his shattered plans. Lucius Everhard soon contacted him with a new offer to establish a clinic in Chicago supported by wealthy backers. Hoxsey formed a common law trust with Everhard and Dr. Miller and moved operations of the National Cancer Research Institute and Clinic to a site a provocative half mile from AMA headquarters. The trust document identified Hoxsey as "the owner and possessor of a secret formula for the compounding of a treatment for cancer, which said treatment is something entirely new in medicine."[1]

When Everhard quickly proved to be a naked exploiter, Hoxsey retreated to Taylorville with Dr. Miller. Backed energetically by the chamber of commerce and local businessmen, Hoxsey renovated and expanded the Moose Lodge into the Hoxide Institute early in 1925. The chamber of commerce mailed thousands of booklets throughout the Midwest trumpeting Hoxide as the "Mayo Brothers of Taylorville" and advertised widely in newspapers. An expectant Taylorville planned on becoming the cancer capital of the world. "All World Will Soon Beat Path to Taylorville" ran banner headlines in the *Breeze*, with local promoter H. T. Morphy, a former theatrical agent, speculating, "They'll come from far and near and each of them will spend money here. I want to boost Taylorville throughout the universe and I'm going to do it."[2] Soon cancer sufferers were streaming into town.

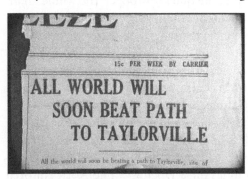

ALL WORLD WILL SOON BEAT PATH TO TAYLORVILLE

15c PER WEEK BY CARRIER

All the world will soon be beating a path to Taylorville, site of

The chamber of commerce is Hoxsey's biggest booster, 1925.

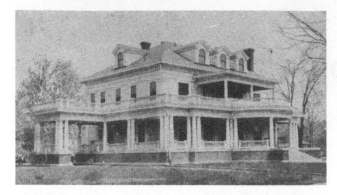

The Hoxide Institute moves into the Moose Lodge, 1925.

The *Breeze* ran breathless articles about the visit of Dr. Homer I. Keeney, a specialist from San Francisco, who visited and reputedly endorsed the treatment. The newspaper followed with reports that Dr. Keeney considered the Hoxsey remedies a specific for cancer, and disclosed that he got the approval of the California State Medical Board to use it. Not long after, Dr. Keeney, who indeed came and investigated the treatment, stated, "I found enough of interest to detain me there for five days."[3] However, he was "prevented from making a speech on Hoxide by the local doctors, under the threat they would break him in California for unethical practices."[4] Caving to added professional pressure from the *Journal*'s negative portrayal of him, he quickly dropped the whole affair. Undeterred, the chamber of commerce continued "circularizing" doctors nationally with pamphlets encouraging them to come see for themselves.[5]

Shortly an agent of the AMA Bureau of Investigation showed up in Taylorville. He queried locals about Hoxsey, his family, and his supposed cures, and was spotted around town poking into any dark corners he could find. He never met with Hoxsey, although Hoxsey said he sought a meeting.

Several months went by quietly before lightning struck. On January 2, 1926, the *Journal* published its first tirade under the banner of Propaganda for Reform: "The Hoxide Cancer 'Cure': A Chamber of Commerce Sponsors the Nostrum of a Horse Doctor."[6] The AMA editorial branded Hoxsey's "cancer cure" a "secret remedy," the surest sign of a quack. By doing so, Dr. Fishbein issued the medical kiss of death. No reputable doctor or researcher could now have any association with it.

Of course, if Hoxsey's charge that the AMA tried to buy his formulas was true, he had every reason to keep their composition between him and the fence post. The coveted recipes became what film director Alfred Hitchcock liked to call the "MacGuffin," the object of desire that drives the plot. Dr. Fishbein would repeatedly try to obtain Hoxsey's MacGuffin, and Hoxsey was constantly on the alert to safeguard his precious legacy.

Henceforth he was observed surreptitiously buying his ingredients one at a time in various drugstores spread around the county, and he always took care to mix the medicines himself.[7]

Dr. Fishbein's editorial made other allegations, ridiculing Hoxsey's father as a "quack who dabbled in veterinary medicine, faith healing and cancer curing." It revealed that Hoxsey senior had been arrested for blackmailing a dentist. It further charged that he had actually *died of cancer*.

The article went on to discredit Lucius O. Everhard as a specialist in "stock-selling schemes with doctors and dentists as its principal victims. Later L. O. V. Everhard was 'President of the Drexel Mutual Life Insurance Company.' The company's offices seemed to have been under Everhard's hat." It investigated Dr. Bruce Miller and found no record of his medical practice for the past thirty years, suggesting that instead he seemed to have been operating a stepladder business.

The editorial quashed "rumors" that the treatment was being used in "high-grade hospitals and by physicians of unquestionable standing." The *Journal* asked rhetorically, "What is the Hoxide cure? Essentially the escharotic treatment with arsenic as its base. Specimens of the stuff used when the Hoxsey outfit was in Chicago were examined in the Association's laboratory and arsenic in large quantities was found. In the case of some of the patients, the arsenic applied to the malignant tissue ate into the blood vessels and the patients bled to death. One of the leading physicians of Taylorville wrote to the *Journal* that the first information he heard 'was from an undertaker who showed enthusiasm about the matter.'"

The editorial conceded that people with "nonmalignant or superficial growths" would have them removed, but with unnecessary pain and expense. It castigated the chamber of commerce for holding out this "false beacon" and predicted tragedy.

Hoxsey replied furiously with a letter to Dr. Fishbein in what would become a lengthy one-sided correspondence. His father had indeed been charged with blackmail but was exonerated. He had not died of cancer, but of erysipelas, and his death certificate was on file in the state capital. Hoxsey further denied that his yellow powder contained toxic arsenic and challenged Dr. Fishbein to verify even one case where anyone bled to death. He demanded the public release of Sergeant Mannix's medical records.[8]

Dr. Fishbein did not have to reply. Hoxsey was now officially stigmatized as a cancer pariah in the medical community, and he was vulnerable indeed. His relationship with the shifty Everhard was merely the first of many such shadowy associations that would undermine his credibility. As Hoxsey's daughter told me, "Dad could be a real sucker if you knew how to stroke him. He had some of the worst business partners you can imagine, and several people took him for a lot of money. If they won his favor, in his eyes, they could do no wrong."

At the time, it appears that Hoxsey was treating mainly external cancers with his escharotic yellow powder. Considerable confusion exists around this pivotal issue. According to several references I found, it appears that Hoxsey mainly relied on the yellow powder and principally promoted his treatment of external cases, although he also used it on some internal cancers through injection. Explicit references to external treatments mention only the yellow powder, not the red paste. I did find two specific mentions of his use of an internal treatment between 1924 and 1930. If he was using the internal tonic in the early days, it was not his focus and certainly was not what he was promoting. By 1930, he definitely had an internal remedy.[9] (The central mystery of just what these remedies are and where they may have come from is explored in depth in chapter 11.)

Nevertheless, his greatest and most spectacular successes clearly came from removing external cancers where the result was visibly undeniable. Dr. Fishbein offered no proof that the yellow powder was causing toxic reactions, but his attacks signaled the onset of a protracted medical controversy that would climax in a surprise ending.

With Dr. Fishbein's rebuke, the Chicago heat was on in the city notorious during Prohibition for its violence and gangsters such as Al Capone. Hoxsey launched a $250,000 suit against the AMA and tried to enlist the illustrious Chicago lawyer Clarence Darrow. "I have been consulted in the case," Darrow said, "but not undertaken it. This institution is engaged in curing cancers. I have seen and heard of so many cures that did not make good that I mean to be sure before I undertake it. Four doctors in regular standing have given me their experience and have the fullest faith in it. I have seen about ten cases that appear to be cured." Darrow ultimately refused the case, and Hoxsey would later say Darrow was "reached" by the AMA.[10] When the AMA later forced the suit to trial, a financially strapped Hoxsey dropped it.[11]

Hoxsey soon found the AMA subverting his relationship with an unnerved Taylorville Chamber of Commerce, which terminated its support. It marked the beginning of a state of siege. Returning from a movie one night in a nearby town, Hoxsey heard newsboys hawking the sensational headline, "Downstate Cancer Mill Raided." He read with amazement that he had been arrested, only to find the clinic intact when he got back to Taylorville.

An investigator from the State Medical Board promptly arrived in town and charged Hoxsey with practicing medicine without a license.

The bust set a pattern in which Hoxsey would go on to be arrested almost continually for the rest of his career. In fact, by working as a medical technician under the aegis of a licensed doctor, Hoxsey was fully within the law. His forensic correctness, however, did nothing to halt the blizzard of warrants burying his practice.

With the typical synchronicity of cancer politics, the local deputy sheriff refused to serve the warrant because Hoxsey was treating him for cancer. When the case finally went to trial, Hoxsey was acquitted. Delivering the verdict was a jury composed of two former patients and ten others who had relatives or friends who believed they had been helped by it. These kinds of intimate connections sown by cancer would reach across serendipitous social pathways to exonerate Hoxsey on many occasions.[12]

Seven more warrants never even reached trial, but Hoxsey soon found himself facing a puzzling half-million-dollar trover suit from eight of his brothers and sisters for illegally appropriating his father's estate: the cancer formulas. The suit cited the formulas that John C. Hoxsey had used "with a great degree of success" and valued them at $500,000.[13] Digging deeper, Hoxsey learned that his relatives had been approached by Chicago lawyers allegedly representing a group of Chicago doctors offering to buy out the relatives' share of the estate when they won the suit. When he grilled one brother on his motivation, Hoxsey was told that "I had stolen those formulas out of dad's bank box, and was making a lot of money. I was going to make a million dollars with it, because the lawyers told him so, and he wanted his part of it."[14]

Faced with having to post a preposterous $500,000 bond, Hoxsey watched his clinic and all his personal assets stripped. When the clinic physician, Dr. Washburn, took his license off the wall and quit, he was stranded again.

Patients under treatment pleaded with Hoxsey to continue helping them. Aware that he was under surveillance and no longer shielded by a doctor's license, he faced an existential dilemma. "What was I to do?" he wondered. "Let these poor unfortunates die?" During the next eighteen months, he moved his clinic to the neighboring towns of Carlinville and Jacksonville and kept treating patients. Arrested repeatedly for practicing medicine without a license, he pleaded guilty to three counts and paid $100 fines for the misdemeanors. "Those cases hung fire for a long time," he later defended himself in court. "It was the cheapest and quickest way out."[15]

When the trover suit finally reached trial in the summer of 1929, it was decided in Hoxsey's favor. Hoxsey's brother Danny confided that the presiding judge pulled some strings because he was raised by a stepaunt whom their father had cured of cancer.

Victorious but broke, with his Taylorville allies exhausted, Hoxsey took an offer from citizens in his nearby hometown of Girard to launch a new clinic. The group bought the Nicolet Hotel, and on July 17, 1929, Girard heralded its native son with "Hoxsey Day." Sponsored by the chamber of commerce, the festive gathering of five hundred onlookers was inaugurated by high school marching bands. Dr. Miller teamed up with Hoxsey again, and they exulted in the emotional procession of Hoxsey patients bearing witness on the stage trimmed with red-white-and-blue bunting.[16]

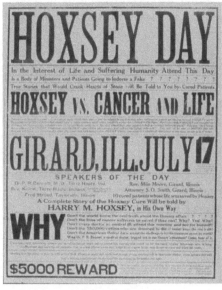

Ad for the prodigal son's triumphant return home, 1929.

The Girard *Gazette* reported on the giddy success of Hoxsey Day. "Applause was accorded the speakers frequently, and when one speaker asked if the audience wished to endorse Hoxsey in his efforts to save lives, the response was so nearly unanimous that those who remained sitting could be counted on the fingers."[17]

Reverend Killion took the podium to tell the story of his lip cancer, which was so severe that he couldn't whistle or even eat at times. "I feel that I owe my life and present good health to the Hoxsey treatment. I went and took the radium treatment. The radium appeared to burn it on top and make it worse. It seemed to stop hurting a little while, then my gums began to bother and pain like the lip did before. I want you to know that Hoxsey deserves the praise for me beginning to continue my work. The old cancer has gone out of my lip and I feel in better health than I have in many years. Praise the Lord and the Hoxsey treatment."[18]

Harry Hoxsey stepped up to address the throng. Never a man of a few words, he electrified the audience with his truculent defiance of the AMA. "I know a lot of faces here and one thing I want to tell you is that this meeting is not a matter for making money, but the purpose of this meeting is to present evidence. There is a lot of knockers who do not know what they are talking about, and especially around a man's hometown, and if those knockers are here today and have the mind of a six-year-old child and don't leave here today a walking, talking, dyed-in-the-wool Hoxsey fan and convinced beyond a reasonable doubt that this treatment is a cure for cancer, they are either deaf, dumb or blind, or else they are crazy.

"My friends, you can see I have had success from the beginning, and the American Medical Association may keep me down for six months, they may keep me down for one year, they may keep me down for five years, but if the public will stick with me like they have, I will whip this organization, because Abraham Lincoln said that a man who can change public opinion can change the government and the laws of the United States.

"How do these doctors drive Packards, Stutz cars, and big automobiles? I will say that if the American Medical Association will sign a contract to treat every cancer sufferer in the world, let him be rich or poor, for nothing, I will immediately give my remedy free of charge to the world."[19]

Hoxsey flaunted his open invitation to Dr. Fishbein, who, of course, failed to show up. "If the American Medical Association had one bit of guts," he taunted his remote enemies, "they would be here, but no, they are thieves in the dark. Friends, why would a bunch of jealous, narrow-minded penny-lovers resort to the dirty tactics that my enemies have resorted to? Why don't the Chicago doctors, who have seen my remedies bring back lives that were almost wiped out by this dreaded disease, endorse it?

"We will let the audience be the jury, as we are for America first, last and always. I thank you and bid you good-bye from the bottom of my heart for coming out and standing for your fellow man who is out to do good for humanity, in jail or not."[20]

Hoxsey offered a bold $5,000 challenge: He would deliver treatment superior to surgery, X-ray, and radium on ten cases. There were no takers.

Hoxsey was certainly not mending any fences at AMA headquarters. Dr. Fishbein's *Journal* struck back immediately in an editorial titled "The Hoxide Quackery Again" deriding the Girard Chamber of Commerce and its citizens. "They will get the doubtful privilege of the reputation of living in a town that fattens off the sufferings of those unfortunates who are lured there by the false hope that an ignorant faker has discovered a 'cure' for one of the most dreadful scourges afflicting the human race."[21]

The AMA jab crumbled the resolve of the Girard backers, and under mounting pressure Hoxsey was relieved when he got an auspicious long-distance phone call in February 1930 from Norman Baker. Baker identified himself as operating a cancer clinic using unorthodox methods in Muscatine, Iowa. Hoxsey had heard Baker on the radio station he

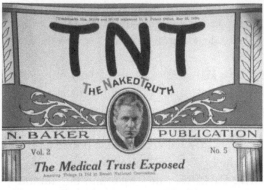

Norman Baker's provocative TNT *magazine attacks "The Medical Trust," 1930.*

owned that broadcast throughout the Midwest. Baker wanted a demonstration of the treatment and offered him a job if it showed results. Hoxsey drove up the next day to the Baker Hospital on the banks of the Mississippi River. Billed as "The Castle in the Air Where Sick Folks Get Well," the facility was part of Baker's home-grown empire comprising Radio K-T-N-T ("Know The Naked Truth") and the KTNT magazine, catalog, gas station, and restaurant.[22]

Baker, a former stage hypnotist, was previously married to Eva Tanguay, the "I Don't Care Girl," with whom he performed a mentalist act in which she used her telepathic powers to read the numbers from playing cards. Baker sported white suits and shoes matched with purple shirts and ties, and was famous for his silver tongue and mesmerist eyes. An inventor, he designed and built the calliaphone, an organlike musical instrument used on top of cars for advertising, which he manufactured and sold nationally.

Hoxsey arrived to find Baker on the air. "The subject of his talk was curing both internal and external cancer at the Baker Institute," Hoxsey later testified. "During his talk he gave a staunch plea for funds for the People's Protective Association which he said would only be used for the purpose of giving the people medical freedom and taking the facts to Washington where he was going to go before the President and show that

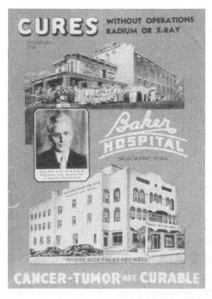

The Baker Hospital: "A cancer cure with cheap cigars and a cheap magazine as sidelines."

cancer was curable and they were curing it in Muscatine. He asked the people to send in donations and made it very plain to the people that the officers of the Association would receive no salaries."[23]

After the broadcast, Hoxsey got a tour of the hospital and met Dr. Statler, Baker's only licensed physician. Baker offered Hoxsey a lucrative salary, but Hoxsey countered that his only deal would be for part of the profits. Baker declaimed that he wasn't interested in making money, only in "busting the Medical Trust." Hoxsey replied, "I told him I was interested in both money and saving lives, but I didn't want one dollar of a poor dying victim's money if we didn't positively think he could be cured." Hoxsey insisted on treating poor people for free and noted shrewdly that his charity cases were often his best advertisements, a good deed that was also good business. During heavy negotiations, Baker finally agreed to give Hoxsey a percentage interest for the cases he treated.[24]

Since Baker was already using an internal "needle" treatment developed by a Dr. Ozias, he put Hoxsey in charge of a new external cancer division. Hoxsey started treatment on several patients, frustrated that he was limited to external cases.

That night Baker summoned Hoxsey to the radio station in the homey upstairs room outfitted with sofas where he was playing his trademark organ while dedicating doleful tunes to his gray-haired mother. When Baker gave over the microphone to Hoxsey, it was love at first sight. Hoxsey held forth, spending an hour at a time several times a day promoting his cures. As Hoxsey commented to Dr. Miller, "My God, it looks like an opportunity of a lifetime. That man has a radio station, and Fishbein can't stop a radio station from talking, regardless of how many dirty articles he runs. He can't get to all the people we talk to. We will have patients come to the radio and do their talking."[25] At the nadir of the Great Depression, he mixed his evangelical oratory of miraculous cures with a drumbeat of populist politics berating the Medical Trust and M.D.'s—"'M.D.' stands for 'More Dough.'"

Within a week the Baker Hospital was overrun with three hundred patients a day spilling over from the Baker hotel into boardinghouses and rented rooms in private homes. Soon came Hoxsey's most sensational and bizarre case. When cancer sufferer Mandus Johnson heard Baker on the radio, he set out for Muscatine in March 1930. His head was bandaged as heavily as a mummy, spooking pedestrians to flee to the other side of the street. Hoxsey called it the worst case of cancer he ever saw. When the retired farmer entered the treatment room, the stench was so overwhelming that Hoxsey insisted, "We got to get this man out in the wind or leave." The entire top of Johnson's head was rotting flesh. The cancer had eaten away the scalp, exposing his skull. Doctors had inserted tubes into holes cut in his skull to drain the pint of pus generated every day. "Either cure me or kill me," the desperate Johnson pleaded.[26]

As Johnson later told his tale, "I had to dress it out about six or three times a day and I couldn't see anything with this eye here. It smelled [like] flesh. I took them rags and put them in the furnace and I go away two blocks and smell the odors then."[27] The farmer had banged his head bringing down a pump handle and it never healed, turning malignant. The doctors operated and gave him eleven X-ray treatments over a three-year period, but it got worse. Then he heard Baker on the radio.

When Baker entered the room and saw the horrible sight, Hoxsey told him, "This man here has got one chance in ten thousand, and that's one chance too many. But if I can get at treating him, I think we'll do a lot of good. If we don't, it will blow you out of the water." Baker decided to take the gamble.[28]

Hoxsey applied the yellow powder under Dr. Statler's supervision, and sent Johnson home. The patient returned ten days later much improved. After going home again, he sent letters through his wife saying that the odor was gone and he could sleep. Baker directly went on the radio and theatrically announced a public demonstration outside the radio station in which the top of Johnson's skull would be removed, and the cancer with it.

Around a covered gazebo on a high hill overlooking the Mississippi River crowded a "human landslide" of 32,000 people, twice the population of Muscatine. Loudspeakers placed about the crowd broadcast the spectacle live. Against a sea of straw hats and parasols bobbing under the

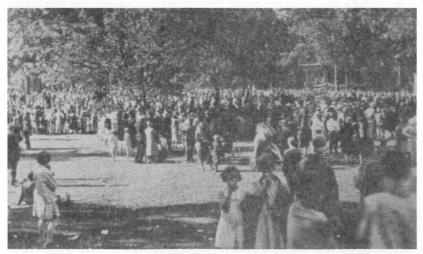

The "resurrection" of Mandus Johnson prompts a turnout of 32,000 spectators.

baking sun, Hoxsey and a doctor removed the now dead tumor composing the entire top of Johnson's skull, temporarily exposing the membrane around his brain. Fourteen people in the audience fainted. A promenade of onlookers was allowed to walk past Johnson to verify the reality of his miraculously improved condition.

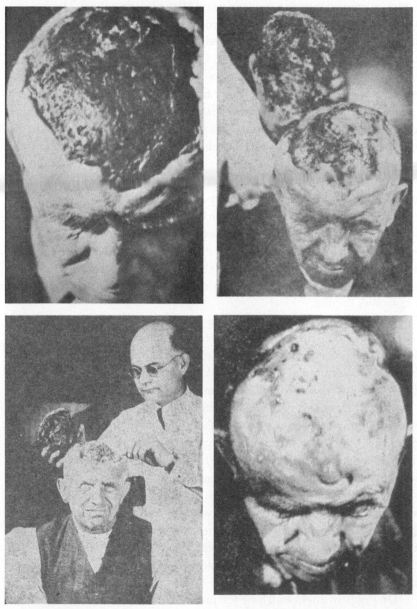

(1) Mandus Johnson's cancerous skull is rotting flesh. (2) and (3) Removing the dead cancer after Hoxsey treatment. (4) Johnson's healed skull.

Baker held up to the crowd a small vial with half a teaspoonful of the yellow powder. It was enough to cure five hundred people, he said, and swallowed some to demonstrate its safety.

The next day, local doctors reported that Mandus Johnson had died horribly at the hands of the "murderers" Hoxsey and Baker. The *Journal* attacked immediately in a polemic titled "Broadcasting Bunk." It charged that one of Baker's supposed cancer cures was a man suffering from nothing more than "barber's itch." The editorial reveled in Hoxsey's association with the notorious Baker as Dr. Fishbein wrote that Baker was selling "a cancer cure with cigars and a cheap magazine as side lines. His cancer cure includes the old Hoxsey fake."[29]

By now, *JAMA* had also unearthed more juicy details on Hoxsey's close associate Dr. Bruce Miller. The physician indeed held a valid medical license, but had not practiced in almost thirty years. During that time he joined his father's woodworking business to help him protect valuable patents, and spent about ten years in Europe where he exhibited a mechanical orchestra of lady dummies he had constructed.

Dr. Miller fully acknowledged the truth of his eccentric past.[30] He got interested in medicine again only after his sister died of cancer. When he began looking for potentially effective treatments, he linked with Hoxsey. It is unclear whether Hoxsey knew about his partner's professional history, although undoubtedly his main concern was the validity of the physician's license.

Dr. Miller did, however, dedicate the next twenty years of his life to working with the Hoxsey treatment. He was convinced of its merit, mainly for external cancers, and started a practice in Los Angeles. By the 1940s, he became a prominent figure as president of the National Medical Association, an alternative to the AMA composed of irregular physicians.

Nevertheless, this time Dr. Fishbein had a live one. Baker and Miller made glorious additions to the AMA's wax museum of quackery, and indeed medical charlatanism was rampant. During the same period, the *Journal* was pursuing the infamous Dr. John Brinkley, who was performing his notorious "goat-gland" transplants in Kansas with promises of restoring virility to a clamoring male clientele. The macabre operation was outright fraud and produced gruesome casualties. The outrageous Brinkley, whose widespread popularity spurred him to run for state office, made a big target for Dr. Fishbein. There was often good cause for the AMA's actions to limit such medical abuses, and it was high tide for quackery at AMA headquarters.

Dr. Fishbein might well have felt justified in using any means necessary to put quacks out of business, especially Hoxsey in light of his budding commercial success, unsavory partners, and newly acquired means to attract patients through the mass media. Hoxsey was boldly stretching the bounds of the battleground and must have known he would invite severe retribution from his enemy.

The same day that "Broadcasting Bunk" appeared, Hoxsey and Baker went on the air at midnight. At Dr. Fishbein's behest, the FCC had by now intervened to limit their hours to non-prime-time: afternoons and the wee hours. After Baker finished deriding "M.D.'s —More Drugs" and "the AMA— the American Meatcutters Association," he signed off emotionally for the night as the "friend of the farmer, the laborer, and the country folks" to wisps of plaintive organ tones. When Hoxsey heard a dog barking outside the window, he moved cautiously to peer from the side of the curtains. There had recently been anonymous threats on their lives, and Baker had posted a permanent watchman, who that night reported a tip-off about a suspicious Buick parked in front of the KTNT restaurant. Hoxsey and Baker were armed, and Hoxsey had his hand on his revolver as he inched his nose to the edge of the fluttering curtains.

Hoxsey spotted a man with a drawn gun and they fired at the same instant. Hoxsey wounded the assailant, but two figures dragged the man away and escaped across the bridge over the Mississippi. Hoxsey raced outside in pursuit while Baker trailed a distant second, terrified and hanging back, according to Hoxsey. While they were scouring the grounds, two bombs exploded nearby at the base of the radio tower in a rain of hot sparks. Hoxsey subsequently claimed that he was fully prepared, forewarned by a Chicago gangster whose mother he had cured.[31] He was a good shot for a Quaker.

The *Chicago Daily Tribune* ran the lurid headline, "Hunt 3 Gunmen Routed by 'Quack' Doctor—Gun Fight Climaxes Fight with Dr. Fishbein," while the *Post* followed with, "Try to Shoot Up KTNT; Attack by Dr. Morris Fishbein."[32]

Hoxsey implied that Dr. Fishbein was behind the attack, but he had no proof, and the accusation was probably spurious.[33] The three gunmen were never caught, but there was no question that it was high noon in the cancer war.

Baker set up machine gun nests around KTNT and sped the publication of a self-aggrandizing book called *Doctors, Dynamiters and Gunmen* portraying himself as a two-fisted hero. Some weeks later, Hoxsey's brother Dan was mysteriously found shot dead execution-style in the backseat of his car in Muscatine. No one was ever charged with the murder, and given the temper of the times, there's no telling what else Dan might have been involved in, from bootlegging to gambling. Hoxsey never spoke further about it.

To quell rumors of Mandus Johnson's death, Hoxsey and Baker went on the radio to announce "The Resurrection of Mandus Johnson" to take place in Weed Park on Decoration Day, May 30. This time, 50,000 people turned out, including the governor of Iowa, who shared the platform. Mandus Johnson appeared, whole and healthy. To explain the stupendous recovery, the *Journal* countered with an editorial claiming that Johnson actually had osteomyelitis, not cancer, which cleared up by itself.[34] Johnson lived on into the 1950s, free from cancer. He had plastic surgery to reconstruct his scalp, and one of the clinic nurses kept his necrosed skull bone as a memento, using it as a workbasket.

The Baker Hospital was now attracting a hefty 365 patients a day, but its prosperity put Hoxsey increasingly at odds with Baker. Hoxsey objected angrily to the use of the other internal treatment, which he believed was worthless, and he bet the nurses a squirrel coat if they could show him even one cure from it. As receipts climbed, Baker started cooking the books and reneged on their percentage contract, which he complained would pay Hoxsey more than the president of the United States. He was stiffing nurses for the salary of dishwashers, and procuring the cheapest ingredients he could find. Finally Hoxsey discovered the greedy Baker turning away impoverished patients, while coercing an elderly woman into selling her farm to pay for treatment.

"The first of September I was through," Hoxsey recalled. "Norman told me to go straight to hell. He wouldn't have me dictating to him. I said, 'Norman, it isn't that I am jealous, but I will be damned if I will see a human slaughterhouse. I think you are nothing less than murderers and I have two-hundred-ten pounds on my frame to back it up.' As far as the People's Protective Association is concerned, there is no other officer, only Norman Baker. You run that like Amos and Andy do their taxi company. You are the financial secretary, the president and the board of directors." After five months and twenty days, Hoxsey and Baker parted ways, climaxing in an angry lawsuit.[35]

The AMA had a field day, harping on Hoxsey's affiliation with Baker for years to come. Baker went on to run for Iowa governor on the Labor Party ticket and kept blasting the AMA from XENT radio in Mexico after the FCC revoked his radio license. Charging the "Medical Trust" with offering him a million dollars for his cancer cure, Baker sued the AMA and lost. After setting up a failed clinic in Arkansas, he was convicted in 1941 of mail fraud for promoting false cures for cancer and other diseases. He served four years in Leavenworth federal penitentiary, and then retired to Florida on a palatial yacht once belonging to robber baron Jay Gould. Baker died in 1958 of liver cancer.

Hoxsey later commented, "Organized medicine has made much of my short-lived association with Norman Baker. It completely ignores the fact that relentless persecution by the AMA made it impossible for me at that time to obtain more reputable collaborators. I had no alternative. If the Devil himself had offered me the facilities and doctors to treat cancer legitimately, and thus save the lives of thousands of victims, I would have accepted."[36] As far as the AMA was concerned, Baker was the devil, and Hoxsey's dance with him cost him dearly.

Muscatine signaled the beginning of Hoxsey's skillful use of the mass media to fight back against Dr. Fishbein. Both men became masters of publicity in their own right and would increasingly wage their highly public battle through the media. Hoxsey proved to be a charismatic promoter at a time when advertising was forbidden to doctors. "I have frequently been accused," he later wrote, "of being a flamboyant showman and promoter, as well as a healer. If I am all of these things, it is because the AMA forced these roles on me. The relentless campaign of innuendo and outright slander against me has been largely a subterranean one. The plain truth is, I had to become both showman and promoter in order to continue to treat cancer by unorthodox means and survive."[37]

Undaunted by his latest blowout, Hoxsey kept up his incessant barrage of letters to the Voice of American Medicine, pleading for a test of his remedies. His entreaties got no response, and he found himself irrevocably exiled to the underworld. An investigation was nowhere in sight.

Following his acrimonious split with the crooked Baker, Hoxsey set up quarters a block away and continued treating patients until he was soon offered an enticing new opportunity by wealthy citizens of Detroit: Ernest Maross, a financier of Henry Ford and founder of the Indianapolis Speedway, and his wife, Maude Slocum, an opera star. The Marosses proposed to set up a free clinic in the Motor City. If Hoxsey could demonstrate results, they pledged to sponsor and fund a free clinic.[38]

Hoxsey moved to Detroit under the aegis of Dr. Homer Van Hyning, Maude's personal physician. On the first day, the clinic hosted 118 patients. But the fix was already in. Two days later, accompanied by Maross, Hoxsey was called into the prosecutor's office. The prosecutor reported the dissatisfaction of the Wayne County Medical Society, but implied that some discreet payments might correct the situation. Hoxsey and his benefactor angrily walked out.

Ten days later Hoxsey was arrested for practicing medicine without a license. Medical authorities had sent a shill into the clinic complaining of cancer who charged that he had been falsely diagnosed with cancer by Dr. Van Hyning, who was then stripped of his medical license. In the trial that followed, Dr. Van Hyning testified that he had indeed been making payoffs to the DA's office and Department of Health. "It is protection money," Hoxsey later testified, "the same as gangsters. The Purple Hand used the same tactics."[39] Maross had already used his political influence to quash some other warrants.

Hoxsey was convicted of practicing medicine without a license, contrary to evidence that he served merely as a technician for the physician. Sentenced to six months in jail and a $200 fine, he was bailed out by Maross and immediately appealed the verdict. Seventeen months later, the Michigan State Supreme Court overturned his conviction and fully exonerated him on December 6, 1932.[40]

But with his license revoked in Michigan, Dr. Van Hyning retired to Ohio, and no other doctor was willing to risk professional censure. Even Maross's formidable political pull couldn't remedy the situation. As Hoxsey later noted, "There's only one thing that organized medicine fears more than unorthodoxy, and that's free medical treatment."[41]

Between 1926 and 1931, Hoxsey had been arrested 119 times.[42] He was convicted only three times on the misdemeanors in Illinois, and once in Ohio, where he got a suspended sentence. He was also permanently enjoined from practicing in Iowa after the Baker fiasco. He spent the next five years "quacking around," as Mildred Nelson termed it, constantly boosted by high hopes that were perpetually punctured by the barbed wire Dr. Fishbein set in his path.

In May 1932 Hoxsey settled in Wheeling, straddling both sides of the Ohio and West Virginia border. He began remodeling an office for a Hoxsey Cancer Clinic in the Hawley Building on the tenth floor next to Radio WWVA, where he bought a broadcasting contract. He invaded the newspapers with ads depicting a folk-art cartoon history of his life, which was smoothly evolving into populist fable. His third wife, a "sassy redhead" named Eva Ruth, opened the offices, while Hoxsey refurbished the furniture and walls, which he striped in black. Before the clinic could open, he was arrested on charges instituted by the Ohio State Medical Society, which had already been in touch with Dr. Cramp at the AMA. The medical society threatened the radio station owner with complaints to the FCC, resulting in the cancellation of his broadcasting contract.[43]

Hoxsey placed bold ads in the local press, touting his famed testimonials and claiming the treatment was now in use in ten states. He also issued a $10,000 challenge to treat twenty-five cases on an equal basis with the doctors and cure twice as many as his rivals. He planned to start a band to help commercialize his cancer cure. When pitching his treatment, he liked to place a jar of yellow powder on the table and tell his shaken audience that, if he should die unexpectedly, enough medicine was there to treat a thousand cases.

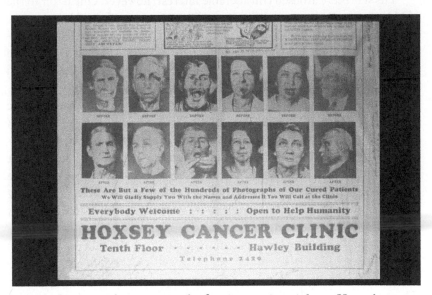

Sensational newspaper ads of patient testimonials are Hoxsey's stock-in-trade, West Virginia, 1932.

A steady stream of interested businessmen and wealthy patrons came by to see for themselves, including reputedly the illustrious doctor who had treated John D. Rockefeller. Hoxsey surreptitiously treated patients himself at night, aided by his wife. Before long, Hoxsey's physician, Dr. Arnold, was harassed, lost his medical license, and quit. Hoxsey was never indicted and was set free, though stripped of doctor and clinic. He fled in the night, carting barrels of medicine over the bridge to the Ohio border.

Hoxsey decided it was time for a vacation. He drove up to Atlantic City, where he met Dr. Willard Mason, a local physician. Dr. Mason, after witnessing the cure of a face cancer of a friend, offered to open a clinic at his home. Among the earliest patients at the International Cancer Institute was Captain Richard Higby, an old seaman who was father of the city's chief of police. He had a hideous cancer spreading across his nose into his eyes and forehead. Hoxsey reputedly cured him as well. Captain Higby, then about seventy-five or eighty years old, lived to be ninety-five, and his wife kept the dead tumor in a jar for all to see.[44]

When the County Medical Society sent an attorney to Police Chief Higby with a warrant for Hoxsey's arrest, the officer told him to drop the charges and stop the harassment of the man who cured his father. Hoxsey escaped legal action for the duration of his stay on the New Jersey coast, with financial backing from the former mayor, Judge C. J. Thompson.

His stay there aroused considerable interest, however. One letter to the AMA protested the apparent stonewalling of a test of the Hoxsey remedies. As Seymour Preston wrote to Dr. Cramp, "I should appreciate knowing how Dr. Willard Mason of Atlantic City has effected the cures that he has made, for I have investigated this also. If the powder now used by him is of an arsenic base, the cures I have seen do not react as you say."[45]

Dr. Cramp replied to another inquiry from the head of the Atlantic City Chamber of Commerce, who had forwarded him a bottle of Hoxsey's tonic. "We cannot undertake to analyze this nostrum. Nothing is to be gained by so doing. The American Medical Association, at the cost of many thousands of dollars, has made clear for anyone to see that Harry Hoxsey is an unscrupulous and ignorant quack. Nothing could be accomplished by analyzing this so-called tonic, and the AMA is not justified in spending its members' money to simply show the composition of one particular bottle of medicine that the faker Hoxsey has dispensed."[46]

The investigation Hoxsey tirelessly sought continued to elude him. He was a tar baby whom reputable doctors scuttled to avoid. As Dr. Mason later reported to a private investigator for Dr. Fishbein, "No one of standing in the medical community would go along with Hoxsey. Hoxsey was his own worst enemy, and if any practitioner persisted in his association with this man, he might just as well take down his shingle and give up his practice. It seemed as though everyone looked at Hoxsey as though a demon trying to sell a witches brew. Our parting was amiable and I gave Hoxsey to understand that I could not continue my association with him and still enjoy the respect and high regard of the community." Dr. Mason remained convinced that Hoxsey did have a real cure, but only for external cancers in early stages.[47]

Hoxsey kept peppering Dr. Fishbein with letters requesting an investigation, even one solely for his external remedies. "If you agree, I will be willing to come to your headquarters and discuss a plan whereby you would select a committee of five or seven of the leading cancer specialists in your Association and to have this committee select fifty patients who are suffering from external cancer—all of this for the purpose of demonstrating to you and your Associates that the Hoxsey treatment is equally effective, if not more effective, than radium, X-ray, or surgery, in the treatment of external cancers."[48] Waiting for an answer from Chicago was, as Hoxsey once put it, "like leaving the landing lights on for Amelia Earhart."[49]

A test, however, was nearer than Hoxsey imagined. Through Dr. Mason, he met Dr. Ira Walton Drew, a respected Philadelphia osteopathic physician who later served three terms as a congressman from the city's blue-stocking district. Dr. Drew also served for twenty years as professor of children's diseases at the Philadelphia Osteopathic College.[50]

As an osteopath, Dr. Drew got his licensing from a separate board, and was not subject to AMA censure. At the time, osteopaths were a school of healing recognized on a par with allopathic doctors. They could perform limited surgery and prescribe some drugs, but principally favored musculoskeletal manipulation as well as a wide variety of natural medicines. As an irregular, Dr. Drew had already been subjected to AMA opposition and sympathized with Hoxsey's status as an outcast. Dr. Drew and his wife, also an osteopathic doctor, invited Hoxsey to stay at their home and join their

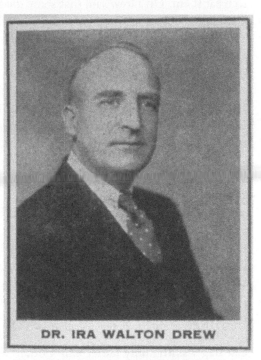

DR. IRA WALTON DREW

The respected Philadelphia osteopathic doctor adopts the Hoxsey treatment.

clinic. They started the Harry M. Hoxsey Foundation to offer the newly dubbed "Hoxin."[51]

Dr. Drew was impressed with Hoxsey's treatment, and their clinic thrived. When they received a visit from Hubert G. Brower of the Endocrine Food Company in New Jersey, Brower told them he knew Dr. Clarence Cook Little, chief of the blue-chip Roscoe B. Jackson Memorial Laboratory in Bar Harbor, Maine, associated with the elite Rockefeller Institute. Dr. Little was also highly influential as managing director of the American Society for the Control of Cancer, later to become the American Cancer Society. He was considered a top cancer researcher, and through Brower agreed to send Hoxsey and Dr. Drew some cancerous laboratory mice for testing. Finally, Hoxsey thought, he had a chance to prove himself.

According to both Hoxsey and Dr. Drew, they successfully treated some of the mice. As the FDA later noted, "According to Dr. Drew, the only experimental work done by Mr. Hoxsey while at the Drew Clinic was with mice sent to him by Dr. Little of the Rockefeller Institute. These mice arrived already inoculated with cancer and Mr. Hoxsey proceeded to treat them. Dr. Drew said that some died, some got better and others were killed at various stages in order to study the progress of the disease and treatment."[52]

The experiment generated a meeting with Dr. Little at the Harvard Club in New York City. Accompanied by Dr. Drew and John Marscher of the *Philadelphia Daily News*, Hoxsey was invited to come to the prestigious Bar Harbor lab to conduct further research. Amid snowdrifts deep enough to swallow a man, Harry Hoxsey arrived in November 1933 to spend a month treating two hundred laboratory mice with the Hoxsey remedies.

The accounts of what happened next conflict sharply. In Hoxsey's version, he claimed to treat the mice successfully, whereupon Dr. Little went away for a meeting at the Rockefeller Institute in New York City. Soon after his return, he informed Hoxsey that he had been unaware of Hoxsey's vendetta with the AMA, which precluded any further association. "The only way I can help you," Hoxsey contended Dr. Little said to him, "is for you to give me your formulas, and you step out of the picture. Or else go to Europe and let this come back as a discovery from Heidelberg, or some reputable place, and you stay over there four or five years and let this be exploited in this country."[53]

Hoxsey was uninterested in the proposition. "I told him that the American flag was the only father and mother I had, and I was not going to leave it to give something I had away."[54] Hoxsey was convinced that Dr. Fishbein was the unseen ventriloquist speaking through Dr. Little to purloin his MacGuffin.

However, in later court depositions and interviews with the FDA, Dr. Little related an entirely different story. He at first acknowledged the possible initial success of the test mice he sent Hoxsey, but later retracted the statement.[55] He also described other alarming problems that set in at Bar Harbor. "Hoxsey had been doing a good deal of loose talking around town both as to his ability to cure cancer and other diseases, his work at the laboratory and his personal situation as regards wealth."[56]

Dr. Little recounted that Hoxsey had illegally treated two people. The first was a boy with a swollen foot, which Hoxsey cut with a razor, making it worse and causing Dr. Little to call in a doctor. The second was the boy's mother, treated for an unspecified ailment, whom Hoxsey told that he had something better than her doctor. He did not charge money for either treatment, and boasted that therefore the authorities couldn't convict him for practicing medicine without a license.[57] It was another lesson from the pages of forensic medicine. By refusing remuneration, he wasn't legally liable.

According to Little, Hoxsey then gave a speech at the Mount Desert Lions Club. "It is evident that he gave the impression he was a doctor," Dr. Little related. "He mentioned his connection with the laboratory. This of course was a public breach of confidence of the terms of the agreement." When the scientist heard about the violation, he severed his tie with Hoxsey. Hoxsey remained in town "talking more loosely than ever." Among other charges, Little claimed Hoxsey said that he and Dr. Little had "rival cancer cures," hence Dr. Little's hostility to him.[58]

"My impression," Little added, "was that he was a skillful promoter, watching for every opportunity to advance himself. He was presentable and ingratiating, and made a very good first impression. This, however, in the days and weeks that followed broke down at every real test to show that he was unreliable."[59]

Dr. Little maintained that the Bar Harbor experiments showed nothing of value and that the yellow powder was a "corrosive agent" that actually injured the mice. He published his uniformly negative findings in the AMA *Journal* in 1935.[60] All records of the experiments were allegedly consumed in a fire at the lab years later, atomizing any documentation to support either side's story.[61]

In later correspondence with Dr. Little, Herbert Brower of the Endocrine Company regretted having made the ill-fated introduction. "My general impression from watching some of the cases treated in Dr. Drew's sanitarium at the time in question was one of extreme interest. I'm certain, temporarily at least, that there were some cases with retrogression of the so-called cancerous growth and improvement in condition. The initial testing [of the mice] showed encouraging results. It was then we arranged for the Harvard Club meeting and subsequent arrangements for further experimental work at your laboratory. From then on the picture changed and I am still sorry for the inconveniences caused you."[62]

Hoxsey returned belatedly to Philadelphia to spend two more years with Dr. Drew. They parted ways in 1934 when Dr. Drew called it quits. "Harry, I have been thinking this thing over," Dr. Drew wrote him. "A man of my age, my standing, I figure getting into politics and running for Congress in 1936. If I get in this thing, it may ruin me politically. It may ruin me every way. I don't think I can stand it. I had rather not start the fight here. I will go ahead and treat these cases, or use your remedy, and do everything I can to help you."[63]

In a later interview with the FDA, Dr. Drew is reported to have had further reasons. "Dr. Drew believes that Mr. Hoxsey has a 'recessive condition,' and is under the impression that he has to be a bigshot, since he was actually only a layman with a little education. He said that Hoxsey is a monumental liar and that you can't believe a thing he says. He won't listen to advice. Hoxsey is the type of man who simply will not play ball with anybody. He is so jealous of his external treatment with yellow powder that he guards it with his life. Hoxsey is a braggart, a liar, a schemer, and a conniver."[64]

The FDA report concluded with a paradoxical summation of Dr. Drew's perspective on Hoxsey. "In spite of Mr. Hoxsey's shortcomings, Dr. Drew claims he likes him and is absolutely sold on his treatment for curing cancer. He said he has seen many of the cures. He said that Mr. Hoxsey was truthful in one respect, and that was he told the patients exactly what were their chances of being cured, and that nine times out of ten he was right. [Dr. Drew was] frank to admit that never once did he catch Hoxsey in a lie pertaining to the success or failure of his treatment in a particular case."[65]

Despite repeated affirmations of at least some merit to his treatment, Hoxsey found himself barred from any official investigation and banished to a medical no-man's-land. Without question, his own inferiority complex and need to be a big shot, as Dr. Drew characterized his personality, contributed mightily to his standing as an untouchable. Yet where Hoxsey was less than trustworthy in many ways, he did seem to draw the line where it came to the real issue: his cases.

Perhaps Hoxsey's abrasive demeanor and latitude with the facts terminally estranged him from the only people who could satisfy the question of the efficacy of his remedies. Nevertheless, a scientific test is not supposed to be a personality contest. Too many objective parties confirmed some value to the treatment to dismiss it out of hand. Why wouldn't Dr. Fishbein's AMA investigate? Was the secrecy of Hoxsey's formulas

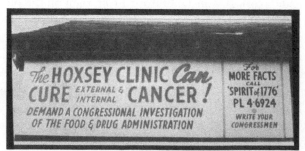

Sign on the side of a New England barn, 1950s.

really the issue or merely a pretext? Wouldn't a test put the matter to rest more expeditiously than the protracted war that served mainly to generate controversy and column inches?

Dr. Cramp, writing in the AMA *Journal* in 1935, was blunt in his assessment. "There is no scientific evidence at the present time to show that any serum, drug or combination of drugs will cure cancer."[66] The AMA was adamant in its conviction that only surgery and radiation were able to cure cancer, even though cancer researchers already knew that these treatments were very limited in their effectiveness. As medical historian Patricia Spain Ward wrote, "Only when it could no longer be denied that cure rates were virtually unaffected by earlier and earlier detection—and greater and greater destruction of tissue by surgery and radiation—did the thrust of 'established' methods shift in the direction of combined therapies, with surgery, radiation and chemotherapy used in various combinations and sequences."[67] Not until the mid-1940s would conventional medicine start to experiment with drug therapies for cancer.

Then again, perhaps there was a more sinister motive behind the AMA's blockade. Was Hoxsey's allegation about the AMA's attempt to buy his formulas entirely a fiction? The truth would never be fully known, but events were yet to unfold that would shed disturbing light on the mystery.

Rootless and married for the fourth time, Hoxsey decamped from Philadelphia back to Illinois. "But I was getting restless," he later wrote. "Time was moving along; I was nearly thirty-five years old, I'd been treating cancer for close to fifteen years and yet my ultimate goal—recognition and acceptance by the medical profession—was as distant as ever. All I had to show for myself was an empty pocketbook, a pregnant wife and a bleak future. Perhaps a change in scenery would help."[68]

When Hoxsey pointed his car south, his fortunes did begin to rise.

Gone to Texas:
The Medical Wild West

"**G**.T.T," said Robert Heath enigmatically as we filmed the gracious history buff and director of the Dallas County Medical Society in the society's downtown headquarters. "If you go to parts of Tennessee and Kentucky and look through files of the sheriff's department, you'll find files marked G.T.T., and that simply means 'Gone to Texas.' In the view of most law enforcement bodies at that time, if you got to Texas, there was nothing anybody could do about you. Things were pretty much free game here."[1] Dallas was flush with oil boomers, slot machines on Main Street, and a Texas taste for hyperbole. Hoxsey felt right at home.[2]

Hoxsey had heard Dallas doctor R. L. Spann promoting several alternative cancer treatments in broadcasts from a Mexican radio station. "I think it was about twenty-five below zero in Chicago," he later recalled. "We got in the car and came to Dallas. I got up the next morning about seven-thirty and called Dr. Spann." Hoxsey cracked open his perennial satchel bulging with case histories to display ghastly before-and-after photographs of astonishing cures. In March 1936 he signed a six-month contract with the Spann Sanitarium, a spacious old southern-style mansion at 4507 Gaston Avenue. Also staffing the clinic was C. M. Hartzog, an aging doctor.[3]

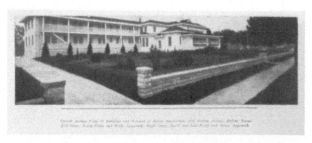

The southern mansion on Gaston Avenue becomes the world's largest privately owned cancer center under Hoxsey.

Hoxsey said he chose Dallas because it had the "strongest medical association" in the country and he wanted to stake his claim where it would stick.[4] The enticing Spann Sanitarium provided a general hospital treating chronic diseases and cancer, including Dr. Spann's "cell-balance" treatment, which he advertised from border station XEPN in Piedras Negras, Mexico, thus evading the ban on ads by the AMA Code of Ethics.[5] Spann was both a medical doctor and former dean of the Physio-Medical College of Texas, a school in the Eclectic tradition that utilized herbs and other natural therapies. (The Eclectic tradition is explored in part 2.) Since coming to Texas in 1899, he watched the small town of 41,000 swell to a burgeoning metropolis of 330,000 residents.[6]

"Don't Give Up Hope," exhorted the clinic's new brochure, amid graphic photographs of compelling Hoxsey external cures.[7] It explicitly characterized cancer as a "constitutional disease," contrary to organized medicine's view of cancer as a local phenomenon. Hoxsey's first patient was Mrs. J. B. Whitehead, who subsequently wrote Dr. Spann a letter about her experience. "Now that I am going back home, I have the mixed feeling of happiness at returning to my family in good health and regret at leaving all those who have been so kind to me during the thirty-three days I have spent at Spann Sanitarium. I have felt more like a guest than a patient."[8]

Mrs. Whitehead described the horror of her illness. "I had suffered severe hemorrhages of the uterus for about two years. In September 1935, the discharge became filled with pus and caused me considerable pain. Last December I consulted Dr. Joseph Elmer Kanatser of Wichita Falls, Texas, who immediately diagnosed my condition as cancer and recommended radium treatments. I was unwilling to accept the judgment of one physician, so went to Dr. Percy King Smith. Dr. Smith confirmed the diagnosis and had me go to Dr. Everett Foster Jones, who also made an examination. Dr. Jones, under the direction of Dr. Smith, gave me eighty-four hours of radium treatment in the Wichita Falls Clinic Hospital. These treatments stopped the flow and gave me temporary relief, but it was not long before I was worse than before. I also had two blood transfusions during this period." Hollow needles packed with fifty milligrams of radium were inserted into Mrs. Whitehead's uterus on two occasions for thirty hours each.

"I then went to the Baker Hospital in Muscatine, Iowa," she continued. "I was told there they would not accept me as a patient because there was nothing they could do for me. I then came to you, and what you have done for me is nothing short of miraculous. If I had not had the experience myself, I would not believe that any treatment could produce such definite results without pain and suffering."[9] Organized medicine couldn't believe it either, and later contended Mrs. Whitehead was cured by the prior radiation and never suffered radium burns.

Following Mrs. Whitehead's apparently successful outcome using Hoxsey's internal tonic, her husband shared his enthusiasm for the treatment with his fellow railroad workers and was soon fired. Hoxsey helped initiate reinstatement proceedings through the National Labor Relations Board. Railroad officials contended that Whitehead was initially reduced to a lower salary, then let go "on furlough" because of a reduction in the workforce. In the interim, the train car repairman was broke, and Hoxsey bought some laundry machines and set him up in business. Whitehead did finally regain his job, but when he was killed in an accident several years later, Hoxsey and his wife took in their son and raised him to alleviate the family's financial burden.[10]

When Hoxsey's contract with Dr. Spann ran out, he joined forces with Dr. Hartzog to set up the Bryan and Peak Cancer Clinic in a small building near downtown.[11] Hoxsey started placing newspaper ads and quickly attracted the ire of Dr. T. J. Crowe, head of the Dallas County Medical Society. Dr. Crowe showed up at the clinic and began haranguing Hoxsey. He threatened Dr. Hartzog with the loss of his license as well as jail and swore he would close the clinic. Hoxsey banished him from the premises.

The next day Dr. Hartzog was ordered to appear before the State Medical Board to show cause why his license shouldn't be revoked. He refused, and several weeks later Dr. Hartzog, Hoxsey, and his wife Martha were arrested and thrown in the Dallas County jail. Hoxsey was enraged at the arrest of his wife, who was put in the tank with prostitutes and slapped around.[12]

What ensued was a Texas tornado of arrests at Dr. Crowe's behest, but the state's "complaining witnesses" turned out to be sympathetic patients who wouldn't cooperate with the authorities, and who didn't even reside in the proper jurisdiction. Mildred Nelson, who would join Hoxsey in 1946, recalled a typical encounter in the protracted vendetta. "I was in Harry's office one day and the phone rang. There was a conversation on the other end, and then Harry said, 'No, I'm not going to do that.' He sat and listened for a while longer and said, 'No, goddammit, you're not going to do that either.' Then there was a long pause again, and he said, 'I tell you what you do—on your way out, stop over at Baylor Hospital and find out how much it would cost to have my boot removed from your ass, 'cause that's what's going to happen!' And I said, 'Harry, who are you talkin' to?' And he said, 'That was Dr. Crowe, head of the County

Medical Society. He was going to come and take the sign on the lawn down, and you heard what I told him.'"

James Wakefield Burke met Hoxsey as a reporter sent to cover the cancer controversy. We found Burke during our research and filmed him in Dallas. A dapper, articulate writer dressed in sporty clothes and a blue tie threaded with silver, he knew Hoxsey for a span of three decades. But when *Esquire* magazine first sent Burke to Dallas to expose Hoxsey around 1937, the journalist was surprised to find that he had already encountered him years before. "When I first met Hoxsey, I was a student at the University of Chicago. I had heard about this man from southern Illinois who was being arrested for curing cancer and I didn't pay much attention. In the summer there was a notice on my fraternity brothers' board that there were jobs to be had. This was in the days of the Depression when it was hard to get a job, and they wanted students from the university to apply for jobs. I went down to a hotel and here was a young, robust, tall man giving a speech about selling pots and pans. I was fascinated by this man's speech and his drive. Why he wanted university students was to set up dates with wealthy families in the suburbs of Chicago, and he would cook a meal and show them what good pots and pans he had. Later on I learned it was Harry Hoxsey, the cancer man. He could sell anything. He could convince anybody of anything. He had power over people that was persuasive. He sounded like he believed in what he was doing.

"About ten years later, World War II was steaming up and I was still going to school, still working my way as a salesman and writing some articles for *Esquire*. By this time there had been a lot of publicity here and there about the quack who was treating people with a tonic in Texas. Arnold Gingrich, my boss, says, 'Hoxsey is getting too big and the American Medical Association would like to put him out of business. You go down there and get acquainted with him, and we'll do a couple of pieces on him and put an end to this.' It was an assignment.

"So it was arranged and I did come to Dallas to meet Hoxsey through a fraternity brother who gave big parties. He was introduced to me and I told him right off, 'I'm down here for *Esquire* magazine to expose you, so we might as well get this thing straight on the table.' He smiled and said, 'What time do you want me to pick you up?'

"Next morning at eight A.M., he was at the door. He took me out to his clinic, which was a converted dog kennel. He had a few old men and women sitting around there, and he led me around and introduced me as 'Doctor Burke from the University of Chicago.' Well, I didn't correct him, so he took me in the back and gave me a white doctor's smock, put it on me, and said, 'I want you to see what I'm doing.' I thought any moment I'm going to get information that he's a quack and be on my way."

Burke followed "Doc," as he was commonly known, on his rounds. "His first patient had been an old gentleman that he had been treating for six or eight weeks who had cancer of the eye. I learned later that he was not supposed to treat people because he wasn't a doctor. He did have an old doctor on the payroll who'd sit around and watch him, but Harry did it all himself. He brought the patient in, took off the bandage, and he says, 'Well, dad, I told you, you were going to get well. Let me take that thing off.' He took his scalpel and peeled it off, and sure enough, the cancer was gone, and he threw it in the wastebasket. He put some medication on it and put a bandage on it.

"The next patient was the wife from a wealthy young couple in their mid-forties. The man was very concerned because the doctors had told him his wife had a melanoma and there was no way to treat her to get well. So this man wanted to talk to Dr. Hoxsey privately. I met with him in another room while his wife was lying on the treating table. This man wanted to know if he could cure her. Harry was positive that he could, so the man wanted to know about what it was going to cost him. Harry said, 'You don't believe I can cure her, and I do believe I can cure your wife. Let's go down to the bank and I'll put $10,000 in escrow, and you put up $10,000. The day your doctor says she's well, I pick up the money.' So that was agreed upon, and he came back for the treatment, and I learned later that doctors never put a scalpel on a melanoma. So Harry looked at this woman. She had it on her navel, a big black one about the size of a walnut. He took his scalpel, slashed it two or three ways, put some of his powder on it, put a bandage over it, and said, 'Go get dressed.' He gave the husband a bottle of his tonic and said, 'Now you come back next week.' So I thought, well, this is pure quackery."

Burke decided to do some further checking of his own. "Six months later, I went over to Fort Worth, saw this woman and she was well. Two years later, I checked on her and she was well. Gradually I became a believer. A believer, not a disciple. I became friends with Hoxsey. He had a great heart, and he was able to cure people as far as I could see.

"I expected to stay about a day, get my information and leave. I became fascinated. I stayed for six weeks. Every day Harry would pick me up and bring me to the clinic. Hoxsey was a fascinating man. He was highly intelligent, but rather crude-talking, but not in an obscene or vulgar way. We'd come in in the morning and he would put his arm around these old men and women, and say 'Dad, them doctors been cutting you up, but I ain't gonna let those sons of bitches kill you.' They'd begin to get better and begin to get well.

"Of course, Arnold Gingrich had sent me down here to write an article exposing Harry Hoxsey as a quack. But now I could no longer do it, so I wrote an outline for a piece which I called, 'The Quack Who Cured Cancer.' I sent it back to the editors, but I guess it was too hot—it never came out."

Meanwhile Hoxsey's splenetic feud with the Dallas County Medical Society escalated. Between 1937 and 1939, he was arrested more than one hundred times.[13] The eager young assistant district attorney Al Templeton brought most of the cases against him. Not one of the charges resulted in a conviction because none of his patients would testify against Hoxsey. As Jim Burke recalled, "He always carried a big roll of money, about $10,000, in his pocket. The authorities would pick him up and put him in jail, and he'd bail himself out. Once in a while he would deliberately stay in jail a few days. He knew what would happen. These old men and women he had cured would come around the jail, bring baskets of chicken, home-cooked pies, and pray and sing. The jailers would turn him out to save themselves the embarrassment."

When Al Templeton's younger brother, Mike, got cancer in 1939, surgeons removed his rectum and performed a colostomy, the removal of his colon, leaving him with a bag at his side to excrete fecal matter. The cancer returned and spread through his body. Down to eighty-three pounds, Mike Templeton was doped up on morphine, waiting to die. The odor became so unbearable that he had to go live with an uncle, where he was attended by private nurse Jack Howard.[14]

When Jack Howard showed up in November at Hoxsey's clinic seeking help, Hoxsey asked if Mike Templeton's D.A. brother knew he was there. The answer was no. Hoxsey agreed to treat Mike secretly.

Within a month, Mike Templeton was off the narcotics and gaining weight. On Christmas morning, he rose from bed, dressed himself, and went to his brother's house. Standing at the door, he asked if he could borrow the shotgun. Al refused, fearing Mike was going to kill himself. Replied Mike, "I've gained forty pounds and I'm off the dope. I want to go rabbit hunting!" He revealed to his stunned sibling that he had been going to Hoxsey.

After a couple days of anguished soul-searching, Al Templeton paid a visit to the clinic. He resigned his post of seven years as assistant D.A. to sign on as Hoxsey's lawyer.[15] When he appeared in court at Hoxsey's next arraignment, Dr. Crowe was shocked at finding his prosecutor now comfortably seated at Hoxsey's table, while the judge informed him he had to drop or refile all the charges prepared by Templeton. Another assistant D.A., Frank Ivey, quit shortly after and also went to work for Hoxsey.[16]

Brother Mike regained his health and lived on for ten years, dying of acute alcoholism. Al Templeton would be elected two years later to three terms as county judge. Suddenly Hoxsey had friends in the courthouse. He began his political ascent in Texas. [17]

Unable to get patients to testify against Hoxsey, the medical society took another tack. In the racially segregated southern city whose newspaper ran headlines such as "Negress Sues for Alimony in Steaks," Hoxsey was already notorious for letting black people in the front door with everyone else. In a confidential letter Hoxsey managed to obtain, W. F. McBride of the Texas State Board of Medical Examiners wrote to the counsel for the board, "It seems that we are having a hard time connecting up a good case on Hoxsey where white people have been treated. I am sending you this for your comment and advice as to whether you think we could stand a chance to stick Hoxsey on evidence which is wholly testified to by Negroes. It seems that these darkeys all have a clean record behind them." [18]

Hoxsey's son and daughter recall accompanying their father on Sunday mornings to black churches where Hoxsey held forth with his own evangelical fervor. He later sponsored meetings at his home for the Progressive Voters League, an early black civil rights organization, and went to bat in Washington, D.C., for Dallas's black community to procure a housing development. [19] "He was the originator of the black vote," asserted his son. "He was as at home in the ghetto as he was uptown. He never shunned anyone. He'd always say that you never knew when you might be down and out, and someone you helped along the way might help you." [20]

Unable to get black patients to testify against Hoxsey, the medical society resorted to other tactics. In 1940 Hoxsey learned that pathologist Dr. Marvin Bell, threatened with the revocation of his medical license, would no longer perform biopsies for him. Since a biopsy is considered the only verifiable proof of cancer, Hoxsey could no longer validate his cures. He soon found himself excluded from obtaining crucial medical records from laboratories, hospitals, and doctors across the country. [21]

Dr. Crowe continued the bombardment of legal cases, but gained only one conviction, which was overturned. In 1940 a beleaguered Dr. Hartzog brought suit against Dr. Crowe. Hoxsey gathered over one hundred patients from all over the Southeast in front of Judge W. L. Thornton, who would play a pivotal role in Hoxsey's legal future. Judge Thornton enjoined Dr. Crowe from "molesting and bothering" the Bryan and Peak Cancer Clinic and from trespassing. [22] In 1942 Judge Joe Brown finally put a decisive end to the flagrant persecution. [23] As Hoxsey related,

"Although my legal battles were far from over, the favorable court decisions in 1942 marked a definite turning point in my twenty-year battle with organized medicine. Our clinic was firmly established; we'd legally won the right to treat cancer by unorthodox methods. Moreover, World War II was in full swing now, the newspapers had little space to devote to the involved controversy between Harry M. Hoxsey and the AMA."[24]

In 1942, however, Dr. Hartzog had a nervous breakdown under the relentless pressure from Dr. Crowe and the medical society, and quit and moved to Louisiana. Hoxsey hired another physician, Dr. Hamlett, who stayed only a year until his father died and left him a small estate. Hoxsey hired and lost a couple of more doctors over the next two years, paying high salaries in hopes of retaining them. He estimated the clinic cleared a modest net profit of $10,000 in 1942, doubling each year to $77,000 by 1945 as the costly court fights and weekly arrests subsided.[25]

Meanwhile, Hoxsey barraged the medical society with loud demands for a fair investigation. He also persisted in filling Dr. Fishbein's mailbox, though his impassioned correspondence went unrequited. In exasperation, he wrote to Dr. W. W. Fowler, chairman of the Dallas Southern Clinical Association, "Doctor, let's forget about ethics or so-called ethics and meet this issue in the face, and let this treatment be compared by actual clinical tests. Doctor, surely suffering humanity comes or should come ahead of everything else. Abraham Lincoln said, 'Taxation without representation is wrong.' Condemnation without being given an opportunity to show our results before your Association is wrong, unjust and unfair and is locking the doors to suffering humanity and mankind."[26] He offered to donate his formulas free to medicine at large, as long as doctors would not exploit the treatment financially.[27] Decrying the greed that was subsuming the profession of healing, he threatened to run for legislative office on a platform of socialized medicine in 1941.[28]

Robert Heath of the Dallas County Medical Society remembered his father's official stance toward Hoxsey's plea for an investigation. "The challenge most often offered was to send a group to come and test our theories. Truthfully, that really never took place because the medical establishment felt that any effort on their part to go and review the work or the material that Mr. Hoxsey might present to them would do little more than give credibility to the program and would not in fact accomplish anything meaningful."

Dr. Harry M. Spence, a patrician figure in the Dallas medical community, contended that Hoxsey's flamboyant challenges for an investigation were nothing but a "publicity ploy."[29] Yet it surely would have been an easy bluff to call, and Hoxsey's apparent sincerity was affirmed by innumerable witnesses over the years, even those who believed he had nothing of value for treating cancer.

One Dallas physician did take up Hoxsey's plea. Dr. Sam L. Scothorn, a respected osteopath and former president of the American Osteopathic Association, took his wife to Hoxsey to treat her ovarian cancer after radiation failed. Introduced by Dr. Drew of Philadelphia, he found Hoxsey willing to treat his wife, but equally interested in getting a fair test. Dr. Scothorn enlisted several osteopaths to review twenty-seven cases using biopsies they conducted themselves. All but three patients lived. In the interim, Mrs. Scothorn got well.

Dr. Crowe angrily ordered Dr. Scothorn to appear before the Medical Board. He refused, indignant at the affront to his credentials, having served on the State Board under three different governors in a state where osteopaths and medical doctors shared equal legal standing. "I have learned that your reason for calling me is because my wife was treated for cancer at the Hoxsey Cancer Clinic, generally considered a quack institution. I use 'quack' purposely because, since your Board was created in 1907, the AMA has looked upon all irregulars as quacks. But because I decided not to let my wife be destroyed by cancer and encouraged her to go to an irregular institution where she got beneficial treatment, I was told to give up my time and go to the expense of appearing before your Board and explaining my personal affairs. I have practiced in Dallas County for thirty-nine years with never a suit against me nor an insinuation of any kind against my practice or character. I feel grossly insulted by your letter and do not intend to appear before the Board, because, in my opinion, the letter smacks of conspiracy."[30]

Dr. Scothorn's charge of a conspiracy would increasingly be echoed by other observers and by Hoxsey himself. Robert Heath of the Dallas County Medical Society discounted the notion. "There really was not a conspiracy in the purest definition of the term *conspiracy*. There was a concerted effort between many concerned individuals and groups of people to attempt to present truthful scientific information about where scientific knowledge was at that present time, and where the information Mr. Hoxsey put forth failed to meet the standard of scientific knowledge."[31]

Nevertheless, the trail of the "concerted effort" Heath acknowledged invariably led back to Chicago, where Dr. Fishbein was acquiring kudos as abundantly as Hoxsey was attracting warrants. As the undisputed Voice of American Medicine, Dr. Fishbein's extravagent personality was synonymous with the AMA. As the *Chicago Daily Times* wryly reported, "Consider the case of Dr. Morris Fishbein—doctor, author, lecturer and one of the most feverishly busy men in town. He is editor of a half dozen magazines, including the *Journal of the American Medical Association*, spokesman for the one hundred thousand members of that organization; author of many books and articles, professor at Rush Medical College and the University of Illinois. He—reads three thousand five hundred manuscripts a year for business purposes—reads ten books a week for pleasure—makes one-hundred-thirty addresses a year—turns out fifteen thousand words a week for publication—keeps four secretaries running to and fro with dictation ('one hundred letters a day correspondence')."[32]

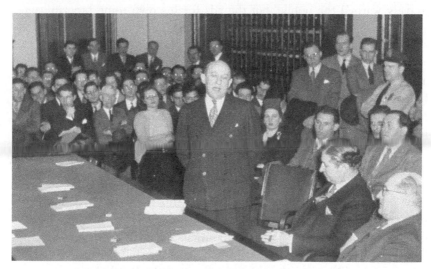

Dr. Fishbein opposes national health insurance, 1940s.

Naturally, no one could possibly accomplish all this, but Dr. Fishbein seemed to believe his own press releases, an alarming signal. He left the technical content of the *Journal* to others, but avidly reported his personal adventures in "Dr. Pepys' Diary," where he was "a man who is doing everything all men want to do, and doing it all the time against a background of frolic and fame," as *Harper's* magazine quipped.[33] In between trips on the fashionable Century express train to Washington to testify against national health insurance, he frequented the glamorous Rainbow Room and Stork Club in New York City and played poker with famed playwright George Kaufman and editor Harold Ross of *The New Yorker*. Hopping back on the Century, he was "called to advise a beauteous lady of filmdom whom an allergist was desensitizing against horse dandruff and who was having an alarming reaction, and discussed orthopedics with the world's greatest orthopedist who happened into the diner." Reportedly the only activity he didn't like was fishing, because of the necessity for keeping quiet.

"Beware the doctor who advertises!" admonished Dr. Fishbein. Yet if doctors were barred from advertising, Dr. Fishbein seemed to be making up for all of them. When he authored the voluminous *Modern Home Medical Advisor* during World War II, the ads were so outrageous—"a substitute for your drafted doctor!"—that he was forced to withdraw the promotions entirely.[34] "Beware the man who guarantees a cure or who promises that he can cure any serious disease on one or two treatments," Fishbein gravely warned the public, but the ads for his own tome breezily suggested readers needed nothing more than clippings from his book to be their own best doctor.[35]

Under Dr. Fishbein's watch, doctordom attained apotheosis. Materially, physicians' wallets were bulging from the fiscal clout of Fishbein's flourishing trade association, although paradoxically Fishbein himself was never interested in the acquisition of personal wealth. He was a true believer in the allopathic mission to bring "scientific" medicine to ascendancy, and tied his own fortunes to it. As *Harper's* noted, "'Some people believe I run the AMA,' he often said. Some people certainly did. In the course of thirty-seven single-minded and single-handed years, he had converted a panty-waist professional society into the most terrifying trade organization on earth."[36] Indeed, the mandatory $25 tithing fee he required from his membership for a "national education campaign" against President Harry Truman's national health insurance bill garnered a breathtaking $2.2 million war chest that sandbagged the legislation.[37]

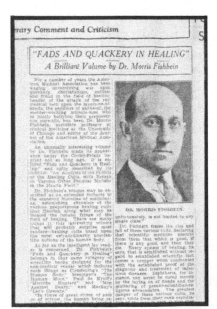

Part of the AMA's success resided in tilting against a sordid enemy—quackery—and from early on Dr. Fishbein staked his highly public image on exposing medical fraud. While still assistant editor to Dr. Simmons, he had established his quackbusting persona with a frothy episode printed in virtually every paper in the country. When a young woman reported an impossible fever of 119 degrees, Fishbein traveled to Michigan to expose the "Hot Girl of Escanaba." He discovered

Dr. Fishbein proves the pen is mightier than the scalpel by exposing medical fraud.

two hot water bottles under her arms, and generated prodigious national heat of his own in 10,000 newspaper clippings, as well as a merry mention in the Ziegfeld Follies.[38]

Fishbein's early success combating quackery revealed to him a gold mine of limitless possibilities. In rapid-fire succession he cranked out three books: *Fads and Quackery, Medical Follies*, and *The New Medical Follies*. "As one reads the rolls of fakirs down through the ages," Fishbein gleefully penned, "one becomes almost convinced of the doctrine of transmigration of souls."[39]

Dr. Fishbein also utilized the "Devil theory of history," as one observer put it, exemplified by his quackdown.[40] In *Medical Follies*, he dubbed the profession of chiropractic a "malignant tumor" whose theory was "so simple that even farm-hands can grasp it. It has been said that osteopathy is essentially a method of entering the practice of medicine by the back door. Chiropractic, by contrast, is an attempt to arrive through the cellar. The man who applies at the back door at least makes himself presentable. The one who comes through the cellar is besmirched with dust and grime; he carries a crowbar and he may wear a mask."[41] Under Dr. Fishbein's direction, the AMA Bureau of Investigation's quack files swelled to a prodigious 300,000 names.[42]

Dr. Fishbein appeared in and consulted on anti-quackery films for Warner Brothers and other Hollywood studios, and reveled in his celebrity.[43] He collaborated on newsreels for the popular *March of Time*, projecting his anti-quackery bulletins through movie houses across the land. Against roiling music, the stern narration warned, "Sole profiteers from cancer have been the quacks against whose fraudulent cures the American Medical Association is constantly crusading. At the Association's headquarters in Chicago, vigilant against quackery is Dr. Morris Fishbein." Cut to Dr. Fishbein's office, where the medical dictator is dictating to an adoring secretary: "There is no serum, drug, or combination of drugs that we know that will definitely cure cancer," he warned, repeating Dr. Cramp's thinly clad jibe at Harry Hoxsey's herbal brew.[44]

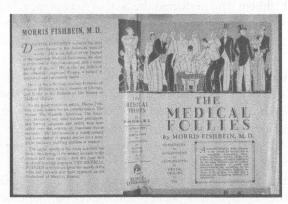

Dr. Fishbein termed chiropractic a "malignant tumor" as part of his quack attack.

Dr. Fishbein's crusade to eliminate the irregulars played no small part in the AMA's financial success by throttling economic competition. While member dues accounted for half the AMA's revenues, the balance flowed from the *Journal*, now the most profitable publication in the world. Flush with revenues, it soon became known as "the tail that wagged the dog."[45] In addition, the *Journal* owned or controlled another half-dozen medical journals along with the thirty-five state society journals, with advertising revenues of over $2 million, a huge sum in those days.[46]

As Milton Mayer wrote for *Harper's* magazine,

> The *Journal* was the heart of the AMA, and the heart of the *Journal* was the AMA Seal of Acceptance. Possession of the Seal certifies that a drug, appliance, food product, cosmetic, or soap has been accepted by a committee of Men in White as advertisable in the *Journal*. The value of the Seal to the manufacturer is incalculable, and the page in the *Journal* is only five hundred dollars or so. Advertising men believe, as a class, that if they are good boys they will go to heaven when they die and get a job soliciting for the *Journal*. "I turn down as much advertising as I accept—over a million a year," the editor said. The Seal is probably the biggest "puller" of advertising ever concocted. The *Journal* was a toll-gate on the highway to recognition of medical research, and the editor was the gatekeeper.[47]

The idea of *Journal* certification of products was originally devised around 1905 by Dr. Fishbein's mentor, George Henry Simmons, but it was Fishbein who perfected the Seal of Acceptance. It positioned the *Journal* as the sole portal to the medical marketplace. Yet the real story behind the money machine it generated was anything but wholesome.

Since it was considered "unethical" to advertise medical products and services directly to the public, all promotions were compelled to traverse a web of arteries flowing directly to organized medicine's heart in Chicago. Inquiries to advertise in disparate county or state medical society journals received a timely reply from the AMA's Cooperative Medical Advertising Bureau. The broad AMA advertising network would cover with no overlap virtually all states as well as the national market. One former *Journal* ad salesman described his job as sizing up candidates for the depth of their pockets and squeezing them for "all the traffic would bear." If they resisted, he hinted at the potentially catastrophic consequences of AMA condemnation of their product. Of two identical products, he reported, the one with an advertising contract would gain the coveted Seal.[48]

Land O' Lakes Butter Company was the first company to receive the Seal of Acceptance from the AMA Committee on Foods, and touted its honor widely. However, the company had a scrolling criminal record rife with dozens of convictions by the federal government and state of Pennsylvania for selling putrid butter and eggs. In 1931 and 1933, Governor Gifford Pinchot of Pennsylvania hauled the company into court for multiple cases of adulterating butter with excessive moisture. In New York and New Jersey, the company admitted that 399 cans of frozen eggs were "filthy, decomposed, and that sugar had been added, presumably to disguise the smell."[49]

Meanwhile, cigarette manufacturer Philip Morris, the *Journal's* biggest single advertiser, also ran into some problems. Blitzing the AMA *Journal* and thirty-one state and regional medical journals, the start-up tobacco company was eager to publicize its innovative use of diethylene glycol as a hygroscopic agent (to retain moisture), in place of the glycerin used by other manufacturers. Philip Morris pegged its campaign on hyping the breakthrough that its cigarettes were consequently "less irritating to the throat."[50]

When the corporation approached the *Journal* with its ads, Dr. Fishbein courteously advised it how to go about conducting acceptable scientific testing to validate its unsubstantiated claims and thereby qualify. The cigarette manufacturer was eager to link its product with health benefits, and Dr. Fishbein saw a vast new opportunity for revenues from nonmedical products, despite the fact that by this time in the 1930s medical journals were already publishing studies associating smoking with lung cancer.

The company completed its testing at the Columbia University College of Physicians and Surgeons with findings that the cigarettes with diethylene glycol caused three times less swelling than other brands. The company used these studies to launch its medical ad campaign, while supplying free smokes to doctors. One *Journal* ad read, "Patients with coughs were instructed to change to Philip Morris cigarettes. In three out of four cases, the coughs disappeared completely. When these patients changed back to cigarettes made by the ordinary method of manufacture, coughs had returned in one third of the cases. This Philip Morris superiority is due to the employment of diethylene glycol."[51]

The campaign was wildly successful and established Philip Morris as a major tobacco player, until, in 1937, seventy-two people died as a result of using a drug called Sulfanalamide Massengill. With help from the AMA itself, the toxic agent was determined to be diethylene glycol. Dr. Fishbein hit the ground backpedaling. He defended his advertiser in an editorial by saying "There is no evidence that the ordinary use of diethylene glycol in industry, or as an ingredient in the manufacture of cigarettes, is harmful."[52] The company was so grateful that it offered him a retainer for his services, which he refused, tipping his editor's public health hat.

Other cigarette manufacturers quickly followed suit in their entry into the medical market using physician testimonials. MORE DOCTORS SMOKE CAMELS THAN ANY OTHER CIGARETTE was the slogan at Camel's exhibit at the 1947 AMA convention. Only in the 1950s, when overwhelming evidence of the causation of lung cancer by smoking reached the public, did the *Journal* stop accepting tobacco ads, though Dr. Fishbein was by then serving as a paid consultant to the Lorillard tobacco company. Through its Members' Retirement Fund, the AMA continued to own tobacco stock in the seven figures until the mid-1980s.[53]

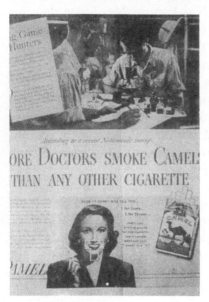

Phillip Morris was the AMA Journal's *biggest advertiser in the 1940s.*

Numerous physicians complained of other high-pressure tactics from Chicago. Dr. George Starr White, a respected physician who lectured extensively to doctors and reputedly had the largest private practice in the country, described how two doctors from AMA headquarters approached him with a proposition. "They told me they knew of the work that I was doing and teaching, and that if I would let certain officers of the AMA in with me so as to get a royalty on my teachings and books, as well as credit for some of my discoveries, that I would have no opposition from them; but if I refused, every obstacle would be put in my way."[54]

So when Dr. Sam Scothorn charged a "conspiracy," his reaction may not have been altogether paranoid. After all, Dr. Fishbein, consonant with his Devil theory of history, had dictated that "anyone claiming to treat cancer by anything other than surgery, radium, and X-ray is an ipso facto quack."[55] Harry Hoxsey was already Public Quack Number One on Dr. Fishbein's most unwanted list, and their battle was about to combust in a firestorm that would singe the loose lips of the Voice of American Medicine.

6

Hoxsey vs. the AMA: "Thrice Is He Armed Who Hath His Quarrel Just"

Intractably blocked by the AMA and Texas medical authorities, Hoxsey sought alternative routes to an investigation. With the world war over, he set his sights on the National Cancer Institute in 1945. Through a friend who was a talent scout for U.S.O. shows, he met three congressmen, Representatives Virgil Chapman of Kentucky and Harold Earthman and J. Percy Priest of Tennessee, who agreed to accompany him to the NCI. Also joining the expedition were Dr. Ira Drew, Dr. and Mrs. Sam Scothorn, two other doctors, and a reporter from the *Dallas Times-Herald*.[1]

The NCI, part of the U.S. Public Health Service, was by now spending a hefty $20 million a year on cancer research, and Hoxsey pleaded his case at the agency's headquarters in Bethesda, Maryland. NCI chief Dr. R. R. Spencer explained that Hoxsey needed to submit fifty case histories of internal cancers only, including verified biopsies.[2]

Dr. Spencer emphasized to Hoxsey that revealing his formulas was a precondition of any evaluation. Ever wary, Hoxsey flinched. He was suspicious that this was merely the latest ploy by Dr. Fishbein to obtain his precious secrets, which he guarded as jealously as drug companies routinely protect their proprietary methods. He did agree to submit the necessary case histories.

Following the meeting, Dr. Spencer fired off a letter to Dr. Morris Fishbein, relating the fact that Hoxsey "did not seem inclined to reveal his formulas." The NCI chief added that "Mr. Hoxsey seems to have a persecution complex and states that he has been treated very unfairly by the AMA many years ago. He says you and a former president of the

American Medical Association, Dr. Harris, thought his remedy to be somewhat worthwhile and would have taken it up if he assigned over to you
personally the entire rights."[3] Dr. Fishbein replied testily by dismissing
Hoxsey as "a liar."[4]

About a month later, Hoxsey supplied the NCI with sixty case histories. But, having been blackballed in the medical community, he was unable to provide biopsies in numerous cases. Instead he supplied the names
of laboratories, hospitals, and doctors where they could be obtained—he
presumed correctly—through the authority of the federal government.

What ensued was a bilious dispute over the state of Hoxsey's records.
The NCI responded with a letter that fifteen of twenty cases of internal
cancer lacked biopsies. It further characterized the other forty cases as
inadmissible since they related to external cancers, and that the majority
of these also lacked biopsies. "Obviously," the terse rejection concluded,
"this does not meet the policy of our Advisory Cancer Council."[5]

Hoxsey adamantly contested the NCI's analysis. What the NCI called
"externals" included cases in which there was evidence of the spread of
the disease. He provided specific records of biopsies from Dallas pathologists, including Dr. Marvin Bell, where the NCI said there were none.
Dr. Bell, however, had changed his tune after being chastised for his association with Hoxsey. Where six years earlier he found cancer, now, he
wrote the NCI, "the slide I find on Mrs. O. G. Brown shows chronic
inflammatory tissues, and I do not know whether I was foolish enough to
call this carcinoma at the time, or if possibly I had another slide which
did show carcinoma and was accidentally discarded at the time."[6] Ostensibly Dr. Bell's brush with the AMA and Texas medical authorities dis-
couraged him from acknowledging any potentially favorable data relating to supposed Hoxsey cures. The status of Hoxsey's cases dissolved into
nebulous confusion.

In fact, there was already in full swing a "concerted effort" against
Hoxsey involving the NCI, AMA, FDA, and Texas medical authorities.
The NCI had been in prior contact with the Dallas County Medical Society since at least 1941, when the agency received a letter seeking help
prosecuting Hoxsey and complaining about his brochure mailings. The
NCI responded that such matters were not under its jurisdiction, and
alternatively suggested enlisting the Post Office Department for fraudulent use of the mails. Meanwhile, the Dallas substation of the federal
Food and Drug Administration, spurred by Dr. Crowe, had been in close
contact with the AMA Bureau of Investigation for years. Dr. Heller's letter to Dr. Fishbein was but the latest instance of the close contact medical
officials maintained in the ingrown world of cancer treatment.[7]

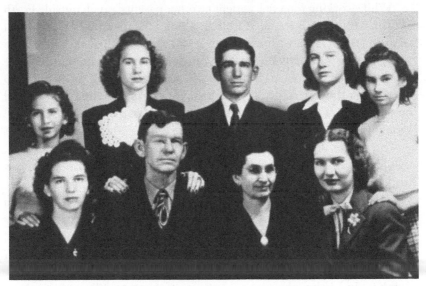

Mildred Nelson (lower right) and family, c. 1945. Mother Della Mae sits next to her and Mildred's father sits next to Della Mae.

Frustrated in his latest efforts for an investigation, Hoxsey returned to his thriving clinic to encounter a case that would permanently alter his fortunes. Ranch wife Della Mae Nelson had uterine cancer that had been extensively treated with twenty units of X-ray and thirty-six hours of radium. She was so badly burned from the radiation that she couldn't even pull a sheet over her body for a year after. Wasted to eighty-six pounds, she was bleeding internally, so severely impaired that she had to learn to walk all over again. Then the cancer recurred.

Della Mae's daugher, Mildred Nelson, was a young home-care nurse at the time, the eldest of her seven children. She bleakly watched her family's hopes fade. "The doctors would look at us," Mildred recalled as we filmed her in 1984, "and say, 'We've done everything we can do, our hands are tied. It's just a matter of time and you're going to lose her.'"

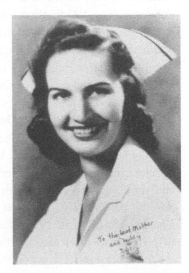

After nursing school, Mildred never expected to join a "quack" clinic, c. 1945.

While working for a sick patient near her parents' ranch outside Forth Worth, Mildred faced a fearful predicament. "Dad, asked me, 'Do you want to go to Dallas with me and drive for me?' And I said, 'Oh, you're going to get some parts for the Caterpillar?' 'Nope, I'm going to see the doctor.' 'What doctor?' 'The cancer doctor.' I said, 'Dad, we're going to see the best there is, so just forget about going to see a damn quack.' And he said, 'Well, I'm going down anyway. If you don't want to go, it's fine.' I said, 'No, I'll go with you.'

"So we get down there," Mildred continued, "and he introduced me, tells Harry I'm a nurse. And Harry said, 'Well, there's the doctors and nurses working in there—go in and talk to anybody you want to. There's the files, get in them if you want to. And would you like a job?' And Dad looked up and said, 'No, she already said you was a damn quack.' I didn't feel very good about that because I thought he shouldn't betray my confidence!

"But anyway, well, I thought I'll talk Mom out of it and get them away from there and then I could talk to them. Well, I couldn't. They didn't budge. I thought, as soon as I get off this case, I'll go down there and go to work and see what's going on, and *then* I can get them out of there. So when I got off that case, I called Harry and asked if he still needed a nurse. He said, 'I sure do, be here in the morning.' I found me a little apartment and went to work."

Positioned in her new job, Mildred was alert for the damning evidence she expected to uncover inside the clinic. "It was probably a year before it really began to set with me what was going on. As the patients would come in—sometimes we didn't see them for three months or six months—then I began to see the changes that would take place and hear their stories of, 'Well, my doctor told me I had thirty days to live,' or 'My doctor gave me three months to live and six months has gone by.' By the end of a year, I began to realize, gee, this does work. Mom had gotten better and to this day is alive and as sassy as can be. And when the doctors look at you and say, 'It's only a matter of time, I've done everything there is to do, our hands are tied, just get prepared'—I know what they're talking about!"

We filmed in 1986 with Della Mae Nelson and Mildred at Mildred's horse ranch outside Dallas. A spry, alert woman about eighty-five years old, Della Mae never did tell her doctor that she went to Hoxsey. "I've outlived the doctor," she reported cheerfully. "Two of the local doctors and the doctor in Fort Worth have also passed away. The nurses, too, have all passed away. As far as I know, I've outlived all of them." Della Mae Nelson died in 1997 of natural causes at the age of ninety-nine, fifty-one years after cancer almost took her life.

After her mother's successful treatment, Mildred surrendered to the

Hoxsey experience. "When I first went to work for Harry, he was on Bryan and Peak, which was a very small building. We had two treatment rooms and an office, and the waiting room was quite small. I couldn't believe that so many people could come to one little building. When the patients arrived, there was no place in the waiting room, so they'd go back to the car. When you got to this particular name on the list, if they didn't answer in the waiting room, you'd go traipsing off down the street to each car. I thought, 'My God, did I go through nurses' training for this?!' But people were so nice about it."

Like James Burke and Al Templeton before her, Mildred converted from a skeptic into a believer. "Harry would tell this wild story about this patient had this and this, and they got well, or he had sent all these records to the Food and Drug or the NCI and they wouldn't check anything, and I'd say, 'My God, he's telling me the biggest lies I ever heard! This couldn't be right.' And I'd listen to this for a few days, and finally I'd pick out the biggest one I thought he'd told me. And I'd go check. And when I got checkin', it was right! The man hadn't lied about it at all. He was tellin' the truth, but it was the wildest stories I'd ever heard in my life when it came to medicine."

Mildred's admiration for Hoxsey increased as she got to know him. "You didn't work for him—you worked with him. He was a big man, big heart, and a fantastic mind. Lots of love and compassion for people. They in return had a lot for him, but I think he actually gave more than they.

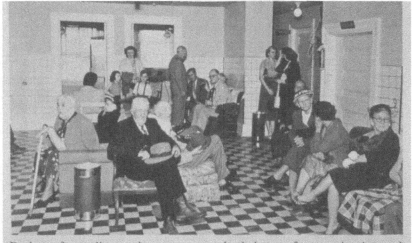

Patients from all over the country await their turn for examination and various clinical tests.

The waiting room overflows at the Dallas Hoxsey cancer clinic, c. 1955.

People would have problems, and in his pocket his hand went. He'd give you the shirt off his back, but don't ever try to take it away from him because you had a helluva fight! He butchered the King's English, and his best friend was an SOB, but he wouldn't have been Harry without it."

Mildred recollected the charisma of Hoxsey's presence in the clinic. "Things would get to rolling along kinda bad and look a little rough, and all of a sudden out of the clear blue sky when everybody's chin was on the floor, Harry would look up and say, 'Well, I believe love is here to stay—what do you think about it? There's too much love in this world for it to ever sink!' Everybody'd laugh, and here we'd go again."

The clinic flourished, and Mildred saw the effect it had on the surrounding community. "A number of taxi drivers bringing people back and forth would say, 'Boy, if I ever get cancer, I'll be here—I've talked to too many people.' The airlines began to wake up to what was going on. The bus drivers knew what was going on. They'd say, 'We don't know anything about medicine, but we see these people getting well like this.' If they heard of somebody, they'd bring them."

Mildred recalled that Hoxsey had a photographic mind and never forgot a patient's face or name, or how much was owed, to the penny. "He was absolutely uncanny in dealing with people. He was left-handed, and it was so strange to see him with his left hand cutting out bandages, but it fit perfect when he got through with it. He had a sixth sense if somebody was sick. He seemed to have almost a psychic thing of what would work for this particular person."

Stepping through the looking glass, Mildred now found herself aligned with the very person she had demonized as a quack. She didn't know how to respond to the same charges now being made against her. Hoxsey invoked the words of his late father. "As far as being called a quack, he said, 'Oh, I've been called a lot worse things than that.' But through the years somebody would say something about it and I would be upset as could be, ranting and raving about it. And he'd say, 'Wait a minute, Millie. Remember one thing: Whatever they think, there's one thing they can't do, and that's put the cancers back on these little people that we have taken 'em off of.'"

Decidedly apolitical, Mildred settled into her role as the Gal Friday of the Hoxsey Cancer Clinic. "You couldn't buy a worker like Millie," observed Hoxsey's son. "She was totally dedicated as a nurse. Everyone loved her." She ran the staff of doctors with an iron hand. Hoxsey would soon trust her with mixing the medicine in the basement, while he increasingly attended to the new rash of trials and cancer politics barring his path to acceptance. "If only they would investigate and see the percentages he was getting well," Mildred remembered him complaining. "If they could prove he wasn't doing this, he'd close the doors himself. I don't know of anyone else that could have ever, ever fought the battles he did for as long a period of time as he did."

After an Oklahoma child was reputedly cured by Hoxsey, the boy's father approached Senator Elmer Thomas. Thomas served in the Oklahoma State Senate from its founding in 1907 to 1920 before ascending to Congress and the Senate. A populist and supporter of the farmer, he backed the New Deal and resisted corporations, and maintained close ties with his grassroots constituents. Yet he was ill prepared for the thorny medical politics about to draw his blood.[8]

When prosperous Oklahoma contractor Tom Chapman shared with Thomas the story of his child's recovery at the Dallas clinic, he also told the senator how the Oklahoma Medical Society rejected his personal offer to sponsor a Hoxsey test of twenty-five patients under its supervision. Following a similar rejection from the American Cancer Society, Chapman approached his senator in consternation.[9]

Senator Thomas visited a dozen Hoxsey patients from the Lawton area and listened to their fantastical cures. Hoxsey wired Senator Thomas to come to Dallas while fifteen osteopaths would be touring the clinic. When the lawmaker arrived on February 2, 1947, Hoxsey brought in 125 allegedly cured patients amid a mock "transcript of proceedings" in a quasi-legal setting. Hoxsey upped the ante with a bold challenge to treat 100 ex-servicemen free of charge. If he failed to cure 80 percent of them, he promised to close the clinic and stop treating cancer.[10] The senator personally interviewed over twenty-five of the cases, focusing on Texans and Oklahomans, and held a press conference with the Associated Press and United Press wire services as well as other reporters on hand for the show.[11]

"I would like to have as much of the record as I can get," Senator Thomas told the assemblage. "I shall present that then to the medical heads of the bureaus in Washington, and I shall ask them to take steps to make an investigation."[12] He went on to say, "I'm not a doctor and don't know cancer when I see it. However, I feel that I have gone into the matter sufficiently to justify asking medical authorities to investigate further. If this is a real cure for cancer, as evidenced here today, then it should at least be given a fair test and made available to the world. If not, the man must be exposed."[13]

Senator Thomas wrote to Surgeon General Thomas Parran, whose authority extended to the NCI, requesting an investigation. The negative reply came bundled with copies of anti-Hoxsey *JAMA* articles and the admonition that it would be imprudent to spend public funds on such a project.[14]

After four months of fruitless efforts, Thomas wrote to Hoxsey. "It seems that the medical fraternity is highly organized and that they have decided to crush you and your institution, if at all possible. I have had a few 'rounds' with the heads of all the medical organizations as well as the Public Health Service here in Washington, and it seems that the public officials are afraid that if they make any move, or say anything antagonistic to the wishes of the medical organization, they will be pounced upon and destroyed. In other words, the public officials seem to be afraid of their jobs and even of their lives."[15]

In the next election, the AMA lobbied heavily against Senator Thomas, and he was defeated, receding into private law practice. He continued to support the treatment, directing numerous patients to Dallas.[16]

Two members of the Oklahoma State Legislature attempted an investigation concurrent with Senator Thomas's efforts. Representative Charles Ozman and Senator Homer Paul introduced a resolution for a joint legislative investigation of Hoxsey. Senator Paul charged from the floor that Dr. Fishbein was personally blocking a test. The AMA vehemently opposed the resolution, which nevertheless passed. A joint committee of ten senators and representatives as well as three medical advisers traveled to Dallas on March 11, 1947. At the start of the hearings, four members were conspicuously absent. Representative Dr. A. E. Henning and the three medical advisers arrived late, because they had been secretly closeted with the Dallas County Medical Society.[17]

Hoxsey trotted out his cured patients and provided sixty case histories of internal cures. He waited several weeks in vain for a response, then made a couple of trips to Oklahoma City to track the matter. The final report from the legislature advised that Hoxsey's refusal to reveal the contents of the medicine "makes it impossible to evaluate its possible effect." It called the case histories "insufficient," and concluded that the medicines had no beneficial effect on cancer and were "toxic."[18]

Senator Paul objected furiously to the report. "We can never get any cooperation on this Dallas cure from the American Medical Association, and I might as well say the Oklahoma Medical Association too. These doctors who went with us down there stayed through the meeting with fear and trembling in their hearts. We tried to get them to help us make out a report but they wouldn't do it until they had contacted the AMA to find out what to do." Senator Paul noted that the stated reason the sixty case histories were deemed inadequate was that the physicians had not examined the patients firsthand. "I know why they say that," he retorted. "They're afraid of having their licenses revoked." Hoxsey claimed that some of the doctors nevertheless covertly "bootlegged" patients to him for many years afterward.[19]

Hoxsey complained bitterly that once again the AMA sandbagged an investigation by coercion and innuendo. "They all say they've been treated unfairly and that medicine won't pay attention to them," the AMA's Oliver Field told our camera about "quacks" in general and Hoxsey in particular. "It's true, because medicine does know that their products are worthless. If they had any merit they would be used. It's a rather unfair thing, really, to expect the AMA to waste its time with something that it knew was absolutely useless."[20]

Undaunted, Hoxsey kept building his clinic. In 1946 he hired Dr. Joseph Durkee, an osteopathic doctor who became the shining star of Hoxsey's staff for the next six years. A sophisticated physician dedicated to natural medicine, Dr. Durkee began to keep the proper records Hoxsey never had and initiated extensive research. Along with Mildred Nelson, he became a trusted associate just as the clinic started its rapid expansion. Hoxsey kept the formulas in a bank safe deposit box in case of his death, while Dr. Durkee swore to carry with him "till the bell rings."[21]

In 1946, Hoxsey moved from his overflowing facilities at Brian and Peak into 4507 Gaston Avenue, the former Spann Sanitarium. He said he bought it from Dr. Spann, but the word on the street was that he won it in a game of dominoes with an unlucky Realtor.[22] An inveterate gambler, Hoxsey also frequented the racetrack, and started holding weekly poker games at his house with prominent local citizens including Judges Al Templeton and Joe Brown. As the clinic grew and receipts rose, he made $10,000 donations to each of their campaigns.[23]

Hoxsey had further cause to celebrate. After years of bad luck wildcatting, the incorrigible gambler struck oil. "Dad and his partner dug thirteen dry holes," recalled his son. "Finally his partner ran out of money and had to bow out. Dad hit a gusher on number fourteen. He gave his partner 50 percent anyway." Hoxsey's daughter added, "Dad always loved a long shot. If it was a sure thing, he wasn't interested."

As Dallas TV newsman Jimmy Kerr observed, "I remember one time I was in Hoxsey's office, and he told this woman who was a cancer patient, 'If I can't cure you in three months—see that Cadillac out the window there?—I'll buy it for you.' As I recall, the woman died and never did get that Cadillac."[24] Hoxsey delighted in buying cars for his friends and donating an organ to his church.[25]

Now Hoxsey could finance his court battles with impunity and lavishly cultivate his Diamond Jim persona. "I don't have to do this kind of work," he bragged about his clinic. "I've got more oil wells than a lot of men who call themselves big producers. I have enough money to burn up a wet mule. So what do I need with money from cancer sufferers? Any man that would traffic on the sick, the dying, the limp, the lame and the blind caused from cancer is the worst scoundrel on earth."[26]

Witnessing Hoxsey's sharp ascent and sudden wealth, Dr. Fishbein once more dipped his pen in crimson ink for the *Journal* with a searing editorial entitled "Hoxsey—Cancer Charlatan." He invoked demons that

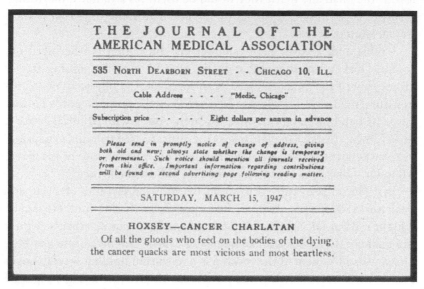

THE JOURNAL OF THE
AMERICAN MEDICAL ASSOCIATION

535 NORTH DEARBORN STREET - - CHICAGO 10, ILL.

Cable Address . . . . "Medic, Chicago"

Subscription price - - - - - Eight dollars per annum in advance

Please send in promptly notice of change of address, giving both old and new; always state whether the change is temporary or permanent. Such notice should mention all journals received from this office. Important information regarding contributions will be found on second advertising page following reading matter.

SATURDAY, MARCH 15, 1947

HOXSEY—CANCER CHARLATAN
Of all the ghouls who feed on the bodies of the dying, the cancer quacks are most vicious and most heartless.

Dr. Fishbein excoriates Hoxsey in the Journal.

would come back to haunt him. "Of all the ghouls who feed on the bodies of the dying, the cancer quacks are the most vicious and most heartless."[27] Fishbein then threw an irritable jab at Senator Thomas and the Oklahoma legislature. "Apparently Hoxsey has been successful in hoodwinking and deceiving eminent jurists and other important persons to the extent that they have given him tacit if not actual support. Apparently his performances and his success have caused him to believe that it is now possible for him to exploit widely his method of treating cancer and that he can get away with it! Harry Hoxsey has had more than twenty years in which to prove such virtues as might have existed in his method. Such proof has never been forthcoming. How long will the complacent authorities of such states as Texas continue to tolerate Harry M. Hoxsey?"

The *Journal* article provoked the Dallas County Medical Society into yet another sensational lawsuit, charging Hoxsey with illegally performing an operation on the breast of a patient who later died as a result of the treatment. The first trial ended in a hung jury, but the woman's husband brought him back into court on a $75,000 civil suit before Judge W. L. Thornton, who had earlier ordered an end to the medical society's harassment of the clinic. Charged with negligence for performing the operation and administering his worthless treatment, Hoxsey was acquitted on all charges. The verdict suggested that the woman's death was related to stopping the Hoxsey treatment and having more surgery and radium, resulting in death from cancer "treated in the manner approved by the AMA."[28] One local paper ran the mercurial headline, "Jury Rules Doctor Finds Cancer Cure."[29]

Addressing the jury after the verdict, Judge Thornton said, "I daresay you will never sit on a case of greater importance or one in which the public is greater concerned."[30] To explain the startling victory, some eyewitnesses said it was the best kept secret in Dallas that Judge Thornton's sister was on the Hoxsey tonic during the trial.[31] "I know most political people in Texas," Hoxsey boasted, "and can control any office."[32]

Aghast at Hoxsey's upset victory, Dr. Fishbein decided to lift the controversy outside medical journals to center stage in the public media. He jointly authored "Blood Money" in the *American Weekly*, the Sunday magazine supplement of the Hearst newspaper chain. The installment on cancer quackery was part of a lavish six-part "Medical Hucksters" series. It strutted Fishbein's purple prose and yellow journalism, lacerating his favorite target, Harry Hoxsey. The tirade smoldered against a lurid four-color painting of a frock-coated Dickensian figure. Wearing white

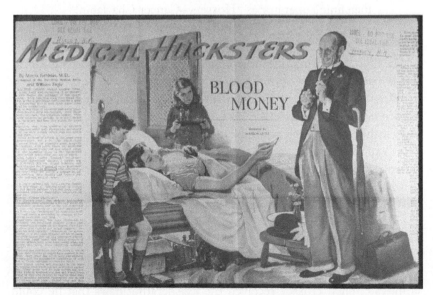

This time Dr. Fishbein went too far, resulting in the Hearst lawsuit defeat.

spats and a diamond stickpin, the nefarious charlatan was taking money from the limp outstretched fingers of a woman on her deathbed while her faithful children looked on with tragically false hope.[33]

"Blood Money" left little to the imagination.

> All the other wicked medical fakes, firing hope and darkening it to despair, pale beside the savagery of the cancer charlatans. They look like men, they speak like men, but in them, pervading them, resides a quality so malevolent that it sets them apart from others of the human race. Even in this time of scientific and social progress, they, brazen, dare the daylight. With Stone Age lures, they call. The credulous believe. They slay their patients as guiltily as if they knifed them in the heart, and they stay within the letter of the law.
>
> The fakers bank blood money. Among today's cancer "healers," the American Medical Association charges, a former coal miner is boldest, has the largest following and even has engaged the interest of some prominent men. He is Harry M. Hoxsey, who inherited a "cancer cure" from his father, a dabbler in veterinary medicine, faith healing and "cancer curing," who himself died of cancer. The American Medical Association condemns the clinic's operator as "Hoxsey—Cancer Charlatan!"

The article went on to recycle Fishbein's previous denunciations against Hoxsey for "hoodwinking eminent jurists" and failing to prove his methods in twenty years of opportunity.

Hoxsey was livid at being defamed and humiliated in the Sunday papers in living rooms across the land. He claimed the article hurt his business at the clinic, which now had 2,000 patients. Though he might have been expected to have developed a rather thick skin by this time, he moaned that the article deeply wounded his feelings. "Every time I read it, where they mention my father's death, or anything else, I have a very nervous lapse, and I have to stay home in bed."[34]

Hoxsey moved to sue the Voice of American Medicine as well as the Hearst newspaper chain and the article's coauthor William Engle. Seeking $1 million for libel and slander, he was taking on not only the nation's most powerful doctor, but also one of the country's formidable media empires.[35] Then Hoxsey received the exasperating news that he could legally sue only the Hearst newspapers, which had published the story in a Texas outlet. The elusive Dr. Fishbein remained inviolate, safely nested in Chicago outside the Texas court's jurisdiction. Fishbein boasted he had been sued for $35 million by quacks without paying a single dollar in damages.[36] Hoxsey didn't seem to stand a chance. Nevertheless, he was determined to lift Dr. Fishbein's "Iron Curtain" and speak truth to power for the world to hear.[37]

While Hoxsey burrowed in, Dr. Fishbein's invulnerability was cracking under mounting notoriety. As Milton Mayer wrote in *Harper's*,

> He had loved the AMA as he loved himself, and greater love had no man. Organized medicine might be a little seedy to its critics; it was always young and fair to Fishbein. The trouble was that under his loving care it was fading fast away. Physicians who were interested in something besides their fees resented their identification with his low-comedy routine. Worse, the routine wasn't stemming the rising tide of protest—in as well as out of the medical profession—against the inaccessibility of medical care to millions of Americans.
>
> Morris Fishbein not only had an American Dream: He was one. In his square-fingered hands he held the priestly power of one hundred forty thousand Men in White. He knew ten thousand practitioners by name, and among those ten thousand were what Fishbein calls "the men who count." The AMA's membership was a model of detail. "We keep track of everything and everybody," said the editor with a small smile. Fishbein did the Association's shoe-leather work. He did its lung-leather work, too, and that was his peculiar genius.
>
> Non-members of the AMA were the scum of Fishbein's earth. Medicine was, and still is, good for limitless exploitation, and when Fishbein set himself up in business it was virgin territory. Medicine needed a spokesman; it got a spieler. The conviction was spreading inside the profession that Morris Fishbein was bad medicine.[38]

Dr. Fishbein's sanctimonious image as guardian of the public health was losing its blush. Writers of the period such as Morris Bealle, a muckraking journalist whose pugnacious prose read more like sportswriting than medical journalism, documented the onset of the corporatization of medicine backing Fishbein's AMA. He chronicled the vertiginous rise of the pharmaceutical industry, whose revenues by the 1940s already exceeded $10 billion, an astronomical sum at the time. It was no secret that the drug industry had long been the advertising mainstay of the *Journal*. Bealle's widely read book *Medical Mussolini* flaunted scathing cartoons satirizing the nation's leading physician as a totalitarian medical dictator with cookie-cutter doctors goosestepping behind him.[39]

Even Warner Brothers movie studio had gotten skittish about escalating public protests over the good doctor's fraud-fighting films. When it was

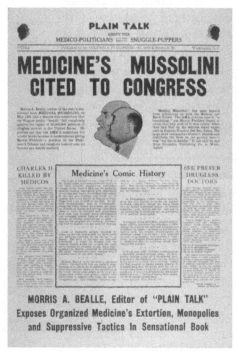

Dr. Fishbein comes under mounting attack, c. 1948.

about to start production on *Your Life Is in Their Hands*, an AMA-sanctioned anti-quackery short, the movie company sent Dr. Fishbein a nervous note. "We are getting hundreds of letters from people all over the country, mostly chiropractors, osteopaths and about seven other kinds of 'paths' and ten or twelve 'isms.' Strangely enough, we have yet to receive a letter from an M.D. encouraging us to go on with this idea, and I hope very soon they balance the scales of fan mail so that we will feel that we have at least a little moral support."[40] The project precipitated such an uproar that the studio abandoned the movie.

When Dr. Fishbein pointed proudly to the AMA Bureau of Investigation's quack files now numbering 300,000 names, he only fueled countercharges of targeting anyone who strayed from the narrow AMA line. His stand against national medical insurance, which he variously called "Communism," "Nazism," and "Socialism," was courting widespread public and professional insurrection.[41]

Dr. Fishbein's AMA was already under pressure from a stunning 1937 court conviction of "conspiracy" for restraint of trade and monopolistic practices, a verdict upheld by the Supreme Court in 1943.[42] The AMA was found guilty of trying to destroy an autonomous doctors' group applying cost-cutting health delivery and insurance in Washington, D.C. Subsequently Dr. Fishbein was muzzled by the national board from speaking publicly on sensitive issues, and his stock was trading low by the time Hoxsey came after him. As *Time* magazine put it, "Last week, as the AMA met in San Francisco, the Californians put on their rubber gloves and prepared at last for a Fishbeinectomy."[43]

Hoxsey was alert to Fishbein's travails and gambled that it was time for the tables to turn. As the trial grew closer, he sent word to Dr. Fishbein through Roy Topper of the *Chicago Herald-American* that he was "sure of winning the case, is a millionaire and does not want the money. He does want to get at the throat of Dr. Fishbein who he claims has constantly lambasted him through the medical association as a quack." Hoxsey offered to drop the charges if Topper could "get the good Doc to come down there to look into his clinic and see for himself." He ended with a challenge to "cure 85 percent of cancer cases or shut the doors forever."[44] Topper got no reply to the message.

As expectations of the epic courtroom confrontation ballooned, Hoxsey started to draw attention from other mainstream medical groups that had scrupulously ignored him for so long. When the influential American Cancer Society, a mainstay of the cancer establishment, sent its representative Pat McGrady Sr. to have a look, he found Hoxsey in a bold mood. "We got a real scientific place," the clinic operator told McGrady with typical bravado, and immediately cut to his obsession with Dr. Fishbein. "I got him this time. I'll have the whole bunch of them come down and testify. And then the world will know what kind of work I'm doing. I'm going to have my witnesses get up and tell how we cured them. What do you say to that!?"[45]

Amid what McGrady described as "country people of modest circumstances," he beheld "great and ugly tumors" mingled with the "stench of cancer." The American Cancer Society official got a garrulous tour from his host. "I know that Fishbein controls your society," Hoxsey taunted him. "You people act under orders from him. This to me is a hobby. I want to cure cancer everywhere. If it's taken up, I'll just wind up business here and get out my fishing rod and gun and spend the rest of my life on my ranch. I got more money than I could use in seventeen million years. If we got something, let's show it. If not, let's expose it. If they can show I'm not curing cancer, I'll close up and go to my ranch. I'll give this place to the blind."[46]

McGrady visited extensively with Dr. Durkee, who had brought rigorous record-keeping to the clinic for the first time and could now address specific concerns about the modalities and success rates for types of cancer. Like Hoxsey, Dr. Durkee claimed an 85 percent success rate for external cancers, and 25 percent for internal cases that had already received the limit of surgery and radiation. For breast cancer, he claimed a 50–60 percent cure. Hoxsey complained that his clinic was a "dumping ground" for the terminal patients of the Dallas doctors and he had to turn away 20 percent, the hopeless cases. He claimed an 80 percent cure rate for patients with internal cancer who had not received prior surgery and radiation.[47]

Dr. Durkee held an exalted position within the National Medical Society, an alternative to the AMA that was growing rapidly with the many M.D.'s, naturopaths, chiropractors, and osteopaths espousing natural medicine practices. Hoxsey's first physician, Dr. Bruce Miller, was now the president of the society, which openly opposed the AMA's monopoly on medical practices and challenged its politically incorrect position blocking national health insurance. As the wide popularity of the National Medical Society attested, the country's mood was less than sympathetic to the AMA's politics of unenlightened self-interest.[48]

While Hoxsey prepared for the trial, Mildred kept the clinic humming. "I'd go crazy," she recalled with a laugh. "I'd be so nervous, but he loved it. He had a ball the whole time. I'd lose ten pounds and Harry would just be putting 'em on, just as happy as he could be. 'We're going to win this! Then they'll have to listen to us!' It was happening every six months, so you'd think I'd get accustomed to it, but I never did. It was always ugly."

The Hearst trial commenced amid whizzing flashbulbs in a thronged courtroom on March 16, 1949, before Judge William Hawley Atwell. A highly respected jurist, Atwell was feared as a hanging judge, a tough, terse figure with forty-seven of his eighty years spent in district court. His customarily saturnine directive to attorneys was, "To the gist."[49]

The trial was a Who's Who of American medicine. It lasted for three days and two night sessions,

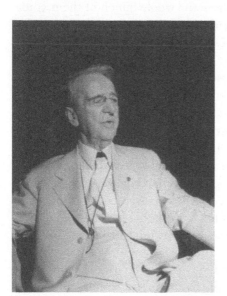

Judge William Hawley Atwell would rule twice in Hoxsey's favor in federal courts.

and produced eighty witnesses, eighty written exhibits, and a numbing two-thousand-page record.[50] Hoxsey sent out penny postcards to all his patients, who packed the courtroom.[51] The Hoxsey plaintiffs opened the proceedings with a scientific explanation of the Hoxsey treatment delivered by Dr. Durkee.

Finally, however, Dr. Fishbein was about to get the MacGuffin. Under court order, the defense compelled Hoxsey to reveal for the first time the ingredients of his three main remedies.[52] He said the internal tonic contained potassium iodide and herbs including cascara sagrada, buckthorn bark, prickly ash bark, red clover, stillingia, alfalfa, and honey drip syrup. He cited all the ingredients as being listed in the homeopathic materia medica, expounding on the philosophical differences between allopathic and homeopathic medicine. In contrast with the allopathic belief, the homeopathic school relied on supporting the body's own defenses to heal itself, which is what Dr. Durkee explained the tonic herbs served to do.[53]

When the Hoxsey team called its first patient witness to the stand, the defense objected strenuously with the rationale that laypeople are not qualified to testify to their own medical condition. "The patient endorsement," agreed Robert Heath of the Dallas County Medical Society, "is really not the best way to evaluate a medical treatment or procedure. Oftentimes these individuals are not knowledgeable enough in their own health to realize that they're not the ones to make the best assessment."[54]

While Hoxsey was intent on proving his cure, the defense was focused on excluding from the record any favorable testimony about the treatment. Their objection to Hoxsey's patient witnesses was ironic, however. In that era, anecdotal case histories were commonly used by the medical profession itself as proof of efficacy. It was not until after World War II that formal clinical testing to prove therapies began and not until the 1960s that it became widespread. By trying to strike the experiences of Hoxsey's patients from the record, organized medicine was employing an obvious double standard.[55]

Judge Atwell overruled the objection and admitted the heart-rending patient testimony. Fifty-seven reputed Hoxsey cures took the stand, replete with graphic before-and-after photographs of grotesque cancers come and gone. Hoxsey noted the fact that he never guaranteed to cure and lost many patients whose cases were too far gone. He further protested that he was not in it for the money, illustrated by the innumerable charity cases he took on.

Hoxsey lawyers Jimmy Martin and Herbert Hyde brought forth disturbing medical testimony on the limitations of conventional cancer treatment, including the fact that radium and X-ray cause cancer. Under cross-examination, several physician witnesses for the defense were forced to concede the dangers of medical radiation.

Jimmy "Trombone" Martin was one of Hoxsey's principal lawyers throughout the 1940s and 1950s. Nearly everyone in Texas has a nick-name, and Martin got his from playing trombone in the orchestra pit of 1920s silent movies such as *The Gish Girls* and *The Ten Commandments*. A former assistant U.S. attor-ney and district attorney, Martin was a skilled court-room tactician, as well as a committed amateur Shake-spearean actor with a Texas twang.[56]

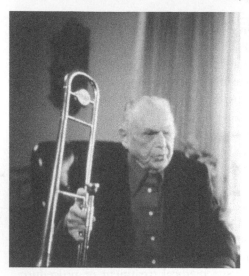

Lawyer Jimmy "Trombone" Martin recalls Hoxsey's court victories, 1986.

We filmed the alert octo-genarian in his Dallas home in 1986. "I'm kinda like Clarence Darrow claimed," Trombone suggested in a measured south-ern drawl, judiciously balanc-ing the scales of justice. "I never speculate on the guilt or innocence of my clients. I just deal with the facts. I heard many, many witnesses testify that they had cancer. Their doctor told them that they did, and said, 'Better get your affairs straight-ened out because you can't live long.' They say they then went to the Hoxsey Clinic and took the medicines and got well. So I asked those doctors, 'How do you explain that?' They'd say, 'He would have gotten well whether he done anything or not. Most cancers cure themselves.' That's what they'd claim. But they don't have any proof of it. All I know is what these witnesses say. They went to this Clinic and took that medi-cine and were cured. I think that's enough to support a verdict, and I'd get a verdict."

The Hearst defense codified Hoxsey's cases into three types of "phony" cures: those who never had cancer in the first place; those who were actu-ally cured by prior conventional treatment; and those who still had can-cer or died. As a last refuge, they suggested any seeming recovery could be the result of spontaneous remission. Unfortunately, Hoxsey's lawyers pointed out, instances of spontaneous remission in cancer are scarce, about one in 100,000 cases. Had all these oddities somehow found their way to

Dallas? If many of these patients never actually had cancer, they went on, there must be an awful lot of misdiagnosis going on. The compelling testimony and homespun honesty of the salt-of-the-earth Hoxsey patients laid bare the transparent maneuverings of the defense.

One witness drew particular publicity. Thomas E. Truman of Waco, Texas, a first cousin of then sitting President Harry Truman, testified he

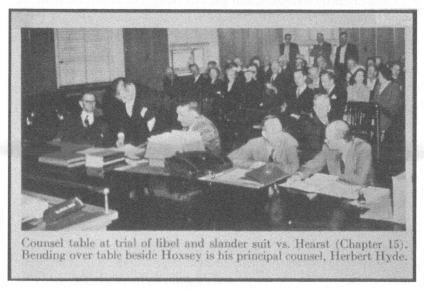

Counsel table at trial of libel and slander suit vs. Hearst (Chapter 15). Bending over table beside Hoxsey is his principal counsel, Herbert Hyde.

Hoxsey faces a Who's Who of American medicine in the Hearst-Fishbein trial.

was twice cured of skin cancers on his face.[57] Mildred Nelson later recalled, "After he was cured, he said, 'Well, I'm going up and talk to the President.' Which he did. But politics and medicine being entwined as they were, there wasn't anything he could do about it. But, the President said to Tom, if he gets in trouble, he knows what to do."[58]

The Hearst defense presented forceful testimony from prestigious cancer specialists that none of the ingredients of the Hoxsey tonic could possibly have any beneficial effect on cancer. They warned that one ingredient, potassium iodide, might actually accelerate the growth of cancer, although it was the only component of the tonic with any known medical use, as a treatment for syphilis.[59]

"They were adamant in their conviction," Jimmy Martin observed. "The doctors claimed that they already knew from their medical education that his remedies had no efficaciousness at all, no cure. They were just set in their ways and adamant in their beliefs, and they never would give it serious consideration. He had a big business. Naturally they were kind of jealous, and thought he was taking business away from them. They never did say that, but that was the motive behind their proceedings."[60]

On the stand, the Hearst lawyers slammed Dr. C. Von Hoover, Hoxsey's chemist, who had submitted extensive "scientific" data on the tonic. They revealed that he had operated under various *noms de plume* around Texas, lied about his medical degrees, and left a weaving trail of alcohol abuse, all of which was true. Once again, Hoxsey was easy to discredit.[61]

Then the Hearst lawyers played the joker in their deck, introducing a death certificate showing that Hoxsey's father died of cancer. They contended John C. Hoxsey had traveled to a St. Louis hospital specializing in cancer, and checked out several days later. They alleged that he had been diagnosed there with cancer of the jaw, and received radium but rejected surgery. All records, however, had been destroyed. The evidentiary death certificate they submitted lacked the signature of an attending doctor, but in its place the Hearst lawyers supplied a sworn affidavit from the widow of a local doctor. However, there was no biopsy, breaching steadfast AMA policy regarding pathological proof.[62]

Although prior *Journal* editorials had repeatedly made the same allegation about John C. Hoxsey's death from cancer, Hoxsey was blindsided by the death certificate.[63] He furiously condemned the document as a crude fake. His own lawyers had been searching for the document for many years since it seemingly disappeared from state and county records shortly after AMA investigators first came to Taylorville in 1925.[64] Hoxsey pointed out that the "fake" certificate had been filed in 1926, seven years after John C. Hoxsey's death, and listed the wrong place of burial. Hoxsey did admit accompanying his father to the Missouri cancer hospital, but said the diagnosis was erysipelas, not cancer, and that his father took no treatment there. Judge Atwell nevertheless permitted the death certificate into evidence.[65]

While Hoxsey was reeling from the shock, the Hearst lawyers riveted the courtroom by unwrapping their "surprise" witness. "I don't know how Harry knew, but he did," chuckled Mildred. "He knew what plane Fishbein was leaving Chicago on, what time he'd arrive in Dallas, and where he was staying." As Hoxsey's son recalled, "Like they used to say, they kept the motor running at Love Field [airport]. He was supposed to leave town right after testifying."[66] Nobody was supposed to know that Fishbein was in town, but Hoxsey knew. In fact, Dr. Fishbein had written a note to a Dallas doctor: "Strictly confidential, it is quite possible that I may spend some time in Dallas in case the Hoxsey law suits come to trial."[67] Somehow, somewhere, the news leaked.

Fishbein confidently took the stand before lunch. He said his purpose for writing "Blood Money" was "the exposé of fraudulent medicine for the protection of the public, and that has been routine practice, in accordance with the principles and ethics of the AMA ever since it was founded in 1847."[68]

Under cross-examination, Fishbein admitted never having administered the Hoxsey treatment, nor any cancer treatment, but defended his authority regarding the disease. An evasive witness, he ducked a protracted volley of tough questions. Dallas TV reporter Jimmy Kerr described his presence. "Fishbein was a real stickler on the stand. He was a fat little arrogant doctor, and made quite a poor impression."[69]

During the lunch recess, Hoxsey slapped Fishbein with a subpoena in the hallway. Now that the doctor had set foot in Texas, he was vulnerable to being served with legal action. He would have to stand trial against Hoxsey after all. The nation's top doctor was visibly unnerved when he took the stand again after lunch.[70]

The very same night the trial concluded, Judge Atwell rendered his oral opinion. Ever circumspect, he reached for the high ground. "I think we may enter this particularly interesting field through the newest part of the greatest Book we have. And, in that great Book, as you will recall,

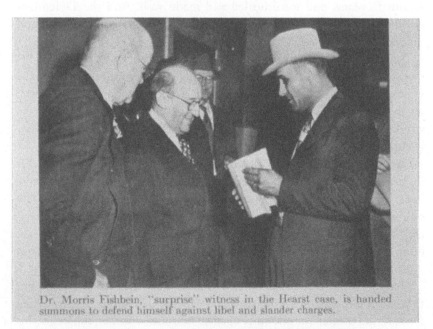

Dr. Morris Fishbein, "surprise" witness in the Hearst case, is handed summons to defend himself against libel and slander charges.

The "surprise" witness Dr. Fishbein is surprised by a subpoena.

there came a stranger. He began to heal the afflicted, and the people did not believe Him; and they came in great numbers to see for themselves. He finally made the big fisherman himself his convert, and his disciple; and one who really believed in Him could enter a pool, when it was being stirred, and be cured, if he had the faith. Not that the curative power was in the water, probably, but it was the faith. So also there were two men who had sat for much time at the doors of the temple. They were blind. They knew whether they were blind or not, and as worshippers would come to enter the temple, they would seek alms from them, and when Peter and John came that way, they sought alms from them. And Peter and John, being disciples of the Great Master, said, 'We have no gold and silver, but such as we have we give unto thee. Arise and go away, and see as you go.' And they arose and went away, and the people said they were not blind at all. 'You don't see at all, do you?' They said, 'All we know is, we were blind, and now we see.'

"That is where we enter here. There are fifty-seven people who have taken this stand, and said they had cancer. It must be granted they are not learned diagnosticians. Some of them have been treated for cancer before, by those who were learned in that particular profession, and their ailment was pronounced cancer. They testified they went out to the Plaintiff's place, and were healed and made well. And the Defendant wanted the Court to not permit that testimony. I could not do that, and that is in here, and must be considered."

Judge Atwell then adroitly sidestepped the snakepit of passing judgment on the efficacy of the Hoxsey remedies. "Pay your money and take your choice. Those who need a doctor, if you think one side is the best, go and get him. If you think the other side is the best, you certainly have a right to go and get him. This is a free country; that is what we stand for in America."

Judge Atwell ruled that "Blood Money" did indeed libel Hoxsey. Yet he mitigated the decision by declaring that it did but nominal damage because the "quick-brained and ingenious" Hoxsey thrived on the publicity and on "such controversies as he can provoke with the American Medical Association, and by making people believe that they are hounding him." The court pronounced that Dr. Fishbein had acted not out of malice, but from "a mistaken sense of public duty."

Judge Atwell further ruled that Hoxsey's father did die of cancer, but that the published statement was nevertheless libelous. He awarded Hoxsey one dollar for the libel against him and another dollar for his father, with court costs against the defendant.[71]

Hoxsey was ec-
static at piercing Dr.
Fishbein's armor at last,
though he drew more
blood than money. He
stood as the first man
labeled a quack to
defeat the AMA on
charges of libel and
slander, and claimed he
never wanted a money
judgment. For years
after, he relished his
court victory over Dr.
Fishbein, adding with
signature Hoxsey hy-

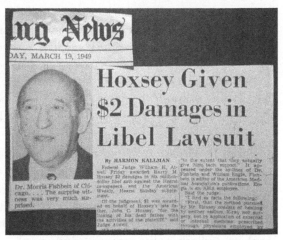

*Hoxsey becomes the first "quack" to beat the AMA
on libel and slander charges.*

perbole, "I have the money in my pocket to prove it." He failed to mention that it was all of two dollars.[72]

Hoxsey was, however, deeply angered by the defamation of his father's
name. He blasted Dr. Fishbein and the AMA as being the real "ghouls"
for digging up his daddy's grave—but he was going to get another chance
to clear his father's name.

For three years, Dr. Fishbein tried to evade the second trial with
Hoxsey. By this time, however, the prognosis was not good for the nation's
premier physician. Only months after his humiliating defeat to Hoxsey,
the AMA flatly dumped him. As Milton Mayer reported in *Harper's*,

> The American Medical Association withdrew its Seal of
> Approval from Morris Fishbein. Then, just so there
> would be no misunderstanding, it beat his head in, cut
> his heart out, and kicked him out into the street. "If the
> atmosphere becomes unpleasant," said the Voice of
> American Medicine, picking himself up and straighten-
> ing his necktie, "I'll quit in five minutes."
>
> Neither he nor anyone else had ever supposed that
> "Dr. AMA" might be fired. To be sure, the deed had to
> be done publicly; there was no other way to persuade
> the public that Fishbein wasn't American Medicine.
> Caesar was stabbed from all sides. Even the trustees of
> the AMA—for twenty-five years his echoes—felt they had

to be shut of him. He had outraged them, too. Presidents
of the Association had come and gone, nameless, face-
less, voiceless before the country. They were as impotent
inside the organization as outside. Fishbein held all the
strings, knew everything, was everywhere, did everything.
The taunt of "the American Fishbein Association" was a
telling one. The knives flashed like satin in the sun.[73]

When finally Hoxsey reeled Fishbein into court in 1952, it was as a private citizen stripped of the bulletproof mantle of organized medicine.
Rejecting eleventh-hour settlement offers, Hoxsey got his third day in
court before Judge W. L. Thornton. He pitted his down-home patients
against the blue-chip array of doctors from the Mayo Clinic, Johns
Hopkins, and other elite cancer institutions.[74]

Tellingly, the defense made no attempt to resubmit the death certificate
of Hoxsey's father. By now Hoxsey and Jimmy Martin had traveled to St.
Louis and Illinois and tracked down the records, including evidence that
the original document had disappeared mysteriously from the official files.
As Martin recalled, "We examined the hospital records and the books where
they had a notation of his father's entry and death. Somebody had tam-
pered with that. It had been written down what he had died from, but they
scratched it out. It was very obvious they inserted the word *cancer*."[75] The
AMA's alleged forgery was equaled, however, by records that Hoxsey himself later provided, which also appear to have been altered. Once again,
conflicting accounts evaporated in the swamp gas of medical politics.[76]

During the testimony of several external cases, Fishbein's lawyer
stopped the proceedings with a staggering admission. The Fishbein defense conceded that the *Hoxsey treatment does cure external cancer*. "We
don't deny that they cure cancer out there at the clinic," attorney Julian
C. Hyer reportedly said.[77] It was a confounding reversal after years of
condemning Hoxsey's "brutal pastes that eat into patient's blood vessels."
However, even this disorienting turnaround was not the most jarring rev-
elation to rock the courtroom.[78]

When Dr. Fishbein took the stand under cross-examination, the digging done by Hoxsey's lawyers paid off. Under oath, Dr. Fishbein made
shocking admissions. He failed anatomy in medical school. He never completed his internship before going to work at the *Journal*. He never practiced a day of medicine or treated a single patient in his entire career. Dr.
Fishbein was sweating profusely by the time he left the stand. His definition of a quack as "one who pretends to medical skill he does not possess"
now reflected back in an unseemly mirror.[79]

After three weeks of testimony, the jury resoundingly decided all issues in favor of Hoxsey. But this time it found that Dr. Fishbein had indeed "acted with malice in doing the things inquired about." Dr. Fishbein was no longer immune, the victim of his own journalistic nostrums.[80]

In his written opinion, Judge W. L. Thornton stated, "This is the second jury of twelve men that has found in my Court that the Hoxsey treatment cures cancer. I am of the firm opinion that Hoxsey has cured these people of cancer. And the fact that this jury has answered all questions proves that Hoxsey has been done a great injustice and that the articles and utterances by defendant Morris Fishbein were false, slanderous, and libelous."

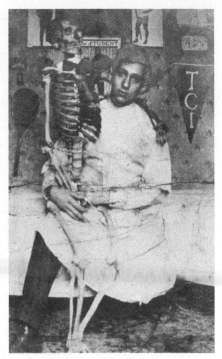

Dr. Fishbein failed anatomy in medical school.

Again the court found that Hoxsey sustained no actual damages from the article, and gave a monetary award of $1.05, with costs to the defendant. "I feel that this will give Hoxsey a clear vindication," decreed the judge, "which I know he was seeking far more than he was a money judgment."[81]

Hoxsey's lawyer Jimmy Martin, reflecting to our camera on Hoxsey's upset victory over the High Priest of Medicine, invoked one of his favorite Shakespeare lines in a throaty Texas accent: "Thrice is he armed who hath his quarrel just."[82]

In some unerring way, Harry Hoxsey and Dr. Morris Fishbein formed a perfectly perverse symmetry. Like Mozart and Salieri, their vexatious relationship magnificently served both their ends while ultimately scotching the professional exaltation they both so desperately yearned for.

Hoxsey did appear to have the "healing tetch" of his ancestry and seemed genuinely moved to be a doctor. It was an aspiration Fishbein was ideally positioned to deny him. Hoxsey had been treating cancer since the age of eight and must have seen more of the disease than almost any physician. If he didn't believe in his remedies, it is hard to see why he would have suffered through the endless arrests, continual prosecutions, incessant jeopardy, and caustic social humiliation. If Fishbein did privately believe that Hoxsey's remedies were authentically valuable, he must have lamented the cosmic curse of finding them in the hands of an ex–coal miner so unworthy of the gift.

As a doctor, Fishbein was a fraud. He exhibited no calling as a healer and never treated a patient. While Hoxsey was practicing medicine without a license, Dr. Fishbein was practicing license without medicine. His legitimate credentials were as a medical journalist and politician, at which he excelled, at least in his milieu. Nevertheless, like Hoxsey, he was unquestionably a true believer in his own brand of medicine.

Many people considered Hoxsey a liar, and he routinely played rather wide with the truth, though apparently not about his medical cases, the central issue. On the other hand, Dr. Fishbein became the master of the Big Lie: Tell a lie big enough, often enough, and people will believe it. His false accusations about Hoxsey's external remedies and subsequent reversal are ample evidence. That his own medical credentials were a fiction buried a painful hypocrisy under the inflammatory tenor he brought to eradicating medical fraud that would fracture medicine for the rest of the century.

Both men desperately wanted fame and recognition, and each got it in his own way. They became masters of publicity, and perfected their respective schtick. Tireless promoters, Hoxsey and Fishbein graced the same pages of *Time, Life,* and *Newsweek*.[83] Yet as a folk healer during an era that condemned herbal and natural medicine as "unscientific" and primitive, Hoxsey was tarred on his forced descent into a Hadean underworld of quackery. His unsavory alliances certainly welded him with spikes and fins that repelled many potential allies. The "recessive" ego that drove him to be a big shot also made an easy target. His rough coal-miner language and vulgar manners further skunked innumerable potential supporters.

The two figures also reflected a deep class division. Always the underdog, Hoxsey adopted a populist persona that seems to have been genuine. His financial largesse toward his patients was an authentic expression of his political bona fides. His explicit battle against the Medical Trust reflected his conscious opposition to the commercialization and monopolization of medicine by the interests of big business. When Hoxsey's father warned his boy about the High Priests of Medicine who would "fight you tooth and nail because you were taking money out of their pockets," the counsel prepared him for the cutting edge of the emerging business of medicine.

As an underdog not unlike Hoxsey, Fishbein was equally hungry for stature. Born in 1889 in St. Louis, Missouri, he was the son of a Jewish immigrant peddler who moved the family to unglamorous Indianapolis.[84] Yet Fishbein went on to gain the social prestige he craved, molting into an urbane sophisticate hobnobbing with the rich and famous.

Dr. Fishbein exemplified the politics of elitism. While Hoxsey was treating poor people for free, Fishbein was fiercely resisting the national medical insurance that would make health care affordable and accessible to millions of disenfranchised citizens. Simultaneously, under his direction doctors became the single richest profession in the country. While Hoxsey was letting black people in the front door in segregated Texas, Dr. Fishbein's AMA was a club of white men that entirely barred blacks (and women) from membership.[85]

The contrast was also very human. One associate reported having dinner with Hoxsey, who ordered the most expensive item on the menu, a filet mignon, and then reproached the waiter for failing to bring ketchup. Dr. Fishbein would surely have ordered just the right cabernet.

Dr. Fishbein once revealed to his daughter his motivation for becoming a doctor. As a high school senior, he was coming home from school one afternoon when he encountered a crowd gathering around a man injured in a street fight. A small child, little Morris was frustrated in his efforts to push his way through the crowd to behold the spectacle. "Soon an ambulance drove up," he recounted, "and a little fellow dressed in white with a black bag jumped out. Immediately the crowd parted for him. I decided to become a doctor."[86]

Morris Fishbein was intent on power. During his quarter-century building the most powerful trade group in the world, the crowd parted for him. At the same time, he used that crowd to block Hoxsey from the recognition he hungered for.

In the end, Hoxsey turned the tables on the High Priest of Medicine. It was a stubborn victory for the populist dark horse hobbled for so long by his medical nemesis. Although the financial penalty was minuscule, the grand symbolism was not lost on the AMA.

It was Hoxsey's spectacular victory over Dr. Fishbein that paradoxically ended up bringing down the house on both men. The AMA was increasingly tremulous over its potential liability in the escalating lawsuits resulting from Fishbein's zealous quarter-century of quack attacks and political escapades. The organization rid itself of him and then deliberately deflected Hoxsey into the fine-toothed gears of the federal government. The AMA retreated from its exposed position at the front lines, instead enlisting the Food and Drug Administration to carry on the fight. Hoxsey would now indeed get an investigation, but it would not be a scientific one.

Uncle Sam's Quackdown: "A Conspiracy Against the Health of the Nation"

Flushed with his monumental defeat of the AMA, Hoxsey was emboldened to knock a second time on the door of the National Cancer Institute in 1950. He submitted seventy-seven case histories, and this time he freely disclosed his formulas, since he'd been forced to reveal them anyway in the Hearst trial, though now he hinted they might not be the actual ingredients.[1]

Once more, the NCI deemed the records insufficient because many lacked biopsies. Hoxsey attempted to remedy the deficiencies, and again supplied the names and addresses of institutions and doctors in possession of the biopsies in question, which the NCI had the authority to obtain. Since Dr. Durkee's arrival four years earlier, Hoxsey was proud of the clinic's greatly improved record-keeping. "Until only recently we have not kept scientific records," Hoxsey complained to the NCI. "We could not. We have been hounded from state to state, hunted as if we were wild beasts, denied every avenue to proper cooperation and recognition."[2]

Hoxsey had reason to be optimistic because the NCI had proactively asked him to resubmit his case histories in 1947, two years after first rejecting them. "It would be appreciated if the same records could be sent to us again for a short time in order that we may permit a number of new people on our staff to review them," the letter stated. What the NCI was not telling him was that its solicitation was prompted by a request for the records by the FDA for the federal case it was preparing against him.[3]

When Hoxsey at last received a reply from NCI Director Dr. J. R. Heller, the terse letter indicated that the agency's review committee, the omnipotent National Advisory Cancer Council, still found the records inadequate. The NCI was therefore closing its consideration of the case. There would be no government investigation.[4]

Hoxsey appealed his predicament to Surgeon General Leonard Sheele, but the NCI's Dr. Gilcin Meadors had already covertly forwarded the new records to the Food and Drug Administration.[5] By November, Hoxsey was facing federal charges from the FDA for "false and misleading labeling" of his tonic shipped in interstate commerce.[6] The Surgeon General therefore responded, "In view particularly of this litigation, no further statement in this matter appears in order pending the outome of this litigation."[7]

The FDA, though legally unable to prevent Hoxsey from operating his clinic, was broadly empowered to stop the interstate shipment of mislabeled medicines. But the government had a problem. "The products are shipped virtually without claims," an internal FDA memo admitted.[8] Therefore the FDA directed the charge at two accompanying pamphlets mailed from the clinic that the government case cited as "labeling." The brochures portrayed case histories, described the treatment, and carried excerpts of patient testimonials from the hearings with Senator Thomas. Behind the scenes, government strategists had decided that an injunction was a less controversial move than another high-profile criminal trial.[9]

The federal dragnet got under way. Facing an unrelenting series of FDA legal actions, Hoxsey was about to be busier than a cat in a roomful of rocking chairs. Ironically, FDA chief Dr. Gordon Granger and his fraud fighters had by now concluded that "although originally he doubtless recognized himself as a charlatan, he has now apparently partly convinced himself."[10]

The FDA sent confiscated samples of Hoxsey's medicines to Dr. Clarence Cook Little at Bar Harbor Laboratory for animal testing. An accompanying letter reminded him of the negative results of his prior 1935 tests published in the AMA *Journal*. The agency withheld the list of ingredients, explicitly to "avoid any accusation that you were biased by reason of your knowledge of the composition of the preparations." The FDA simultaneously informed the supposedly unbiased researcher that its "purpose is to terminate, within the provisions of the Federal Food, Drug and Cosmetics Act, the illegal shipment of this material in interstate commerce." It didn't take reading between the lines to get to the gist.[11]

Since Dr. Little had already had an ugly run-in with Hoxsey, his objectivity was compromised in the first place. Nor had the eminent cancer research scientist's career been progressing smoothly of late. He had been unceremoniously relieved of his prestigious position at the American Cancer Society, and was now working as a tobacco lobbyist as well as medical researcher. Under the circumstances, it was highly unlikely that he was going to rock the FDA boat.[12]

The case came to trial in November 1950 in U.S. District Court in Texas before the same Judge William Atwell. This time the Hoxsey tonic was unavoidably on trial, and the government was set on using the courts to eliminate it from interstate commerce. Again Hoxsey faced off against the aristocracy of American medicine. The doctors testified that his medicine couldn't have any positive effect on cancer and might make it worse. Dr. Little's latest negative findings were introduced as evidence. Bolstered by the testimony of prominent physicians, the government asserted that the only acceptable methods for treating cancer were surgery and radiation.

Among those testifying was Dr. Gilcin Meadors, chief of Technical Services at the NCI, who reiterated the agency's position that Hoxsey's submissions to the agency did not meet its most basic criteria for a test. However, under cross-examination, Dr. Meadors acknowledged that the NCI could have obtained the biopsy records in question. But, he said, doing so would constitute an investigation, which it was not authorized to conduct without the prerequisite records. It was a textbook case of bureaucratic Catch-22.[13]

When Hoxsey called his panoply of cures to the stand, the prosecution once more objected vociferously to admitting the testimony of laypeople. Judge Atwell overruled yet again and permitted the witnesses to describe their dramatic recoveries.

The Hoxsey defense vigorously attacked the limitations of conventional cancer treatments. At the time, the American Cancer Society was claiming about a 32 percent five-year survival rate using conventional treatments. However, as local treatments, surgery and radiation treatments could be applied to only about 25 percent of cancers.[14]

After six days of testimony, Judge Atwell retired to his chambers, returning the next afternoon to an overflowing courtroom to present his "Findings of Fact and Conclusions of Law."[15] This time the judge did not sidestep passing judgment on the efficacy of Hoxsey's medicines. He found: "That the respondents' treatment is not injurious. Some it cures and some it does not cure, and some it relieves somewhat. That respondents do not guarantee to cure. That the percentage of efficient and beneficial treatments by respondents is reasonably comparable to the efficiency and success of surgery and radium, and without the physical suffering and dire consequences of radium, if improperly administered, and surgery if not successful in completely removing the entire malignant portion."

Judge Atwell declared Hoxsey not guilty of false and misleading labeling essentially because he did have a real cure, though not a cure-all. The bursting courtroom exploded in pandemonium, and the judge seemed to be banging a silent gavel amid the din of Hoxsey's triumph over the government. With his cure validated for a second time by a federal court, Hoxsey was on a roll.

The AMA *Journal* struck back instantly with an editorial headlined, "Comment on Court Opinion That Internal Cancer Can Be Cured by Medicine." The editorial decried the admission of the lay testimony of patients, and called for an immediate appeal.[16]

The government appeal took place without a jury in November 1951 in the Fifth U.S. Circuit Court in Fort Worth. It was handled as a kind of modern star chamber in which the case was based solely on the prior trial record. No witnesses or further testimony were allowed. In a rare judicial upset, the higher court reversed Judge Atwell, pointedly handing down its verdict in the middle of Hoxsey's second trial against Dr. Fishbein in the summer of 1952.

The court opinion adhered to the AMA's position that lay witnesses were unqualified to testify regarding cancer and entirely eliminated their testimony from consideration. The court found: "The evidence as a whole does not support the findings of the trial that 'some it cures, and some it does not cure, and some it relieves somewhat.'" The ruling stated, "Qualified experts recognize in the treatment of internal cancer only the methods of surgery, x-ray, radium and some of the radioactive byproducts of atomic bomb production. This is so even though the ghastly truth is that these methods frequently fail and are in many cases themselves unsatisfactory. But it is true, nevertheless, that with present enlightenment they are our sole defense against the scourge of cancer."[17]

The court ordered Judge Atwell to issue an injunction against Hoxsey's interstate shipment of medicines. Atwell was outraged, having been reversed but twice in his twenty-seven years on the bench.

The two sides met to work out a deal. Government lawyers provided Judge Atwell with a proposed injunction, while Hoxsey's lawyers countered with an alternative, agreeing to an injunction with explanatory language containing "appropriate qualifying statements revealing the conflict of medical opinion as to the truth of such representations."[18] In other words, there was a legitimate difference of medical viewpoints, to be represented as such on the labeling. The amended language fit the original purpose of Congress in chartering the FDA in full knowledge that such disagreements are common in medicine. The founding legislation's real intent was to prevent competing medical factions from skewing the law to their own ideological bias to the disadvantage of the public health.[19]

An irritated Judge Atwell considered the dilemma. "There is nothing to do here but to prepare a judgment," he said, "and the one submitted by the government is a little too broad. I think the other [Hoxsey] judgment covers it all right. You gentlemen have had a hard time agreeing, and I have signed this order, and if you don't like it, you know what you can do."[20] Judge Atwell signed the decree using Hoxsey's language allowing for a difference of medical opinion on the tonic.

In an unusual move skirting normal judicial boundaries, the higher court retaliated with a writ of mandamus flatly commanding Judge Atwell to sign the government's more restrictive decree.[21] The court said it had "ruled that claims that the Hoxsey medicines will cure cancer are false in fact, thus leaving no room for asserted differences of medical opinion."[22] Atwell still resisted and was severely castigated by the higher court. Left with no other choice, a livid Judge Atwell signed the government injunction. Hoxsey's appeal was denied.[23] NCI Director Dr. J. R. Heller sent a prompt thank-you letter to the commissioner of the FDA.[24]

The FDA was now deliberately using the courts to settle medical questions. It politicized a legitimate difference of medical opinion, a disagreement whose rightful resolution is in a laboratory or clinic. The act also initiated a crucial stratagem that the FDA would continue to employ up to the present day of using labeling laws to restrict or ban treatments not conforming to orthodox views. The ruling amounted to a gag order on one of the loudest mouths around.

Hoxsey was forced to jettison his literature and stop shipping medicines to the ten states where doctors were administering the Hoxsey treatment.[25] All patients would now be compelled to travel to Dallas to get the remedies by prescription from the clinic. But when the FDA sent agents to Dallas to inspect the clinic in 1954, they found Hoxsey unrepentant. "We were invited quite graciously into his office," wrote Inspector Prillmayer. "We were notified by Hoxsey that he had nothing to hide and wished to cooperate with us in every way. Hoxsey was quite erratic in his conversation as he would divert the subject time and again about his recent oil strikes that were bringing him in millions. Hoxsey began his usual story of how he welcomed any investigation. Hoxsey launched into quite an animated spiel of how he was helping mankind, how the profit motive had never entered into his mind, how he had cured thousands of cancer cases given up as hopeless by the medical practitioners, how he intended to do so in the face of all the difficulties until 'they lay me out on a slab or bring in the militia,' as that is the only way he could be prevented from operating."[26]

Hoxsey bragged to the FDA agents about his latest suitors. Dictator Juan Peron of Argentina as well as the Mexican government were interested in his treatment. Mexican doctors from the National College of Medicine in Mexico City had spent time at the clinic, and an article in a mainstream Mexican newspaper had caused an avalanche of interest south of the border resulting in its use at the Mexican Army Hospital and at three clinics under the Mexican Surgeon General.[27] When he completed pending arrangements to transfer the clinic into a nonprofit foundation, he boasted, the country's richest man, H. L. Hunt, would be joining his board of directors along with other powerful people including Tom Braniff, founder of Braniff airlines. The FDA closed its report on the meeting by saying Hoxsey "would defy any attempt made to prevent the distribution of the treatment in spite of the injunction. With his added wealth and influence, his egomania has become more uncontrollable than before, if possible."[28]

Boosted by the federal court victory, the AMA published a pointed editorial suggesting that Texas authorities now needed to take care of business in their own backyard.[29] But while organized medicine moved to start tightening the noose around Dallas, Harry Hoxsey was fastening a diamond pin on his necktie and mapping his expansion plans.

Hoxsey continued implacably pursuing every available avenue for an investigation, and found several takers. In 1951, Senator William Langer of North Dakota visited the Dallas clinic and took patient testimony. After studying the FDA trial records, Langer introduced two resolutions in the U.S. Senate, the first calling for an investigation of Hoxsey and the second for a broader investigation of any clinic or hospital in existence for ten years treating pathologically proven cases of cancer. Both resolutions were stifled in committee.[30]

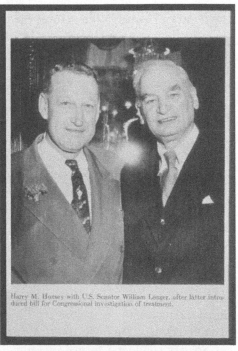

Harry M. Hoxsey with U.S. Senator William Langer, after latter introduced bill for Congressional investigation of treatment.

"The medical fraternity is out to get you," Senator Langer told Hoxsey after Congress rejected his bills for an investigation.

Another investigation was in the works, too. Dr. L. T. Coggeshall, a highly respected Chicago doctor and dean of the Division of Biological Sciences of the University of Chicago Medical School, had been contacted by a local Hoxsey patient seeking his attention about the alleged cure of his son. Dr. Coggeshall in turn called the American Cancer Society, which encouraged him to go to Dallas and report back. Dr. Coggeshall agreed conditionally if Dr. Andrew C. Ivy would accompany him because of his "prominence in the national cancer program."[31]

As vice president of the University of Illinois and head of its medical school, the largest in the country, Dr. Ivy was among the most venerated cancer researchers in the nation. He was former executive director of the elite National Advisory Cancer Council at the NCI and former board member of the American Cancer Society. The organizer of the Naval Medical Research Institute, he had presided on behalf of the United States at the Nuremberg trials on the question of medical ethics, at the recommendation of the AMA itself.

As a committed cancer man, Dr. Ivy agreed to join Dr. Coggeshall to look over the clinic.[32] Dr. Coggeshall also wanted Dr. Ivy along because he was trying to immunize himself against the contagious controversy surrounding Hoxsey. When Oliver Field, director of the AMA Bureau of Investigation, first caught wind in 1948 that the esteemed Chicago doctor was considering an investigation of the Hoxsey Clinic, he wrote, "I advised him that he would get himself in trouble."[33] Dr. Coggeshall understood that venturing to Dallas was a perilous act, even for the top figures in medicine.

Drs. Ivy and Coggeshall arrived at the clinic on February 10, 1949, and met with Dr. Durkee, who explained the remedies and freely discussed their constituents. He conceded that poor or no records had been kept until his arrival, and their investigation of various cases left them unimpressed. "We told Mr. Hoxsey that we had seen nothing which convinced us that any internal cancers or metastases had been cured," Dr. Ivy later wrote, "and that we were not particularly interested in the results of treatment of skin cancers with escharotics, because we knew that they worked in some cases and that by radiology and surgery 95 percent could be cured." Dr. Ivy concluded that Hoxsey's reputed cures were either cases of wrong diagnosis or the result of a delayed reaction to conventional treatment.[34]

Nevertheless, Dr. Ivy strongly recommended that the American Cancer Society conduct a formal investigation. He observed that Hoxsey's "business quite obviously improves on high-grade opposition, since it seems to cause some patients and some prominent lay persons to believe that Mr. Hoxsey is being persecuted. It would be an interesting experience to try a new approach to test and prove early the truth or falsity of an alleged cancer cure and in this way attempt to prevent the exploitation of the cancer patient."[35] Dr. Coggeshall concurred. "There is absolutely no way to determine whether he has anything of merit other than by a carefully supervised study in his clinic. In my opinion, Mr. Hoxsey is a very clever man. He seemed genuinely interested in having his method of treatment evaluated by experts, and was completely willing to show the records of every case, including failures."[36] As part of the terms, Dr. Ivy obtained Hoxsey's firm agreement not to advertise any test that might be arranged.

This strong prompting by the eminent doctors did not lead to an investigation, but Dr. Ivy soon found himself embroiled in his own controversy. If he was suspicious of Hoxsey's tall tales of persecution, he was about to get a crash course in medical politics that would derail his career and test his faith in the medical institutions he dearly loved and himself helped build.

Dr. Ivy had been fascinated with cancer since his earliest medical education, first developing a theory about it as a graduate student in 1917 at the University of Chicago. He suspected that decreased resistance or a deficiency of some sort in the body led to the disease's development. He concentrated his research on a natural substance in the liver that might inhibit the growth of the disease. He was approached in 1950 by another scientist working along similar lines. Dr. Stefan Durovic, a Yugoslavian researcher who had emigrated to Argentina, conducted experiments there with government support, isolating an immune-boosting natural substance. Dr. Durovic injected horses with actinomyces, the organism that causes lumpy jaw, a cancerlike disease in animals, in hopes of stimulating their bodies to produce an immune reaction. He then extracted what he believed was the immune-boosting factor from their blood.[37]

Dr. Ivy worked quietly with Dr. Durovic at the University of Illinois medical school and in private Chicago hospitals for eighteen months, testing what they called Krebiozen. On March 26, 1951, Dr. Ivy held a press conference at the Drake Hotel before one hundred scientists, physicians, and researchers in Chicago to discuss Krebiozen as a possible agent for a new cancer drug. He related his observations of twenty-two cancer cases that were terminal when Krebiozen was given to them. Fourteen were still alive, and two no longer had any evidence of the disease. Always fastidiously conservative in his projections, he was adamant in making no claims for the drug.

"It is my opinion," Dr. Ivy wrote in a press release inviting the select medical group to review his data, "that the substance merits a thorough clinical study and evaluation since I believe it shows much promise in the management of the cancer patient."[38] To the electrified gathering, he circumspectly stated, "Krebiozen is not to be viewed as a final goal in the chemotherapy of cancer, but I believe it is an important step in that direction. I could hardly believe my eyes when measurements showed an effect on humans sometimes in twenty-four hours."[39]

Dr. Ivy was immediately discredited by the medical profession. He was suspended by the Chicago Medical Society for three months for using a "worthless drug" for cancer. He was stripped of his post as vice president of the University of Illinois, and voluntarily resigned from the American Medical Association. Incredulous, he found himself cast down from the acme of his profession. Yet there were other, more disturbing circumstances besides outright intellectual suppression, and like Hoxsey, Dr. Ivy now charged a conspiracy.

Illinois legislators in 1953 appointed a commission to determine whether there was a conspiracy against Krebiozen and its sponsors. The target of the most alarming accusations was Dr. J. J. Moore, treasurer of the AMA and a prominent Chicago pathologist. Dr. Durovic and Dr. Ivy alleged that Dr. Moore approached them with an offer for $2.5 million for the drug's distribution rights for two businessmen, associates of Dr. Moore. Dr. Ivy said he advised Dr. Moore that he first needed to complete his testing. If Krebiozen proved effective, Dr. Ivy told him, he then planned to offer the drug nonexclusively in commerce to prevent price gouging. He contended that his refusal resulted in Dr. Moore's threat to destroy Krebiozen and ruin both him and Dr. Durovic through his influence with the AMA and the university.[40]

An article derogatory to Krebiozen quickly surfaced in the AMA *Journal*, asserting that ninety-eight of the one hundred Krebiozen patients had died.[41] Its claim was quickly repudiated when ten patients termed dead or dying wrote letters to the Krebiozen Investigating Committee certifying they were alive and well.[42] Dr. Ivy charged that his records had been deliberately falsified.

Senator Paul Douglas of Illinois headed up the legislative inquiry, which found that FDA reports attacking Krebiozen were "based on unfair, inaccurate, and prejudiced statements." At a press conference, Senator Douglas commented, "Medical people are highly conservative, and the pundits in medicine—the medical politicians—do not like innovation. There are a lot of other circumstances in this particular Krebiozen case which may implicate the American Medical Association itself, but I shall not mention them. I'll merely say that this is too important a subject to be left purely to medical politicians."[43]

The similarity of Dr. Ivy's charges to those of Hoxsey was unmistakable: a failed attempt by an AMA official to buy his formulas, followed by black-balling and a refusal to test the therapy. Where Hoxsey fit the image of a quack, Dr. Ivy surely did not. By echoing the allegations of conspiracy and dirty deals, Dr. Ivy gave weight to Hoxsey's seemingly incredible story.

"After Dr. Ivy got started with Krebiozen," recalled Mildred Nelson, "they almost buried him. He called Harry. I was in the office when this call for outside help came in. 'What do you do? [Dr. Ivy asked.] How can I get out of this so I can go on?' As soon as Harry gets off the phone, he said, 'Millie, make me a reservation for Chicago. I've got to help Dr. Ivy.' And Harry flies to Chicago to help him."[44]

Thousands of patients anxiously sought to obtain Krebiozen while thousands of doctors prescribed it as an "investigational new drug." Dr. Ivy waged a bitter battle for the next thirteen years against the AMA and FDA to get a fair test and combat criminal charges brought against him, Dr. Durovic, and other associates.

Hoxsey and Dr. Ivy, however, were far from the only ones to land on organized medicine's "index" for their pursuit of alternative approaches to cancer. Serial condemnation over the course of the century left a trail of shattered careers and untested therapies. Prominent among them was William Frederick Koch, M.D., Ph.D., a reputable laboratory scientist and professor of physiology at the Detroit College of Medicine. Dr. Koch built on the seminal discovery of Dr. Otto Warburg in the early twenti-eth century that cancer arises as an anaerobic condition in the absence or deficiency of oxygen. He believed that the chemistry of natural immunity in the body is able to destroy the toxicity of germs, and hypothesized that the body's oxidation mechanism is the key to burning off an excess of poisons. He devised two injectible drugs, Glyoxilide and Benzoquinone, synthetic antitoxins that, he conjectured, act as oxidation catalysts to help the body both build cell tissues and burn up waste products. He also be-lieved strongly in the importance of diet and intestinal cleansing. When another practitioner applied his work to human patients, the drugs showed impressive results not only in cancer but also in tuberculosis and other diseases.[45]

Dr. Koch's work was highly praised in an AMA *Journal* editorial in 1913, and then condemned in 1919 after he claimed to treat eight cancer cases successfully, while simultaneously criticizing surgery and radiation. An ill-fated test ensued before the Wayne County Cancer Committee, composed of surgeons and radiologists, and was terminated acrimoniously before its completion. Dr. Cramp of the AMA Propaganda Department called for an immediate end to any such efforts.[46]

Dr. Koch also maintained that he was approached by business interests closely allied with organized medicine with an offer for the rights to his drugs. Refusing, he was demonized, and doctors associating with him were expelled from medical societies or lost their licenses. Dr. A. R. Mitchell, chairman of the Board of Trustees of the AMA and a supporter of Dr. Koch, advised the researcher against any further publication in order to safeguard his formulas and methods.[47]

Because Dr. Koch had never bothered to conduct the requisite animal studies with his drugs, the remedies were distributed widely through Canadian stockmen and cattlemen in British Columbia to obtain documentation. Cattlemen in Brazil also took a strong interest. As pragmatic ranchers seeking tangible results, they were impervious to medical ideology. For over twenty years, the veterinary community carried out dramatic cures with the Koch remedies on animals with cancer, tumors, and other afflictions, keeping careful data. Doctors across the United States continued to use the preparations on people, and also claimed impressive results in a broad array of diseases. Tests in Mexico and Brazil included success with leprosy and dementia.[48]

While conducting experiments with human beings in Brazil in 1941, Koch alleged, he angered a representative of Parke-Davis pharmaceutical company with his successes. Dr. Koch shortly received a communication from the FDA regarding problems with his labeling. He cut short his trip and voluntarily returned to the United States to clear the matter up. He was immediately arrested upon his arrival in Miami and jailed in April 1942 on FDA charges of false labeling, a case for which Dr. Fishbein took personal credit.[49] The FDA's Wallace Janssen reflected the government's view when he quoted a federal prosecutor on the Koch remedies, which were highly diluted and contained only fractional amounts of the "active" ingredients: "This dilution was like dumping a cocktail into the Detroit River and expecting to get a kick from the water flowing over Niagara Falls."[50]

After five months, the jury set Dr. Koch free. In 1948, he faced new charges, ending in a mistrial. During the trials he was supported actively by William Merrill Dow and Dr. Charles Hale, founders of Dow Chemical Company, who provided a thousand-page scientific testimony documenting the success of the Koch cancer remedy. Dr. Hale called Dr. Koch a "modern Pasteur."[51]

Government attorneys dropped the charges in 1948 amid a national controversy in which Dr. Koch, a devout Christian, had now gained widespread public support as well as the representation of the Christian Medical Research League, a large national nonprofit foundation to which Koch donated his formulas.[52] Senator William Langer supported him in Congress, to no avail.[53] Amid rumors of another aggressive government case in the works, Dr. Koch expatriated to Brazil in disgust. A permanent FDA injunction against the Koch remedies was granted in 1950, and a succession of doctors among the estimated 2,000 daring to use the therapy lost their licenses. Years later, Nobel laureate Dr. Albert Szent-Györgyi, who developed the free-radical theory of cancer with Dr. Linus Pauling, credited Dr. Koch as a seminal precursor of his work.[54]

Mildred Nelson visited Dr. Koch in Brazil in the early 1960s, and recalled being stumped by his biochemical erudition. By the early 1950s, the Hoxsey clinic accommodated patients who requested both the Koch remedies and Krebiozen.[55]

Meanwhile, outside Boston in Medford, Massachusetts, Dr. Robert E. Lincoln was making another discovery. An obscure general practitioner and research scientist, he had conducted research at Harvard's Laboratory of Applied Physics on supersonic energy in medicine, and invented a celebrated mechanical heart pump during his tenure there. When Dr. Lincoln took an interest in studying the germ *Staphylococcus aureus*, that causes infection, he fell across two strains of a virus that, he believed, attacked and killed the harmful bacterium. He started administering these two "bacteriophages" (bacteria-killers) to treat sinusitis and grippe and got "apparent cures" in an astounding 95 percent of cases. Serendipitously he noticed that the treatment seemed to clear up a variety of secondary conditions, including arthritis, angina, deafness, and blindness. Also among these was cancer, and his clinic was soon overrun with desperate cancer patients.[56]

A modest man, Dr. Lincoln said there was nothing new about his method except the therapy itself. He sought to destroy bacterial hosts for viruses in the body by using a virus developed to extreme potency. The application itself was simple: patients sat in a chair and breathed the strains through a tube. Dr. Lincoln charged from one dollar to five dollars, and accepted charity cases free. He set up the nonprofit Lincoln Foundation to dispense the therapy. It should have been great news, but his woes had already begun several years earlier.

The AMA *Journal* first rejected Dr. Lincoln's 1946 paper detailing clinical case histories. When he resubmitted it in 1948 to *The New England Journal of Medicine*, it was declined for "lack of space," although there was room in the publication for an article on "The Vitamin D Content of Mare's Milk." Dr. Lincoln invited a research committee from a large Boston hospital to study his work, and was snubbed. In 1949 he contacted the Massachusetts Medical Society requesting meetings, which were scheduled and then indefinitely postponed. The society meanwhile sent out derogatory letters in response to queries about the treatment. By 1949, the president of the AMA flatly refused to assist Dr. Lincoln in his efforts to publish.

Among Dr. Lincoln's cancer patients was Charles Tobey Jr., who experienced a complete remission. The patient's father was Senator Charles Tobey Sr. of New Hampshire, who became impatient over the apparent neglect of Dr. Lincoln's work. The legislator used his clout to demand a formal investigation by the Veterans Administration. A month later the Veterans Administration responded that the National Research Council (NRC), the decision-making body at the NCI, opposed such a test. The senator went directly to the NRC and demanded an investigation. The NRC deflected it back to the Massachusetts Medical Society. Despite an angry meeting in the senator's office, the federal agency insisted on deferring the important investigation to the middling state society.[57]

The Massachusetts Medical Society set about its "investigation" by sending doctors to interview Lincoln patients on the back porch of the physician's home. Society representatives made another visit a month later and promised a hospital study, which never materialized. Subsequently, the supply of Lincoln antibiotics was severed by the labs of Boston University Medical School, where they were manufactured. Six weeks later, when the supply resumed, Dr. Lincoln discovered suspiciously that his original strain was not present in the drugs. He had wisely retained cultures of the strains, and was able to reconstruct the medicines.

In March 1952, after eight months of study, the Massachusetts Medical Society released its report rejecting the Lincoln method. It attributed the cure of Charles Tobey Jr. to prior surgery and radiation. It stated that "equally beneficial results from X-ray and surgical treatment in this disease have been reported on patients who did not receive Dr. Lincoln's treatment."[58] The medical society exclusively advocated surgery and radiation as the treatments "of choice." It peremptorily dismissed Dr. Lincoln's bacteriophage.

After Dr. Lincoln criticized "the high degree of stupidity that has been maintained by this segment of the American Medical Association," the medical society demanded his resignation. After he refused, he was expelled in April 1952.[59]

Senator Tobey, enraged over the seeming suppression of Dr. Lincoln's work, brought the matter before the Senate, where the high-visibility debacle was generating sweaty pressure. Now familiar with the larger pattern of repression around unconventional cancer treatments, he opted for drastic action.[60]

As head of the Senate Interstate and Foreign Commerce Committee, Senator Tobey secretly hired a young Justice Department lawyer, Benedict FitzGerald, to conduct a covert investigation into the possible suppression of unconventional cancer therapies. A graduate of Boston University Law School, FitzGerald had a background as a tough investigator, trying federal malpractice cases both for and against doctors. Having also served in 1950 as chief counsel to the chairman of the House Committee to investigate lobbying activities, he knew that the AMA was the biggest lobby in the nation's capital. Well schooled in the inner workings of hardball Washington politics, FitzGerald began scouring the country, interviewing Dr. Lincoln, Dr. Ivy, Harry Hoxsey, and a half-dozen other similar individuals. He also peered into the recesses of organized medicine's own war on cancer, but cautiously avoided letting the AMA know what he was up to.[61]

FitzGerald's operative passage through the underbelly of cancer politics led him to produce an explosive exposé for the Senate Committee, titled *A Conspiracy Against the Health of the American People*.[62] It focused in depth on Harry Hoxsey and Dr. Andrew C. Ivy, while naming a raft of other cancer treatments systematically sunk by organized medicine without fair investigation. FitzGerald affirmed Hoxsey's court victories and noted Judge Atwell's decisions that the Hoxsey treatments were in some ways "superior to X-ray, radium, and surgery and do have therapeutic merit." Specifying Hoxsey patient witnesses by name and address, he stated, "It has been determined by pathology, in a great many instances by laboratories wholly disconnected from the Hoxsey Cancer Clinic, that they were suffering from different types of cancer, both internal and external, and following treatment they testified they were cured." After scrupulous detective work, FitzGerald confirmed the validity of Hoxsey's records of reputed cures.

FitzGerald then examined Hoxsey's failed attempts at a federal investigation. "No such investigation was made. In fact, every effort was made to avoid and evade the investigation by the Surgeon General's office. The record will reveal that this clinic did furnish sixty-two complete case histories, including pathology, names of hospitals, physicians, etc. in 1945. Again in June, 1950, seventy-seven case histories, which included the names of the patients, pathological reports in many instances, and in the absence thereof, the names of the pathologists, hospitals and physicians who had treated these patients before being treated at the Hoxsey Cancer Clinic. The Council of the National Cancer Institute, without investigation, in October 1950, refused to order an investigation. The record in the Federal Court discloses that this agency of the Federal Government took sides and sought in every way to hinder, suppress and restrict this institution in their treatment of cancer."

Turning his attention to the case of Dr. Ivy, FitzGerald wrote, "There is reason to believe that the AMA has been hasty, capricious, arbitrary and outright dishonest, and the alleged machinations of Dr. J. J. Moore (for the past ten years treasurer of the AMA) could involve the AMA in an interstate conspiracy of alarming proportions.

"It is my profound conviction," FitzGerald continued, "that Krebiozen is one of the most promising materials yet isolated for the management of cancer. It is biologically active. This substance and the theory behind it deserve the most full and complete scientific study. Dr. Andrew C. Ivy is absolutely honest intellectually, scientifically, and in every other way. Moreover, he appears to be one of the most competent and unbiased cancer experts that I have ever come in contact with. Behind all this is the weirdest conglomeration of corrupt motives, intrigue, selfishness, jealousy, obstruction and conspiracy I have ever seen." FitzGerald also saw the Lincoln treatment fitting the same ominous pattern of obstruction.

The government investigator summarized his report by concluding, "My investigation to date should convince this Committee that a conspiracy does exist to stop the free flow and use of drugs in interstate commerce which allegedly have therapeutic value. Public and private funds have been thrown around like confetti at a country fair to close up and destroy clinics, hospitals and scientific research laboratories which do not conform to the viewpoint of medical associations."

FitzGerald further directed severe criticism at the limitations of surgery, X-ray, and radium. He cited the radical difference of opinion within the medical profession itself as to both their utility and harm. He demanded an investigation into the abuse of the AMA's Seal of Acceptance, and duly noted the organization's previous conviction on conspiracy charges. His far-reaching probe turned up a morass of corrupt medical politics infiltrating the highest offices in the land. FitzGerald's conclusion of a wide-ranging conspiracy implicating the AMA, FDA, NCI, and Surgeon General affirmed the allegations of Hoxsey, Dr. Ivy, and the others.

The report lit a fuse that was about to explode in the halls of Congress when Senator Tobey died suddenly of a heart ailment. Taking over the Interstate Commerce Committee was Ohio Senator John Bricker, dubbed "Mr. AMA" in the Senate. Because the report's existence had been kept entirely secret, Bricker only learned of it directly from FitzGerald. The investigator alleged that Senator Bricker told him to file just a brief report and offered him a good job if he would lie low and not talk to the press. FitzGerald submitted the report nonetheless, which was inserted into the Congressional Record in August 1953. Senator Bricker immediately decreed the report not within the jurisdiction of his committee and snuffed it. Two weeks later, FitzGerald was relieved of his job at the Justice Department, while Senator Bricker was guest speaker at the next AMA convention.[63]

Oliver Field, director of the AMA Bureau of Investigation, penned an angry letter to an Oregon doctor about FitzGerald's tactics. "It is obvious," complained the AMA official, who never visited the Hoxsey clinic, "that Mr. FitzGerald engaged in the rather peculiar stunt of having investigated the American Medical Association without coming anywhere near it."[64]

With support from Charles Tobey Jr., FitzGerald appealed to Senator William Langer, head of the Senate Judiciary Committee, whose two earlier Resolutions to the Senate to investigate Hoxsey and other alternative cancer treatments had already been smothered in committee. In a lengthy letter to Senator Langer, FitzGerald reiterated his findings of a "giant conspiracy," and revisited allegations Hoxsey had long ago made. "From the evidence I have gathered," FitzGerald wrote, "it appears that as early as 1924 the Hoxsey method of treating cancer was considered so effective by a former president of a medical association that he personally presented its sponsor with a written proposal, which, among other things, provided for the relinquishment of valuable property rights in the Hoxsey method and medicines and formulae to the same official. The evidence indicates that when the proposition was spurned, Hoxsey was advised to sign and accept the proposal or face ruination. Such tactics, if true, constitute blackmail of the rankest order and this evidence should be examined closely to ascertain its credibility." FitzGerald had seen enough of the seamy side of organized medicine to conclude that both Hoxsey and Dr. Ivy might well be telling the truth.[65]

FitzGerald closed by noting the prisoner's dilemma he suddenly found himself confronting. "The fact that various agencies of the Federal government are manned by officials who are also active in medical associations requires a consideration as to whether or not these officials are directing their first allegiance to the citizens and government of America— or to these same medical associations."[66]

Besides its obscure insertion into the Congressional Record, the FitzGerald Report did manage to reach many citizens through energetic distribution by advocates including Charles Tobey Jr., who printed 22,000 copies and began disseminating them nationally in his crusade against the "Un-American Medical Association." He personally canvassed the 389 doctors of his hometown, Concord, New Hampshire, to visit Dr. Lincoln and review his reputed 5,000 cured patients. Not one replied, although the state medical association did ask him for copies of any future correspondence. The sole doctor in Concord who braved testing the remedy was warned he would face immediate removal of his license, and quit the pursuit.[67]

Tobey attended a public meeting that Senator Bricker held with high cancer officials, where both Dr. Ivy and Dr. Lincoln were in the audience. The floor refused to recognize Tobey, and the officials threatened to walk out if he persisted in interrupting. There would be no dialogue on the matter.

Along with Hoxsey, practitioners such as Ivy, Koch, and Lincoln, most of them respected medical men prior to their transgressions, were pointing to a new therapeutic direction for cancer: immunology. Their theories would not be embraced by mainstream medicine for over thirty years, and in 1953 a dark wind of extreme political polarization was sweeping through the nation's capital. Senator Joseph McCarthy was gearing up the communist witchhunt, a mentality easily extended to "quacks." "Anticancer ideology became an article of scientific faith," wrote Alex Jack. "The disease was an irrational attack, a viral, bacterial or unidentifiable conspiracy subversive to the human body, which must be hunted down and rooted out, whatever the cost." Clearly there was no room for a difference of medical opinion.[68]

Benedict FitzGerald went on to become an attorney for various unorthodox cancer practitioners including Harry Hoxsey. Among other cases, he managed to free a Maine doctor from an insane asylum where he had been committed without having had legal counsel for administering the Koch remedies in his practice. The message was clear: A doctor offering alternative cancer therapies had to be crazy.[69]

The FitzGerald Report exploded organized medicine's dubious refusal to investigate unconventional cancer therapies. FitzGerald's disturbing charges would continue to reverberate for decades to come in serial scandals displaying a similar pattern.

Hoxsey's charge of a medical conspiracy could no longer be discounted as the publicity ploy of a lone crank. By 1954 even the staid *Yale Law Journal* would publicly criticize the AMA's monopolistic practices.[70] Against the chorus of protest rising across the country from credible doctors, senators, and federal officials, Harry Hoxsey pumped up the volume.

Twelve Thousand Patients in Dallas: "You Couldn't Run Me Out of Here with a Gatling Gun"

Back in Dallas, Hoxsey was flying as high as the booming oil industry's famed neon winged horse atop the tallest building in town. The clinic now boasted a whopping 5,000 patients, three osteopathic physicians, fifteen nurses, and twelve technicians. And Hoxsey was just getting going.[1]

Allen Bernard, a reporter for the pulp *Man's Magazine* whose wife had died of cancer, set out for Dallas to expose Hoxsey as a quack. Instead, he too was converted.[2] Bernard's provocative feature story garnered the largest reader response the magazine ever had, drawing 15,000 letters.[3] There soon followed a spate of favorable profiles in *Male, Sir,* and a host of tabloid publications.[4]

The melodrama attracted *Time* magazine, which predictably roasted Hoxsey. "For a fellow who ended his formal schooling after the eighth grade, Harry M. (for Mathias) Hoxsey, 52, has made quite a name for himself in medicine. His formula for success: a mixture

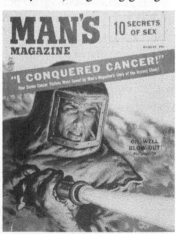

The pulp Man's Magazine *inspired an astounding 15,000 letters with its positive Hoxsey story.*

of roots, water and licorice labeled the Hoxsey Tonic and sold in 16 oz. bottles to thousands as a remedy for cancer." But Hoxsey got the last word in the piece, bellowing, "You couldn't run me out of here with a Gatling gun."[5]

The leering article caught the attention of an old friend. In the intervening years, journalist James Wakefield Burke had served as a test pilot in World War II, after which *Esquire* commissioned him to write a series of articles covering the Nuremberg trials, including an interview with the infamous Hermann Goering, deputy to Hitler and chief of the Luftwaffe. Burke stayed on in Europe for sixteen years, and wrote *The Big Rape*, a book about the German invasion of Russia.[6]

"General Lucius D. Clay, the military governor, discovered that I was his cousin," Burke recounted to our camera, "and he asked me to take a leave of absence from *Esquire* and join his staff, which I did. It was a lot of fun, it was a lot of power. We were like the Roman conquerors back in the old days. I was very comfortable in a requisitioned mansion in Berlin. One day I picked up *Time* magazine, and here was this article about the high priest of quackery, Harry Hoxsey. I smiled and read it. He was in Texas, according to the article, curing cancer and being put in jail for it. But he was making a lot of money and the AMA was in an uproar.

"Well, I picked up the phone and called him. It was just like no time had passed between. We had become real good friends. I liked the man, thought he was a great personality, a great human being with a big heart. He was such a salesman, so persuasive, that he convinced me to give up this luxurious conqueror's life in Berlin and return to Dallas to assist him in his battle with the AMA."

Burke returned to find Hoxsey thriving. "He was no longer at his old dog kennel. He had converted an old mansion on Gaston Avenue with about seventy rooms. He had at least ten doctors and a bevy of nurses. He was really in the cancer-curing business. He was making so much money, about $17,000 a day, and he had a lot of patients coming in from all over the world. This had apparently attracted the Texas Medical Association as well as the AMA, and he was having a fierce battle with the FDA and the AMA. He had a brilliant mind, but he was handling it badly. He was writing tough, crudely written letters in his coal-miner language to government people, trying to defend himself and his cure.

"He wanted to put me on the payroll, but I didn't want that because I realized that once I was on the payroll my effectiveness for him would diminish because I would be just as guilty as he was. I said, 'Look, I'm not going to charge you anything, but I'm going to help you because I believe in what you're doing, and I believe these people are unjustly persecuting you. I'll help you all I can.' I'd already been convinced that he did cure cancer. But being a big-hearted fella like he was, he said, 'Look, I'm in the oil business, and I'm going to put you in the oil business.' When he would strike a well, he'd draw a line on that lease right next to that well and sell me the adjoining acreage for a dollar an acre. All I had to do was hire somebody to go drill the well. I never got a dry hole."

Burke took stock of Hoxsey's situation and launched a new battle plan. He went through the files and quickly concluded he had better take over any official correspondence to important officials. Burke's assessment was that Hoxsey needed a thorough makeover, starting with his own quarters. "His office looked more like a bookie joint than it did a medical office," Burke recollected with bemusement. "It had a little bronze sign on his desk that said, 'There are two kinds of people in this world: Dem that gets and dem that gets took.' He had pictures of racehorses, and a couple of pictures of women which I would say he got from the back of a bar. It was coal-miner stuff.

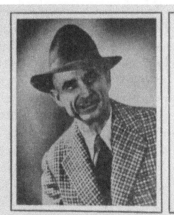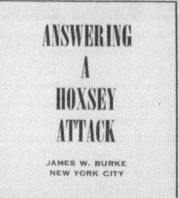

ANSWERING
A
HOXSEY
ATTACK

JAMES W. BURKE
NEW YORK CITY

For some unexplained reason the widely read magazine, Consumer Reports, has opened its columns to a vicious attack on the Hoxsey cancer treatment. Just why the editors teamed up with Commissioner George Larrick of the Food and Drug Administration in promoting the Big Smear is not clear. It is known, however, that they have received many letters of protest from persons reading the damaging articles ... of which the following by Mr. James W. Burke is an example.

James Burke goes to bat for Hoxsey in the Defender, *1954.*

"He was very proud of these defensive, belligerent letters he'd been writing to government officials, the head of the FDA, the head of this one and that. I said 'Now Harry, you've got yourself in the fire. If I'm going to be here with you, you've got to listen to me. I'm going to try to get you out of the fire.' So he turned everything over to me. From then on we became a pretty good team. Some months later, he said, 'How are we doing?' I said, 'The best I can do is put you back in the frying pan.'"

The cash pouring into the clinic inflamed hostile accusations that Hoxsey was in it for the money. From behind owlish glasses, William Grigg, a public information officer for the FDA, represented these sentiments to our camera. "Like some of the best salesmen, he was very convincing. He was what one of our people called a blackguard, the worst kind of scoundrel who had no feeling that he was harming anybody. They've probably been all the way back to early man, people that would take other people's clamshells or their dollars. He was certainly a master at it. He was a great liar, and he was able to make people think he was taking money from his oil interests and plowing it into the clinic out of the goodness of his heart. The IRS records, which we tried and were not able to get into one of the court cases, showed that he was doing the reverse. He was actually taking the money from these poor patients and trying to make a buck in the oil business with that money."[7]

The FDA failed to produce any documentation to back up its assertion. But the very fact of Hoxsey's financial winnings was enough to rankle government officials, a portfolio that included a 1,500-acre ranch, a dairy products company, manufacturing businesses, and a gold mine in Mexico.[8] A confidential FDA memo revealed a close and secret collaboration between the agency and the IRS. "The Intelligence Unit of the Internal Revenue Service has always been very cooperative," the 1954 memo described. "One of the agents was working on Hoxsey at this time, but he wished it to be understood that any information they passed on to us was to be held in the greatest confidence and that we were under no circumstances to divulge the source. I felt that we then could take other means of obtaining it so that they would not be suspected. The Internal Revenue agents stated that they were quite perturbed over Hoxsey's bragging manner over his having 'beaten the government' in the Food and Drug case, and that 'they knew they were beaten.'"[9]

Oliver Field of the AMA Bureau of Investigation cut to the bottom line. "The money! That's what all of them are in business for. There is no charity in their hearts, believe me." Dr. Harry Spence of Dallas concurred. "He made millions, and that was a lot of money for those times. He might have deluded himself, but frankly I think that he was avaricious and in it for the money."[10]

Jim Burke disagreed flatly. "I don't think money was uppermost in his mind. I went into that very thoroughly before I even agreed to help, to see how much greed he had. I don't think he had any greed at all. If patients could pay ten dollars, that's all he'd charge—for a lifetime treatment. If they could pay one thousand dollars, he would only charge them four hundred dollars. They could pay nothing. In would come an old mother or an old aunt, given up to die. After being interviewed, they said, 'We only have enough money to get here.' Harry would personally take that old lady or old woman in his car down the street, put them in a boardinghouse or hotel, and pay all their bills, treat them the six or eight weeks until they were cured, send them home, pay their bus fare or airplane fare back, with enough medicine to last them. 'And if you need to come back, write me a letter and I'll send for you.' How could you not help a man like that?"

Hoxsey unremittingly broadcast his call for an investigation while organized medicine tried to disconnect the microphone. In 1954 ten medical doctors from around the country dared to make a three-day investigation of the clinic. The physicians held a press conference at the close of their visit and made a joint statement, which Hoxsey published as "Ten Doctors Declare 'Quack' Cures Cancer." "We find as fact that our investigation has demonstrated to our satisfaction that the Hoxsey Cancer Clinic is successfully treating pathologically proven cases of cancer, both internal and external. We as a committee feel that the Hoxsey treatment is superior to such conventional methods of treatment as X-ray, radium, and surgery. We are willing to use it in our office, in our practice on our own patients, when at our discretion it is deemed necessary."

In private letters, the ten doctors made additional comments about their impressions: "That place does the best work in the field of curing cancer and many kindred conditions." "I am convinced that he has something for cancer." "They are doing more to relieve suffering humanity among cancer sufferers than all the other doctors in that city." "Doing very good work—the Hoxsey Clinic is genuine." "Curing about 50 percent of the cases." "The Hoxsey cancer cure is all it claims and more, for if the public knew the real facts of its value, there would be an uprising."[11]

The doctors' press conference was blacked out in the media. Oliver Field had been busy blanketing the nation's press with letters advising reporters against promoting quackery. "I'm sure you've heard about Hoxsey's 'medical jury' publicity stunt in Dallas over the weekend," he wrote the science editor of United Press Associations.[12] As the science editor replied to the AMA, "Nor do I have to tell you that the United Press carried nothing and won't."[13]

Oliver Field supplied the media with a damning dossier on the ten doctors. He challenged their credentials, pointedly underscoring the fact that most did not belong to the AMA or state medical societies. All but two, he noted emphatically, were users of the Koch remedy, and several were associated with the Lincoln treatment. "It appears fair to say that the majority of those who served on the 'jury' were cancer quacks. It is obvious that if he [Hoxsey] had anything of value in the treatment of cancer, he certainly wouldn't need to advertise."[14]

Part of Dr. Fishbein's enduring legacy was a pact with the journalistic profession to report exclusively on medical treatments officially approved by the AMA. The *Journal* in 1940 boasted that the United Press wire service at its behest would now "clear" any stories on cures and human health with its "science editor," who had an open line to the AMA.[15] Thanks to Dr. Fishbein's efforts, this legitimate media concern about endangering the public health was now deeply ingrained in the press, but distorted by the AMA's partisan medical-political lens.

When Hoxsey did manage to get on national TV and radio shows, more often than not the AMA had gotten there first. Internal correspondence between the AMA and news organizations revealed carefully scripted programs designed to discredit Hoxsey, with copious back story supplied by the Bureau of Investigation.[16] In other cases, the pressure was less subtle. After Hoxsey appeared on a public debate on KCOP-TV in Los Angeles, a member of the AMA legislative committee suggested he would speak to friends in Congress about having the Federal Communications Commission revoke the station's license.[17]

While the mainstream press was slighting Hoxsey, he found another ally who had his own private media kingdom. The notorious Reverend Gerald Winrod was the "rabble-rousing publisher-preacher-radio orator of Wichita, Kansas," as Oliver Field tagged him.[18] Head of the Defenders of the Christian Faith, Winrod was a fire-and-brimstone fundamentalist preacher whose Defenders had been founded in Kansas by his minister father. Winrod had a large national flock, and beamed his evangelical message of apocalypse and redemption through a widely syndicated radio show and his popular *The Defender* magazine, whose forgotten archives we unexpectedly unearthed in Kansas through one of our investors in Wichita.[19]

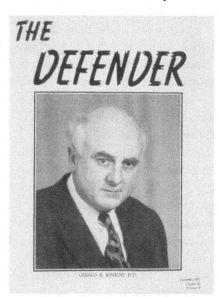

Notorious evangelist Winrod takes up Hoxsey's cause with religious fervor.

Winrod was a prominent advocate for Hoxsey as well as Drs. Koch, Lincoln, and Ivy. He mollified his sermon of hellfire with the balm of godly natural healing, and often ended his windy broadcasts by intoning, "God bless the quacks, the only quacks who are curing cancer."[20] Winrod maintained that the Hoxsey treatment cured him as a child of a horrible neck cancer under the care of a Dr. Rochelle of Wichita, a friend of Hoxsey's father. He saw it as nothing less than an act of divine intervention that he was now situated to lift Hoxsey's righteous banner.[21]

In many ways the granddaddy of modern televangelism, Winrod was a voluble demagogue with a tainted past. He had visited Nazi Germany in 1934 and returned home to herald its advances. After nearly winning the 1938 Republican nomination for Kansas governor amid allegations of German funding, he was brought up on charges of sedition during World War II for his Nazi associations. He evaded the trial when a sympathetic right-wing congressman killed the investigation from behind the scenes.[22] An overt racist, anti-Catholic, and anti-Semite dubbed the "Prairie Pogromist," Winrod served as the model for Buzz Windrip, the minister of vengeful salvation in Sinclair Lewis's novel *It Can't Happen Here*.[23] At the height of the McCarthy era, Winrod was at one with the zeitgeist, proudly publishing "Senator Joseph McCarthy: A Speech That Will Live" in *The Defender* magazine.[24] Not that his credibility was ever much of an issue, but *The Defender* also heralded "Flying Saucers Considered Prophetically."[25]

Following in the ugly tracks of Norman Baker, Winrod was the latest in Hoxsey's rogues' gallery of ignoble partners. Paradoxically, while close to Winrod, Hoxsey continued to consort openly with black and Jewish friends who were aghast at this repellent bedfellow. Hoxsey took comfort where he found it. Paradoxically, the issue of medical freedom of choice united the libertarian wings of both left and right in common cause, a strange de facto alliance that continues to exist today. I have met Hoxsey supporters among left-wing radicals, middle-American fundamentalists, flower-child hippies, and card-carrying John Birch Society stalwarts.

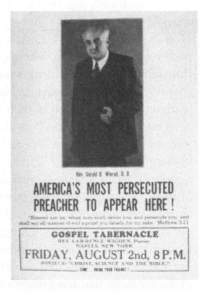

Rev. Gerald B. Winrod, D. D.

AMERICA'S MOST PERSECUTED PREACHER TO APPEAR HERE !

"Blessed are ye, when men shall revile you, and persecute you, and shall say all manner of evil against you falsely, for my sake." Matthew 5:11

GOSPEL TABERNACLE
REV. LAWRENCE WIGDEN, Pastor
NAPLES, NEW YORK

FRIDAY, AUGUST 2nd, 8 P.M.
SUBJECT: "CHRIST, SCIENCE AND THE BIBLE."
COME   BRING YOUR FRIEND

Winrod escapes a sedition trial for his past Nazi associations.

Winrod broadcast Hoxsey's praises far and wide from the flatlands of Kansas. Zealously proclaiming the Hoxsey clinic as the "Medical Mecca for cancer sufferers," he painted organized medicine as an infernal force.[26] When a subsequent FDA investigation uncovered Hoxsey making over $80,000 in payments to Winrod, Hoxsey weakly defended them as legitimate donations to a religious organization.[27]

It was not the only media manipulation Hoxsey attempted. After *Man's Magazine* continued to publish a torrid series of articles promoting Hoxsey cures, the FDA dug up a fistful of "expense" checks Hoxsey paid to writer Allen Bernard following his first article. It was war, and Hoxsey obviously knew how to fight dirty, too.[28]

The FDA decided it was time to lift its investigative magnifying glass to the sun to incinerate Hoxsey. The agency instigated a broad probe into his affairs to put an end to his activities by any means necessary. The government again cast a national dragnet, discharging dozens of agents to scour the country to discredit his alleged cures, reviewing a reputed four hundred cases.[29] One agent drove 17,000 miles, knocking on patients' doors, interrogating them, and demanding "samples" of their medicine. "We were met with almost universal opposition by the Hoxsey patients whom we visited to obtain samples and labeling," reported an agent in frustration. It was the same pattern of satisfied Hoxsey customers that had stymied authorities since the 1920s.[30]

One such case, reported in a letter from FDA Commissioner George Larrick, stemmed from visits by FDA agent Gordy Johnston to three Hoxsey patients. Agent Johnston soon received a visit from Hoxsey supporter Harold Edwards, who "was abusive, intemperate, profane, and threatening. He warned Inspector Johnston that he would get his skull split open with a meat ax, if, as Mr. Edwards put it, he continued his 'rat work under the direction of the rat outfit' he worked for."[31]

Another case was James Powell, the husband of a Hoxsey patient. Powell was so disturbed by the visit of an FDA agent to his home that he wrote to his Virginia congressional representative. His wife's health was failing after a cancer operation, and she was despondent when they decided to go to Hoxsey. "She began to feel better almost immediately, and in one month, an amazing change for the better occurred. Shortly after returning from our first visit to the Hoxsey Clinic, a representative of the Food and Drug Commission [sic] called at my house while I was at work and began asking my wife numerous questions about the treatment and also requested samples of the medicine that was prescribed for her. The approach and manner in which the representative presented himself and the remarks he made to my wife about the clinic upset her so much that it gave her an awful setback."[32]

When the FDA agent was rebuffed in his second attempt to get a sample of the tonic, he aggressively demanded to buy it. Mr. Powell said that the agent then made "even stronger remarks against the clinic, even going so far as to insinuate that we were breaking the law by bringing the medicines home for my wife to use in fighting this most dreaded of all diseases. These unnecessary visits by the Pure Food and Drug representative have upset my wife to the extent that they have undone everything that has been done for her, have left her in doubt as to whether or not she is improving, and she is losing confidence in the treatment and herself.

"I would appreciate it," the anguished constituent implored his representative, "if you would kindly take immediate actions to prevent reoccurrence of similar actions to my wife and to others they are now visiting all over the country. If not, I will be forced to take such action as may be necessary to protect her from further annoyance of this type."[33] FDA Commissioner George Larrick himself replied to the congressman's inquiry about "harassment of a citizen" by saying that there was "nothing to suggest that the inspector acted improperly."[34]

Mildred Nelson observed numerous skirmishes between Hoxsey patients and federal agents. "The Food and Drug have always been famous for harassing the Hoxsey patients, usually doing it to find something to harass Harry with. Their basic intention was not to harass the patient, yet scare them enough that they didn't remain a patient. There was a number of times that I know the tables really turned on them. A little woman in Arizona was on treatment and her husband had called up and said, 'I cannot get in there and I don't think she's able to travel at this time. She's doing better, but please send us some medicine. We're close to being out.' When the postman delivered the package, the Food and Drug man was standing right behind him, and as the postman handed it to the man, the Food and Drug man said, 'I'll take that.' And the man said, 'This is my wife's medicine.'

"The Food and Drug man followed him on in the door, and the man reached behind the door and picked up a shotgun and he said, 'I can't keep you from taking it, but I'll guarantee you if you do, you will go with my wife, because I'm going to blow your head off!' When he looked up in a minute, there was no Food and Drug man. He didn't even know which way he went on the street, whether he went up it or down it. He immediately got on the phone and called Harry and said, 'The Food and Drug Department was just here wanting to take my wife's medicine, and so I told the man I was going to kill him. Had the gun in my hand.' Harry said, 'I don't think you'll have any more trouble with him, but if you do, pull the trigger next time. No, really I don't mean that, but if he comes back, don't give it to him. He's not entitled to come into your house unless he gets a search warrant.'"[35]

The FDA staked out the Dallas clinic parking lot to record license plates to track down patients. Agents set wiretaps and had the post office monitor mail.[36] "The FDA never investigated," Mildred commented dryly, "except in a criminal type of way, to see what Harry might be doing wrong. Go to people's houses, talk to them, tell them they were doing wrong, take their medicine. We'd catch them in the parking areas, writing down numbers."

Despite the government's operations, Hoxsey kept magnetizing supporters. The *Man's Magazine* articles attracted hundreds, perhaps thousands, of patients to Dallas. Among them was Verne Haluska Kielbowick. As she told the magazine, after six months of vaginal bleeding, she consulted her family physician, who found a tumor of the cervix and called for an operation. Her brother, Pennsylvania State Senator John J. Haluska, administrator of the Miners' Hospital, made arrangements at a Pittsburgh hospital. The surgeon there decided against a hysterectomy because her condition was so fragile. She received eight treatments of deep X-ray at the hospital, and thirty more back at the Miners' Hospital. The radiation made her ill, and she returned home too weak to do her housework. When her nephew picked up a copy of *Man's Magazine*, her brother the senator decided it was time to take her to Hoxsey.

"Two weeks after I started the treatment," Verne Haluska Kielbowick reported, "the bleeding halted and I haven't had any hemorrhages since. I've gained eight pounds, feel much stronger, do all my own housework, cook and bake for my husband and four children. I'm in good condition and have no complaints."[37] In a characteristic Ping-Pong, the doctors countered that they had in fact performed an operation, and claimed that the cure was the result of X-ray treatment and surgery.[38]

Following his sister's improvement, Senator Haluska loudly boarded the Hoxsey bandwagon. For Hoxsey it was a bit of a homecoming, since Haluska was also a former coal miner and presided over a coal-mining district. The senator tried to enlist the support of the Miners' Hospital, which he had served since 1932, to take up the Hoxsey cause at a former nursing home nearby.[39] The Cambria County Medical Society issued a surprising statement "wholeheartedly endorsing" Haluska's investigation of the AMA "conspiracy" against Hoxsey.[40] The medical society joined Haluska in writing Senator Langer, demanding such an investigation, while preparing to dispatch a team of physicians to investigate the Hoxsey Clinic in Texas on *Man's* dime.[41]

The AMA intervened and stopped the doctors' delegation from visiting Dallas, while spurring the Miners' Hospital staff to call for Haluska's resignation. Haluska threatened to sue, and, from the AMA convention in San Francisco, the Pennsylvania State Medical Association staff issued a statement endorsing the hospital's anti-Hoxsey position.[42] "There will be bloodshed, marches on the hospital," Haluska told *Time* magazine. "Labor is inflamed."[43]

Senator Haluska delivered a stinging speech in the front of the Pennsylvania State Senate on February 7, 1954, to a packed house that included his sister, Harry Hoxsey, and Dr. Ira Drew, the former congressman from Philadelphia who remained a Hoxsey supporter. The senator invoked his personal tragedy of losing his eight-year-old son to cancer and then confronting his sister's looming mortality. To loud applause, he summoned his recovering sister to rise from the gallery.[44]

Decrying the "carnage" of conventional treatments, Haluska also signaled little Kathy Allison to stand in the gallery. The five-year-old girl suffered from a tumor in her chest, and, after radical surgery and radiation, she was preparing to "meet Jesus and the angels" when her parents took her to Hoxsey. Clutching her giant doll, little Kathy waved bashfully from the audience, blushing with health thanks to Hoxsey.

Swirling with emotion, Haluska motioned Hoxsey to rise. "Mr. President, permit me now to introduce to you that great humanitarian, a man who needs a critic like I need a hole in my head; a man devoted to suffering humanity; the man who wants to give this treatment to America; the man who has been put in jail because the AMA says he was practicing unorthodox methods." Hoxsey basked in the standing ovation from the floor of the State Senate.[45]

Amid charges he tried to extract a $10,000 payoff to bow out of the Miners' Hospital, Haluska resigned in a fury and launched his own Hoxsey Clinic in March 1954, attracting over 7,000 people during a two-day open house.[46] Technically unaffiliated with the Dallas headquarters, the clinic hired Dr. Newton Allen, an ordained minister, osteopath, naturopath, and M.D. with experience with cancer who was impressed after a visit to Dallas. The clinic quickly drew streams of clients amid a firestorm of controversy.[47]

Haluska feted the town of Portage in June 1954 with "Hoxsey Day." Over

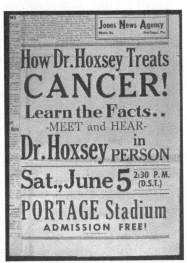

It's Hoxsey Day again in Pennsylvania, 1954.

2,500 onlookers lined the rain-soaked parade route to cheer the open convertible escorted by state police. Hoxsey and Haluska waved triumphantly at another 1,700 spectators who withstood the drizzling rain for two hours at Portage Stadium to hear Hoxsey promise he would defy the FDA injunction against interstate shipment of his medicines. Hoxsey was now substituting pills for tonic as a tactical technicality to circumvent the federal injunction against shipping his tonic, though the pill's effectiveness was uncertain.[48]

In local newspaper interviews, Hoxsey blasted the medical authorities with characteristic vigor. Questioned as to his own medical credentials, he defended himself with 80/20 embellishment. "The extent of my medical training consists of assisting and working with my father from the time I was eight years old until his death. Then I started studying and I went to the Bar Harbor. I did my animal experimental work on a group of mice in Philadelphia for the cancer work for the Bar Harbor Institute in Bar Harbor, Maine. I was successful in treating thirteen cases of cancer, seven internals and six externals, for that group."[49]

Hoxsey's only legitimate medical credential was a degree from the Western Texas Naturopathic College in Dallas in 1942. He was licensed in Texas in 1949 when the practice was legally recognized.[50] As a naturopath, he was fully licensed by the State of Texas to practice. Hoxsey described naturopathy as "the art and science of treating human ailments without the use of coal-tar preparations. With roots, herbs, foods, diets, light and water."[51] By now, the AMA was also waging a full-throttle national campaign against naturopathy hatched at its 1953 convention. South Carolina, where there were only forty-eight naturopathic physicians, was the proving ground for the AMA's intensive lobbying in the state legislature, and only a last-ditch filibuster had put a temporary stop to it.[52]

"In my experience," Hoxsey wrote, freely mixing his metaphors, "I have seen outstanding naturopathic physicians arrested, humiliated, and browbeaten because they have persisted in the belief that medical science was not supreme and have refused to bow and scrape to the dictation of the medical octopus whose tentacles have slowly but surely been wrapping the American public in a strait-jacket."[53]

Within a year, the FDA invaded the Pennsylvania clinic without a search warrant. Agents vainly commanded Dr. Allen to cease and desist his practice there.[54] Soon after, U.S. marshals seized half a million pills along with clinic brochures and reprints of *Man's Magazine* and Winrod's *The Defender*. Sensational newspaper headlines blared, "U.S. Raids Hoxsey Cancer Clinic."[55]

Once again the FDA's charge was the misbranding of medicines that were ineffective against cancer and shipped in interstate commerce.[56] In an internal FDA memorandum, the agents described the surprise attack, to which they had surreptitiously alerted the media in advance.[57] They portrayed Dr. Allen as scarlet, railing furiously at the government raiders, "If I couldn't get a better job, I'd get a job driving a garbage truck. That's the kind of punks we have working for the government."[58]

Haluska, who was present during the raid, immediately picked up the phone and in rapid succession called his attorney Benedict FitzGerald and Hoxsey. Haluska and Allen defied the agents to remove the medicines "over their dead bodies." The agents proceeded to remove the pills and litera-

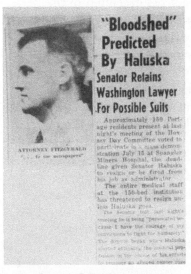

U. S. Raided Their Clinic

Left, State Sen. J. Haluska, right, Harry M. Hoxsey.

Pennsylvania Senator Haluska opens a Hoxsey clinic under fire, 1954.

ture while Haluska protested against the violations of his constitutional rights. "We'll open Monday morning as usual," he barked stubbornly.[59]

"Bloodshed" Predicted By Haluska
Senator Retains Washington Lawyer For Possible Suits

The former federal investigator becomes the lawyer for Hoxsey and Senator Haluska.

A week later, agents privately informed the press that they would invade Dr. Allen's office that same afternoon. They arrested the physician on charges of criminal violations of the Pennsylvania Medical Practice Act. Publicly accused of not having a valid medical license, Dr. Allen lunged at the clot of news reporters while Haluska threatened to punch them out. As an osteopath, Dr. Allen was fully accredited to practice, and in fact did have a valid M.D. license, although he had not registered in Pennsylvania.[60] The raids exemplified a campaign of terror skirting the bounds of both the law and the facts.

As lawyers prepared feverishly for the trial, the FDA struck again in a landmark action. Exasperated with its inability to nail Hoxsey in court, the agency resorted to an obscure federal statute permitting extreme measures in a case where there is "imminent danger to health or gross deception to the consumer." Wallace Janssen, an FDA Public Affairs officer, devised the famed "Public Warning" against Hoxsey. Signed by FDA Commissioner George Larrick, it saturated the country initially as a press release in April 1956, and then in January 1957 as a sensational black-and-red poster tacked in 46,000 post offices across the country and distributed to all the hospitals that agents could reach, along with farm, lodge, and church groups.[61]

When I visited Wallace Janssen in the Kafkaesque steel-and-glass hive of FDA headquarters near Washington, D.C., I met a small suspicious man with a neatly trimmed mustache and bow tie. In a trembling voice he told me that the dire action was justified because Hoxsey was a "murderer."[62] Proudly he pulled from his fastidious files the poster of which he was the author:[63]

> Sufferers from cancer, their families, physicians and all concerned with the care of cancer patients are hereby warned that the Hoxsey treatment for internal cancer has been found by the United States Court of Appeals for the Fifth Circuit, on the basis of evidence presented by the Food and Drug Administration, to be a worthless treatment. Its sale represents a gross deception to the consumer. The Food and Drug Administration has conducted a thorough and long-continuing investigation of Hoxsey's treatment. In addition, the National Cancer Institute has reviewed case histories submitted by Hoxsey and advised him that the cases provided no scientific evidence that the Hoxsey treatment has any value in the treatment of internal cancer. Those afflicted with cancer are warned not to be misled by the false promise that the Hoxsey cancer treatment will cure or alleviate their condition. Cancer can be cured only through surgery or radiation. Death from cancer is inevitable when cancer patients fail to obtain proper medical treatment because of the lure of a painless cure "without the use of surgery, X-ray, or radium," as claimed by Hoxsey.[64]

The FDA gloated over its ingenious legal maneuver, as government agents monitoring Hoxsey's clinic parking lot witnessed a 50 percent decline in patients.[65] Gordon Granger, associate medical director of the FDA, wrote to Oliver Field at the AMA, "I am enclosing for your information, education and benefit, a work of art which is soon to be displayed in every Post Office in the United States."[66] FDA representatives visited Oliver Field at AMA headquarters to relish their victory.[67] Several years later, a gratified Wallace Janssen sent a personal memento of the poster with an admiring letter to Dr. Morris Fishbein.[68] Janssen estimated that the warning dissuaded at least 3,000 people from trying the Hoxsey treatment.[69]

We were originally scheduled to film with Wallace Janssen, Oliver Field, and the federal prosecutor who tried Hoxsey in Pittsburgh, but just days before the crew was scheduled to leave, I got a dramatic telegram from Janssen calling it off. He had been in communication with his former colleagues. "Regretfully, I am recommending that you cancel your travel arrangements for filming me, since I am not convinced that the project can be productive of more good than harm. Specifically, it seems increasingly clear that to re-publicize the Hoxsey cases, which were decisively concluded over thirty years ago, will result in causing some cancer patients to again seek a treatment that was found both worthless and fraudulent. The proposed film will inevitably advertise the Mexican clinic, and this will be irresistible to some of the many thousands of people who are fearful about cancer. I do not wish to collaborate in this."[70]

After months of distraught negotiations, I was unable to convince Janssen and the federal prosecutor to film with us, but I did finally prevail on Oliver Field and the FDA's William Grigg, who was familiar with the Hoxsey case although never personally involved in it. Clearly, however, the core team behind the "concerted effort" was still intact and ever vigilant.

Hoxsey was sitting in his office, unaware, when word came that the warning was broadcast nationally over the radio.[71] He immediately made the rounds of local TV and radio stations, and protested to the FDA commissioner against "this un-American persecution. It is the apparent objective of your department to give the general public the impression that I am, in the eyes of the government, a criminal, since most of the posters in the post offices are of wanted criminals." He went on to say, "This is the kind of behavior I understand stems from behind the Iron Curtain, government officials using their office to 'liquidate' an individual. You stated that you have sent investigators to my clinic. You meant, didn't you, that you sent several policemen or flat-foots to do some snooping? The louder the voices against me, and the more hostile my enemies become, the more cancer sufferers come to my clinic."[72]

As Hoxsey implored the *New York Times*, "I want an investigation—not in test tubes or guinea pigs or mice. I want it made on the 11,000 patients that we now have under treatment. If we are the largest cancer clinic in the world, why isn't this the place to make an investigation?"[73] Indeed, the Hoxsey clinic was now the world's biggest privately owned cancer center.[74] Hoxsey marshaled his forces to retaliate against what he called the government's Stalinist tactics.[75]

The Public Warning against Hoxsey generated passionate resistance. "We began getting calls from all over the country," Mildred Nelson remembered with a smirk, "that there was this poster to beware in every post office in the United States. One patient called me and said, 'May I take it down?' The next one called and said, 'I'm going to get it down.' And then they'd begin calling to tell how they got them down! Some of them would walk in and be fighting mad and yank it right off the wall with everybody standing there."[76]

Gerald Winrod fought back with a massive "Call to Prayer." Broadcasting on the radio, he reassured his flock, "I honestly believe that Hoxsey's survival must be attributed to answered prayer. Millions of Christians are at this hour interested and concerned that the treatment shall be saved. The power of God must be released, and this can be accomplished only through prayer."[77] He launched a drive that landed a whopping two million petitions on the FDA's doorstep demanding an investigation of the agency.[78]

Hoxsey appealed the Public Warning in court, but lost.[79] The noose was tightening, and James Burke was concerned. "They were closing in, and we realized, if we didn't have a diversion right quick, that it might be closed up soon, and he might go to the penitentiary."

Burke devised a creative distraction. "At this time there were sixteen candidates running for governor. One morning I said to Harry—not seriously—'You up for governor? You're a public figure—everybody knows you. The church people and the black people love you, and the poor people love you. Announce you are going to get in the race and let's take some of this heat off!'"[80]

Burke saw that Hoxsey was frightened by the prospect of running for office. "He didn't want to go for that. That scared him a little bit. Remember, he was a coal miner and he realized that he wasn't too well educated. But then I convinced him that we're going to be all right. First of all, I cleaned out his office desk, took care of all this racehorse paraphernalia, and I put a large picture in back of his desk of Christ on the cross, and pictures of his family, his children, and the babies, and some nice Christian sayings on his desk.

"The next day I called a press conference. The press was always eager to come hear something Hoxsey had to say, and that morning I said to my wife, 'I've got to write something for Harry to say.' I sat down and wrote something, and I took it down to him and said, 'Now Harry, you're going to say exactly what I say. Stick to this and say nothing more.' I had brought down some notes and I told him to write them down. I told him, 'You want to say, "Caesar's enemies murdered him too," very calmly.' Harry asked, 'Caesar? Who is Caesar?' I said, 'Don't worry about it. It's a metaphor.' 'Metaphor? What's that?' Anyway, he got the idea."

Burke's ploy caught Hoxsey's fancy, and the happy warrior embraced electoral politics with gusto. "The press appeared," Burke went on, "and Harry made his little statement. 'Now,' he says, 'the only way I can keep curing people is I'm going to run for governor and I'm going to win. Then we'll go right on curing people.' The press reacted very well to it, and Harry got carried away with himself. He had more power over an audience than any man I ever saw except Churchill. He could make a speech and spellbind an audience, and he had this group spellbound. He saw that and he ended—I'll never forget—he's a big man, powerful man, and I don't know whether he did it deliberately or instinctively—he stood up before that picture of Christ on the cross, and he says, 'They crucified Jesus Christ, didn't they?' Cameras went off. We went off flying for the governorship."

Hoxsey told the eager press that he was running to "bring pressure to investigate the Federal Food and Drug Adminstration and bust up the monopoly of the American Medical Association. I've run out of patience and everything but money."[81]

While Hoxsey's left-handed run for the Texas governorship was gaining momentum, Burke watched with bemused concern. "I had no idea that putting Harry up in this race for governor would create such a sensation, but it did. As time went on, this became a serious matter. It never was serious with me, and I presumed it wasn't serious with Hoxsey. One day somebody in the press called me and said, 'Look, you've been making a lot of fuss around here. What the hell is Hoxsey's platform?' I hadn't given that a thought because we didn't expect to get that far along. I had no idea what to do, so I woke up in the morning, and I had set a press conference where Hoxsey would give his platform. Even the morning of the press conference, I didn't know what to do. It occurred to me that, when I was on General Clay's staff and the Soviets were pushing to communize Berlin, they came up with Ten Points of Socialism. I rushed around in my files and I found a copy of this. So I sat down very quickly, converting those to Ten Points of Democracy for Texas.

"I brought them down and told Harry, 'Now, this is your platform. You just follow these ten points.' Harry read them off very soberly, and I remember one dealt with the transfer of wealth to the poor. But the way that Harry had interpreted it, with his hyperbole, he expanded on my note. He said, 'A farmer comes into the city of Dallas, and he buys an automobile. He pays the taxes on it. He buys some gasoline to drive it home. Then he comes back into town with that car and then he parks it, and he puts a nickel in this meter to park it. That ain't right,' he says. 'When I'm governor, I'm going to take those sons of bitches up. Why give it to them people down in the white towers. That poor farmer, he don't have to pay a nickel—not to drive his car.' The reporter sitting next to me said, 'You know, I'm going to vote for that fellow.'"

As the Hoxsey campaign snowballed in the Texas desert, the unorthodox candidate's gambling instincts kicked in. Burke slipped his candidate a famous line from Davy Crockett, about whom the journalist had written a popular biography. Hoxsey resurrected Crockett's pledge to voters during his run for Congress: "Whatever my opponent promises, I will double." When the only serious competitor dropped out of the race, Hoxsey actually had a shot at winning.

Kingmaker Burke was edgy about the political monster he had animated, which was starting to lead an eccentric life of its own. "It came time to put up or shut up. We had to make a formal register and go through the rites of which party, so I called another press conference and I didn't say what it was about. This was the moment that Harry had to withdraw. I met with him in the office and I said, 'Harry, now your statement is really going to be a tearjerker. You're going to tell them that you know you could be governor, but that's not the place for you, because these poor people dying of cancer deserve all your attention.' Say, 'I was guilty of ambition and I don't want to be that way. I want to serve these poor people. I'm going to withdraw.' I saw this shocked look on Hoxsey's face, and he says, 'Jimmy, we can beat them sons of bitches! We're going to run. We're going to beat 'em!'

"I saw Harry had caught the bug too. So I said, 'You dumb ass—if you do run and win, I myself am liable to assassinate you. You can't be governor of this state.' We called it off. For the rest of his life, I don't think he ever forgave me for that. Sometimes in the middle of talking about something, Harry'd get a faraway look and say, 'Jimmy, we could have beat them sons of bitches!'"

For now, Hoxsey had more pressing matters to attend to. The government was gearing up for its final campaign to put him out of business just as the Dallas Hoxsey Clinic was spreading branches into seventeen states.[82] As high as Hoxsey had climbed, it was going to be a long way down.

Endgame:
The Government
"Liquidates" Hoxsey

T he government watched anxiously as it suffered yet a fourth dramatic court upset on the heels of Hoxsey's high-profile victories against Hearst, Dr. Fishbein, and the FDA. When Hoxsey beat the rap by the Texas Board of Medical Examiners to revoke the licenses of all seven of his clinic doctors, the federal government played out an endgame that would devolve into a calculated war of technicalities.

"We have the time and we have the money," stated the confident federal prosecutor, William Goodrich, going into the clamorous Pittsburgh trial known as the "Hoxsey Pill Case" in October 1956.[1] Although the baseless charges against Dr. Allen were dropped, matters did not augur well for Hoxsey in Pennsylvania. The besieged Senator Haluska had just lost his Senate election under heavy lobbying by the AMA and the Pennysylvania state medical society.[2]

The government prosecution set out to "prove" the worthlessness of the Hoxsey treatment once and for all. The Hoxsey forces vainly objected that such medical matters could not be settled in a courtroom, but only through the legitimate scientific investigation Hoxsey had now been denied for thirty years.

The Portage Hoxsey Clinic faced off against a firmament of star allopathic physicians well rehearsed to testify to the inefficacy of the internal tonic. All external cases were to be excluded from consideration. Top medical witnesses including NCI chief Dr. J. R. Heller again maintained that the Hoxsey internal medicines were worthless at best, or might actually accelerate the cancer.[3] The Hoxsey defense retaliated with blistering attacks on the destructive effects of surgery and radiation, and strutted Hoxsey's famed cures before the jury. By now, prominent medical researchers were also experimenting widely with the new field of chemo-therapy, and Hoxsey had taken to challenging organized medicine by call-ing his approach "nontoxic chemotherapy."

This time the prosecution was taking no chances in discrediting Hoxsey's "phony" cures. The government unveiled secret evidence gath-ered during an underground sting operation. The FDA had sent two agents posing as patients into both the Texas and Pennsylvania clinics. Neither had cancer, yet both testified they were diagnosed with the disease. Dr. Harry Spence of Dallas confirmed on the stand that he had examined FDA agent Euclid Gulledge prior to his visit to the clinic and found him in perfect health. Gulledge said that Hoxsey himself examined him and diagnosed prostate cancer.[4] The government also reveled in the recent death of one of Hoxsey's prize "cures," little Kathy Allison, who had suc-cumbed to her cancer after all. Meanwhile in Texas, one of Hoxsey's own doctors died of cancer after a failed trip to the Mayo Brothers Clinic.[5] The credibility of Hoxsey's cures was badly undermined, although he countered with the testimony of two medical doctors reputedly cured of cancer in Dallas, including Dr. Eva Hill of New Zealand.[6]

The trial was thick with skullduggery. A Dallas physician subpoenaed to testify about patients who died after taking the Hoxsey treatment had instructed his office to ship the medical records to the hotel where he would be staying. The night he arrived, he laid the records out on his bed next to his briefcase and left for dinner. When he came back, the records were gone. Following his testimony the next day, he returned to his hotel room to find the documents mysteriously reconstituted on his bed.[7]

The government again cited Hoxsey's pamphlets as false labeling, but this time there was a strange twist. The prosecution focused on the clinic brochure's faithful reproduction of a report critical of surgery and radia-tion. The study was originally published by the Government Printing Office and Hoxsey reprinted it verbatim from the Congressional Record.[8] His fate would ride on this controversial document.

The story behind the government-issue report was tangled indeed. Dr. George Miley, director of the Gotham Hospital in New York, had previously testified before a congressional committee in 1946 about a survey conducted by his close associate, Dr. Stanley Riemann of Pennsyl-vania. Dr. Miley's summary of the survey revealed that over a long period of time cancer patients lived longer if they did not receive surgery, X-ray, and radium treatments. The study further showed that the use of surgery and radiation did "more harm than good" to cancer patients.[9] Benedict FitzGerald quoted it in his report to Congress, exactly as it had been entered into the Congressional Record.

Dr. Riemann subsequently changed his tune, protesting that his survey was never completed or published, and was thus invalid. He said he informed the Senate committee of his objections and was told that his refutation would be published as an addendum. But it never did appear in the Senate report or anywhere else.[10]

Under cross-examination in Pittsburgh, Dr. Riemann revealed that, following Dr. Miley's Senate testimony, he came under attack from the American Cancer Society and other physicians who disputed his findings.[11] Was Dr. Riemann altering his conclusions because of peer pressure and the threat of professional censure?

An internal FDA memorandum revealed yet another layer of the controversy gleaned from an FDA visit to Dr. Miley in his New York office. The physician observed that surgery was often used when it should not have been, causing the disease to spread. He noted that Dr. Riemann was also concerned about the presence of extensive X-ray burns in many cancer cases and had wanted the abuse of X-ray therapy brought out at the hearing.[12]

However, Dr. Miley confessed that the attendant publicity about the disconcerting survey "caused havoc in the medical profession. X-ray physicians were vexed about it." He added that "Dr. Riemann got hell from the X-ray men." It was only then that Dr. Riemann disavowed the study. Both doctors retreated to saying that it was just the *abuse* of surgery and radiation to which they objected, not the treatments themselves.

The FDA did not disclose the extenuating context that the doctors were under intense professional pressure not to criticize conventional cancer treatments publicly. Because Dr. Riemann's retraction was never inserted into the official record, Hoxsey could not have known about it when he republished it in his literature.[13]

When the polarized sides finally rested their cases, the judge made a highly unorthodox charge to the jury. He stated that Hoxsey's representation of Dr. Riemann's study should be considered false labeling because the doctor disclaimed the report. The judge further directed the jury that the validity of only *one* count was needed for a guilty verdict.[14] His instructions ensured a conviction.

Bad omens were abounding for Hoxsey in Pittsburgh. After Haluska's election loss, the ex-lawmaker ominously announced he was going to make some kind of deal with the government. Then on the Sunday night before the jury was to go into deliberations, General Electric Theater broadcast a national TV program called *The Charlatan*, starring George Sanders, who bore an uncanny physical resemblance to Hoxsey. The drama told the tale of a quack who knew all the angles, won a big jury trial, then got cancer and underwent the very surgery he told his patients to refuse.[15] Later that week, the Portage Hoxsey Clinic was found guilty of false labeling in interstate commerce.[16]

A dizzying round of legal skirmishes followed, resulting first in an injunction against shipping the medicines from the Pennsylvania clinic. It also forbade treating out-of-state patients if the clinic continued advertising its treatment as a cure.[17] Ultimately, the clinic burned all its literature and kept treating patients from all over the country. Hoxsey's request for a new trial was denied, and by 1958, Haluska decided to close the clinic.[18] Yet another crusading legislator folded under the sheer tonnage of medical politics. Only the Los Angeles and Dallas clinics were left standing.

In the wake of its victory, organized medicine zeroed in on Dallas while Hoxsey struggled to reach out nationally. He released his incendiary autobiography, ghostwritten by *Man's Magazine* writer Allen Bernard, who was now writing for *Life* and *Newsweek* as well.[19] Eternally optimistic, Hoxsey wrote, "I am fifty-four years young. For thirty-five of those years I have been kicked, hounded, persecuted and prosecuted because I've treated cancer with medicine and without the use of surgery, X-ray or radium. As the poet says, I've stood 'like a beaten anvil' on the theory

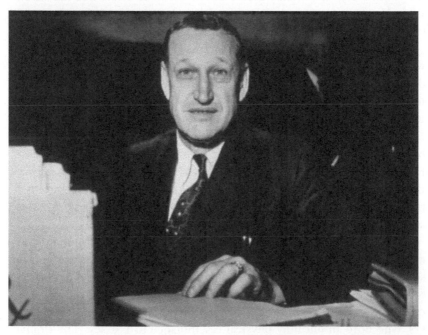

Ever optimistic, Hoxsey finds the legal tide about to turn against him.

that the more they beat, the louder the noise; the louder the noise, the bigger the audience; and the bigger the audience, the sooner the truth shall be known. 'The anvil wears out the hammers,' you know."[20]

But now it seemed the hammers were wearing out the anvil. Desperate to get the word out, Hoxsey made his own movie at the Dallas clinic. Battle-worn and ill, he roared to the camera, "I'm swimming in blood now. They've done everything they possibly can to try to humiliate me. They've had me in court many, many times. But do I care about that? I'm not thinking about what they're doing to me. I'm thinking about the twelve thousand patients under treatment and observation here at this clinic. I'm only thinking of one thing: suffering humanity."[21]

Mildred Nelson recollected that while the film was being made, the sympathetic cameraman came to Hoxsey and warned him that it was too hot to handle and would never see the light of day. "Give me $7,000, and I'll get you a print of it," the cameraman reportedly propositioned him. Hoxsey paid up, got the print, and sure enough the film negative disappeared. He charged that the AMA had purchased the negative for $1 million.[22]

Hoxsey attracted further derision with the commencement of his latest enterprise: "bonded eggs" from chickens fed the tonic. He claimed that cancer was at times a virus, and that chicken eggs were a principal

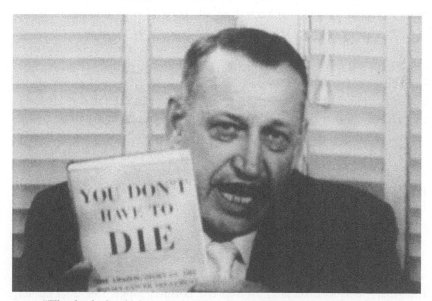

"This book should have been printed on asbestos paper," says Hoxsey of his incendiary autobiography, 1954.

disease vector. His North Carolina farm was set to supply the nation with virus-free, tonic-fed eggs.[23]

Arguably the largest natural health movement in modern times swelled around the unorthodox healer. Two Hoxsey clinics were getting under way in Los Angeles, where Hoxsey addressed rallies of 10,000 people sponsored by the National Health Federation, a large alternative medical rights group he helped finance.[24] Ubiquitous FDA agents scanned license plates and tapped phones.[25] They tried to block his increasing appearances on national TV talk shows and radio broadcasts.[26] *Time, Newsweek, Life*, and Walter Winchell blasted him in acerbic articles.[27] Hoxsey lashed back from a San Diego gospel radio station at the doctors who "cut, burn, bake, and bar-b-que" cancer patients.[28] He rallied his agitated audiences against the FDA, which he charged was "dominated, controlled and dictated to by the Drug Trust," and vowed to "fight them and beat their brains out."[29] In frustration, he threatened to market the tonic as a patent medicine without making any curative claims for it.[30]

There was no doubt it was a full-on firefight. Hoxsey's son remembered leaving the clinic with his father for a hunting trip up to Colorado. Several blocks down the road, bullets shattered their windshield. Badly shaken, they turned back and went home. No suspects were ever named.[31]

Organized medicine's war of technicalities expanded into a bold series of new stratagems to get Hoxsey. When the Texas Board of Medical Examiners canceled the medical licenses of all seven Hoxsey doctors in 1955, Hoxsey challenged the action.[32] Judge Thornton, slated to hear the case, had to disqualify himself because of his prior rulings favoring Hoxsey, saying, "I agreed with the jury's findings that these particular witnesses had been cured [of cancer]."[33] Instead, the hostile Judge Charles Long stepped in. To the judge's chagrin, the jury found in favor of the Hoxsey clinic in the trial of the first doctor, permitting him to keep practicing there.[34]

Judge Long then unilaterally reversed the favorable jury decision. He cited an obscure precedent barring doctors from working for a layperson.[35] He applied the statute to the other Hoxsey doctors, denied them jury trials, and uniformly suspended their licenses for eighteen months.[36] In principle, the same law should have put most hospitals out of business, since they are owned and operated by laypeople. It was enforced only against Hoxsey.

In another lateral swipe, the Texas Attorney General declared the 1949 state statute legalizing naturopathy to be unconstitutional, a judgment the AMA had been seeking around the country since 1949.[37] The act negated Hoxsey's only legitimate medical credential. Without it, he could no longer operate his clinic.

Hoxsey abruptly found himself out of the cancer business. To comply with the law, he was compelled to lease the clinic to one of his physicians, Dr. Harry Taylor.[38] "The main reason," Hoxsey said, "was that I was interested in those patients having attention, and to treat those patients out. I'm telling you and I'm telling everybody that they will never be turned out, even if I have to start a free clinic and do it with the Hoxsey Oil Company. I'm never going to see those twelve thousand people turned out in the street. I love them. They might die today, and they are American citizens and have a right to live just like anybody else."[39]

The FDA immediately slapped Dr. Taylor with an injunctive decree against shipping medicines or literature interstate. He protested that he was doing neither, but the government responded that his treating out-of-state patients violated the "spirit of the injunction," and ridiculed the doctor as a "crybaby." An internal FDA memorandum stated, "Dr. Taylor is beating the bushes for osteopaths. He is getting desperate."[40] All the Hoxsey doctors except Taylor lost the battle to retain their licenses, and the Texas Supreme Court refused to hear their appeal. The nation's Supreme Court also shunned the case.[41]

The dice were going cold for Hoxsey. His supporter Gerald Winrod died suddenly of pneumonia in 1957 just as the Winrod-sponsored Fremont Christian Clinic in Los Angeles opened in the old Hollywood Mineral Baths on Melrose Avenue under a permanent stakeout by the FDA and California health authorities. Hoxsey helped inaugurate a twenty-six-room clinic in nearby Monrovia.[42] With Winrod buried, Hoxsey adopted yet another notorious man of the cloth, the infamous Kenneth Goff. Together they addressed huge rallies.[43] At one such gathering in Santa Ana, California, according to an FDA surveillance report, Goff "in his own rancorous way attacked the Jews, the Food and Drug Administration, the American Medical Association, Paul Coates, communists, Eleanor Roosevelt, the UN, and the general state of government today, casting a spell of doom on the assemblage."[44]

Challenging local doctors to a debate, Hoxsey was rebuffed by the president of the Los Angeles County Medical Association. "We would never go out and debate with a man like Hoxsey, as such a debate implies there are two sides to a question."[45]

By 1958 the historically permissive California medical climate was convulsing with sharp political contractions. State Attorney General Caspar Weinberger introduced a bill sponsored by the American Cancer Society to outlaw all unconventional cancer treatments.[46] The hearings turned into a ferocious altercation as a horde of incensed unorthodox practitioners and cancer patients packed the halls. Hoxsey refused to testify because he was allotted only one hour.[47] Many others did speak in ardent protest against the exclusionary regulations, including Dr. Andrew Ivy, who denounced the FDA's investigation of Krebiozen. For the first time, he publicly revealed his confidential visit to Hoxsey's clinic many years before, and although he still doubted the treatment's value, he called for its fair investigation. He suggested that one or two ingredients might have anticancer effects, and acknowledged that he had personally seen two or three patients whose cancers disappeared, possibly a result of the treatment.[48]

Under California's new anti-quackery laws in 1959, it became a crime to treat cancer with anything but surgery, radiation, and the emerging chemotherapy.[49] The only exemption was for religious beliefs and prayer, since Weinberger had Christian Scientists in his family. (Weinberger later became Secretary of Health, Education, and Welfare, which oversaw the FDA, and then Secretary of Defense under Ronald Reagan.) The restrictive California laws were soon adopted by other states.

In 1958 a delegation of doctors from British Columbia came to the Taylor Clinic to investigate after a member of Parliament became a Hoxsey enthusiast.[50] The delegation first stopped by the AMA and National Cancer Institute, and after visiting Dallas went on to meet with the American Cancer Society and FDA.[51] The report found "no evidence whatsoever of a cure."[52] For decades to come, the American Cancer Society's influential pamphlet, "Unproven Methods of Cancer Management," listed this visit as its sole citation of a definitive scientific investigation of Hoxsey.[53]

On September 16, 1960, Dr. Harry Taylor signed a consent order mandating the "complete and final discontinuation of the Hoxsey Treatment."[54] He was ordered to tell all 10,270 Hoxsey patients that the treatment was no longer available. At the time, the clinic had over 25,000 case histories of cancer patients on file.[55] The government issued a statement that the federal court had terminated "the last remaining major source of the worthless and discredited Hoxsey Cancer Treatment."[56]

In December, FDA agents raided the Taylor Clinic and seized 22,500 capsules "being illegally used in the treatment of internal cancer." Tabbed "Dr. Taylor's Special Formula 'L,'" the capsules contained laetrile, an extract of apricot pits purported to contain an anticancer substance.[57] Laetrile would soon replace the Hoxsey tonic as the next poster child of cancer quackery in organized medicine's ongoing campaign against unconventional therapies.

"Harry fought 'em longer and harder than anyone," Mildred Nelson told our camera. "He had a big mouth, and he did a lot of talking. But it didn't do any good. Politics is bigger than one man any day."[58]

As the 1950s drew to a close, the government quackdown was nearly complete. It had taken the full power of the state apparatus to eliminate Hoxsey and the host of other unorthodox cancer practitioners from the medical playing field. Employing its virtually unlimited resources, the government politicized the courts to determine medical questions. In the aftermath of the McCarthy era, the political theater of demagoguery cast quacks as the subhuman "ghouls" populating Dr. Fishbein's Devil theory of history. There was simply no room for a difference of medical opinion.

Those politicians who had dared support Hoxsey, such as Senators Thomas, Langer, and Haluska, were systematically driven from office by AMA political action. Respected judges like William Atwell had their decisions reversed in star chambers, while juries saw their verdicts unilaterally overturned by partisan judges. Doctors such as Miley and Riemann suffered professional censure for pointing out the limitations of conventional cancer treatments or suggesting new directions in research.

The ingrown configuration of the AMA, FDA, NCI, FDA, and federal prosecutors bound the weave tight in the monocultural blanket smothering the diversity of potentially promising medical approaches to cancer. Even the fact that the government and AMA conceded that Hoxsey's external remedies are effective did not lead to a test or acceptance. Admissions don't get much more tacit. Nor did the acknowledged fact of the salves' efficacy spark any curiosity that the internal tonic just might be worth looking into.

Organized medicine's scorched-earth campaign to eradicate unorthodox cancer therapies was a success by 1960, when the last tattered vestige of the Hoxsey Cancer Clinic closed its doors forever in the United States. Or so it seemed.

Mexican Standoff

While filming at the Tijuana Hoxsey clinic, we met Fred Walsh, a patient first treated in Dallas in 1958 for cancer of the forehead and nose. He recalled going over to see the now absent former owner, Harry Hoxsey. "I met him in the Oilman's Building on the expressway, and I had quite a visit. I was surprised to find that his office, instead of being filled with oil reports, was filled with filing cabinets. He remembered who I was immediately, and went to the files, which I figured were oil leases. Instead he pulled out my medical records. He wasn't a man you could turn back easily."[1]

Hoxsey continued quietly treating a few patients himself on the sly, despite heavy surveillance. The FDA tried to entrap him at least once in 1961, but he cannily evaded the phony request for treatment.[2] Dr. Taylor may have kept using the Hoxsey treatment under the table, and Dr. Joseph Durkee had gone underground with it years before.[3]

"Harry was wrecked out totally when he had to leave the clinic," Mildred recalled. "Physically and mentally, very, very distraught about it. His whole life had been spent trying to put this to the people so that they could get well if they wanted to. It took about three or four years for him to even begin to get his feet on the ground solid. He was bitter, because nowhere had he done anything wrong. There were many, many people across the whole country who were well as a result of it, and he was proud of it. He always said, 'Someday this will be accepted.' He never doubted it one moment. Certainly he thought his whole life had been wrecked out by not being able to go on with it. He was the most miserable person I'd ever seen."[4]

Hoxsey dispatched Mildred Nelson Cates, still carrying the name of her former husband, on the road, first to Reno, Nevada, and then to Long Beach, California, to work with a Dr. Nelson Mathisen. Mildred sent out a discreet Christmas card to former Hoxsey patients informing them that the "original form of Chemotherapy" was now being offered in Long Beach.

"Know this will be a shock to all," she wrote to a patient, "but we are carrying on in the same old manner. Suggest you contact Harry if any doubt."[5]

For Mildred it was a daunting new game. "When I left Dallas around 1959, I was totally lost. I had never thought there'd be a day when I couldn't go next door and say, 'Harry, what do we do about this or that?' I was on my own. It was frightening to have all this responsibility dumped on you all of a sudden."

Mildred's peregrinations did not go unnoticed. "The [California] State people have the [Long Beach] office under surveillance," read an FDA internal memorandum, "and are checking out the license plates of visitors. People leave the premises with brown paper bags, in the manner the Hoxsey treatment was distributed in Dallas. Purpose of the broad State efforts is to work up a case under California's new cancer quackery law."[6] Another memo stated that "Mildred Cates, one of Hoxsey's former nurses, appears to be the moving spirit behind these enterprises and we have some evidence that she in turn may be Hoxsey's personal representative."[7]

The FDA also started using a "mail cover," cooperating with the U.S. Post Office to monitor correspondence. The FDA was unable, however, to obtain sufficient evidence for prosecution or an injunction, despite being "prepared to make the same kind of lengthy and expensive investigation which we had to make in Dallas if it were necessary to stop the duping of the public by Mildred Cates and the osteopaths she employs."[8]

When Dr. Mathisen had a heart attack, Mildred motored to Bountiful, Utah.[9] The state had long been a haven of Hoxsey support because of the Mormon community's commitment to the use of herbs as biblical medicines. Mildred said the head of the Mormon church used to send hundreds of patients to Dallas. (Utah is today the largest herb-producing state in the country.)

Working with a Dr. Homer Cate, Mildred set up shop in Bountiful in 1962. Once again, the FDA found patients "extremely uncooperative" in government efforts to bust the clinic.[10] One agent proposed sending his own wife as an informer along with another FDA investigator, since she had nonmalignant lumps on her breast.[11] The FDA collected license plate numbers in the parking lot and at the nearby Dreamland Motel, and monitored all correspondence.[12]

In a mix-up worthy of the Marx Brothers, at one point the FDA, Bountiful police, the FBI, and Army Intelligence discovered each other staked out around the clinic. The Army was looking for a hot car used by a deserter and had noticed unusual traffic at the remote spot. The FBI was also suspicious of the anomalous activity, surmising it might involve the white slave trade.[13]

In Utah the FDA was surreptitiously contacted by J. J. Cates, Mildred's ex-husband, who volunteered to inform on her. An FDA internal memo reported that "'they' had cut him out of the money and he was a fellow to which the saying 'misery loves company' applies." But Cates never showed up for a clandestine airport meeting, leaving word that his mother got sick, and he had to leave town.[14]

In 1962, while visiting Utah, Hoxsey ordered Mildred back to Dallas. She loaded up her car and hit the road, followed by the moving truck transporting the clinic belongings. Five days after she reached Dallas, the truck finally showed up, accompanied by FDA agents who had sequestered the driver in Salt Lake City and cataloged all the contents.

The FDA then tried to entrap Mildred. "I went down to where we were going to unload in a storage room," Mildred recalled, "and as I get out of the car to go over to the building, here comes two this way, two that way, and two from over there. I said, 'Well, have you boys had a nice trip?' They nearly fell over. And as the boys were unloading, he asked me, 'Are these your products?' And I said, 'No, they're on the truck that I brought my things on, but as you see, there're bills from Dr. Cate to Dr. Lowell. I'm just a dumb nurse, and there's no way I can buy or sell a vitamin or anything else, and you know it.' 'But they're yours.' 'No, they're not mine.'

"They stood around and they said, 'Don't bother these until we tell you you can.' We got everything in the office unloaded there, and I was going out to the house to unload. They followed me to the house and the truck. And here they stand in the way, and finally I told them, 'I'm going to tell you something. Either, goddamn it, you start unloading furniture or you leave. Either one you want to do, but you've been in the way all day and I'm tired of it and I'm moving in right here. So you can tap the phone, you can do any damn thing you want to do, but this is where I live."[15]

The FDA seized the "misbranded drugs" and noted in its report a permanent injunction against Mildred Cates from practicing nursing in Utah.[16] By this time the outlaw nurse was familiar with the rules of the road, but says she could never get used to the life.

Mildred went to work briefly with Dr. Durkee in Dallas, who was by now an alcoholic. It was a disaster. Then Harry Hoxsey called her into his office in the Hoxsey Oil Company. "I was the most surprised person you ever saw when he said, 'You've got it to go from here on. I've gone as far as I can go. They've wanted us in Mexico for a long time. Get off your butt and find somebody to help you because these people have got to be taken care of.' He was just about that kind about it. He always said things very point-blank. Up until then, it was always, 'We'll do this and we'll do that.' But that time it was 'You.' I was as lost as could be. Horrified. Can you imagine having that responsibility dumped in your lap? I couldn't believe it!"

Then came the bombshell. "And he said, 'The one thing I want you to do is drop the Hoxsey name. Change the name.' I said, 'Harry, people won't even know what it is if we do that!' 'No, the problem has been the Hoxsey name. Drop the name and it will be easier for you.' Well, I dropped the name, but the patients didn't. It's still to them, 'Hoxsey.'"[17]

On May Day 1963, Mildred Nelson crossed the border into Mexico. She had been in every other border town from Matamoros to Mexicali, but never Tijuana. She got a tiny office building near the downtown bull ring when the city was small and personal, and started offering the treatment at the Biochemical Research Institute. Later renamed the Bio Medical Center, it moved to another small perch high atop Avenida General Ferreira. Mildred Bell Nelson now applied to the Mexican authorities for a nursing license, and married a Mexican to get working papers. Nurse Mildred Zamora was in business in Mexico.

The FDA continued its surveillance of "the Hoxsey business thriving in Tijuana." Expecting runners to be bringing the medication for distribution on the American side, agents alerted customs officers and arrested two patients at the border.[18]

In 1965 FDA agents and officers of the sheriff's department posing as patients showed up at San Diego's Singing Wheels Trailer Park. An undercover agent told Mrs. Edith Crampton, "Mildred sent me for my medicine," and asked if it was the genuine article. The unsuspecting resident replied that it was the real thing and "that my husband had been cured of cancer with it." Mrs. Crampton was immediately arrested by police descending from all directions. They found only the one bottle of tonic in an exhaustive search. "Mrs. Crampton then became very uncooperative," the FDA report stated, "and refused to answer additional questions. The search lasted approximately one-and-a-half hours, and Mrs. Crampton spent the majority of this time loudly reading from the Bible and singing hymns." Another arrest was made later at the trailer park.[19]

Then Mildred's ex-husband, the duplicitous Johnny Cates, turned up again, offering to help the FDA entrap her. On two years' probation for a customs violation, he was looking to lighten his sentence. Cates informed the agents that a German physician friend of Hoxsey's, Dr. Schultz, was now handling diagnosis and physical exams. "Mildred lives in Tijuana and rarely crosses the border," Cates went on. He displayed stolen receipt books, and confided that Mildred "flatly refuses to ship drugs either via mail or common carrier." He added that Mildred paid off a Mexican health inspector $100 a month.

According to an FDA memo, Cates suggested that "the easiest way to close the clinic would be to offer the local health inspector more money than he received from Mildred. Another approach would be the arrest of Mildred by customs officials at the border in a car containing non-declared drugs. Johnny Cates was certain Mildred would not cross the border even under an emergency situation to treat a patient. He did say, however, that he personally might be able to induce her to cross the border in a car with the Hoxsey medicine for a big sale on this side." It never happened.[20]

Mildred settled comfortably into Tijuana. She especially liked being able to double-park without consequences. She found the medical community welcoming and open. Patients began to come to the Bio Medical Center, but to them it was still "Hoxsey."

In 1967 *Medical World News*, a prominent AMA publication, ran a sensational piece on the new spate of Tijuana clinics. Featuring a photo of nurse Mildred Zamora, "Cancer Victims" set a seamy scene. "Like most Mexican border towns, Tijuana is a place where *gringos* come to cut loose. Pandering to this fact, men and boys swarm along the Avenida Revolución, furtively offering an astonishing variety of wares and services. Depending on taste and need, the visitor can buy cheap liquor, a quickie marriage or divorce, marijuana, or a pornographic movie.

"But one other item blatantly offered in Tijuana has nothing to do with pleasure. 'Cancer treatments,' with a variety of preparations and regimens that have been discredited or legally banned in the U.S., are available in a number of store-front clinics scattered among the town's scrubby streets. For desperate Americans with confirmed or imaginary cancer, Tijuana is the end of the line.

"A statuesque red-haired RN, Mrs. Zamora used to be chief nurse at the Dallas clinic run by Harry M. Hoxsey, whose 'cancer remedy' first appeared in the early 1920s and managed to survive a succession of exposures by medical authorities over the years."[21]

If the purple prose had a familiar ring to it, it should come as no surprise. The editor of *Medical World News* in 1967 was Dr. Morris Fishbein. Following a spell in Europe after he was deposed by the AMA, he returned to resume an illustrious career as a medical writer and professor at the University of Chicago. Several of his popular books (coauthor of twenty-seven and editor of sixteen) remain in print today, and a chair at the University of Chicago memorializes his name. He died a revered figure at the age of eighty-seven in 1976.[22]

Dr. Fishbein's legacy of quackbusting proved to be eminently durable. By the mid-1960s, the Hoxsey and Koch treatments had been permanently driven out of the United States. Dr. Lincoln's treatment disappeared from view, as did at least a dozen other promising unorthodox cancer therapies that never got a scientific investigation.

Only Dr. Ivy kept up the fight. A featherweight boxing champion in the Army, he was not one to quit. In 1963 the FDA conducted a "test" of Krebiozen by analyzing its chemistry. The agency identified it as creatine monohydrate, an amino acid present in all animal tissue and "without value in the treatment of cancer." Other FDA laboratory analyses claimed it to be nothing more than mineral oil. [23] A National Cancer Institute committee of twenty-four experts reviewed 504 case records and found unanimously that Krebiozen was worthless.[24]

The FDA followed with a forty-nine-count federal indictment for fraud and conspiracy against Dr. Ivy and his compatriots Dr. Stefan Durovic and his brother, a business manager.[25] Because the drug was unapproved, its interstate distribution was illegal. A jury trial dragged on for nine months in 1965 in federal court in Chicago. Dr. Ivy appeared in court every day because, he said, "this has become a way of life."[26]

Krebiozen advocates turned out in great numbers to block the door to the FDA commissioner's office with vocal sit-ins. Eleven U.S. senators called for another investigation of the promising drug, but the FDA rejected the plea, saying, "Data from tests conducted in animals was totally inadequate to justify FDA approval to test Krebiozen in humans."[27]

The defendants were acquitted on all counts. Dr. Ivy, then seventy-two years old, vowed he would "wait until the smoke of battle clears" before seeking another test.[28] "I have no regrets because I have seen a lot of people relieved of pain and their lives apparently prolonged by the use of this drug. I have no regrets because my first objective as a scientist is to hang on to this theory of the existence of an anticancer substance in the bodies of all multicellular animals, and all *multicellular plants*," a coded reference endorsing Hoxsey's herbs, after all.[29]

Dr. Ivy remained philosophical to the end. "When you come forward with a committee opinion to kill a scientific theory or destroy scientific observations, you're living in the past, in the dark ages of medicine. It is high time that when something new comes on the horizon which apparently is going to prolong life or alleviate suffering, we should all get together and work on it to try to decrease the scientific lag."[30]

Following the national television airing of a high-profile special about Dr. Ivy's struggle, Krebiozen sympathizer Reverend Virgil A. Kraft preached to his Chicago congregation. "Man's deadliest cancer is the selfishness of any man or any group of men who tremble at the prospect of putting any investigation or discovery which might benefit mankind to a fair test, simply because such a test might cost them a little prestige, or a little power, or a little money."[31]

Other Ivy supporters were considerably less kind in their assessment of the FDA. They estimated the costs of the criminal trial alone at over $1 million, with a total of $20 million spent by organized medicine to prevent a Krebiozen test over the fifteen-year ordeal. As an Ivy support group wrote, "There has been displayed in the whole of this sordid transaction a wantonness of additional persecution and ruffian-like ferocity by the United States attorney, rarely incident to the most depraved and obdurate of our species. On an indictment admittedly grounded on vicious, illegal and unconstitutional procedures involving spurious and faked letters by inspectors of the Food and Drug Administration, spurious and faked clinical records of imaginary cancer victims by unscrupulous physicians deliberately manufactured in a concerted conspiracy with the scalawags of the Food and Drug Administration to entrap and ensnare the proponents of Krebiozen into alleged and manufactured felonies, the United States Attorney General put on trial Dr. Andrew C. Ivy, Dr. Stefan Durovic, and Dr. William F. P. Phillips. The purpose of this trial was not really to legally convict these great scientists, but to bankrupt them financially and spiritually. There could be no conviction on the evidence presented."[32]

Dr. Durovic, whose health was destroyed by the tribulations, emigrated to Switzerland. Dr. Ivy continued working through the Ivy Cancer Research Foundation on Carcalon, as he now called it, supported by wealthy and prominent allies. Krebiozen disappeared with Dr. Ivy's death a decade later in 1977.

When Mildred Nelson went into exile in Tijuana, Harry Hoxsey stayed in Dallas. As his son told me, "He was from a different era. He lived three lives in one. By the end he was like a wore-out car. Everything just broke down at once."[33] After suffering a heart attack in 1958, he was never fully well again. A teetotaler, he nevertheless remained a confirmed steak-and-potatoes man and a smoker.

James Burke remained close with him.[34] "After Harry finally was driven out of business into retirement, he was such a restless, driving man that he could not be happy in retirement. He developed cancer of the prostate. He refused to see a surgeon, and he applied his own medicine, believing thoroughly that he was going to cure himself. He did it a long time and it did not cure him. Finally, his wife took him to the surgeon and they operated on him, but it was too late to make him well. He lingered on about seven years as an invalid in bed. He contradicted his main thesis, as he told his patients, 'Don't let them doctors cut on you because that won't cure you.'

"I never asked him what he thought about having taken the tonic for himself. He never told me he tried to cure himself. His wife told me. He kept his counsel to himself. I would say, if you asked me to venture a guess, that he went to his grave believing in it, because it didn't work with everybody. He probably thought, 'Well, it didn't work with me, but it worked on others. I'm just the unlucky one it didn't work on.' He was rather bitter at the doctors who operated on him. There was some suspicion in his mind that because he was Harry Hoxsey, the high priest of quacks in their view, that they deliberately cut a little too much on him. I never believed that."

Then James Burke faced an existential test of fire. "Coincidentally, I too developed the exact same cancer. With Harry being like a brother to me all these years, I discussed it with him. He kept his counsel to himself. But day after day I'd bring it up and I'd say, 'Harry, what shall I do?' He never once told me to take his pills or his medicine. Finally, one day I said, 'Harry, they're going to give me a maximum of two years, and I've got to decide. What do you say?' He thought for a long time and said, 'Jimmy, go let them sons of bitches cut it out.'"

Harry Hoxsey then closed the curtain on a Shakespearean fifth act. As Burke recalled, "After I had my cancer and was cured, I arranged to have my doctor, who is one of the most famous neurologists in the world—he's called on to go to Tokyo, Brazil—to attend Hoxsey, and that was Hoxsey's last doctor of record. Dr. Paul Peters told me that Hoxsey was free of cancer. But Hoxsey had a weak heart and he was an aging man, and he couldn't last very long. I pinned my doctor down, and he said it was liver trouble and a weak heart. He stated over and over that Hoxsey was free of cancer, and this man came to his house and treated him about every other day.

"Hoxsey died when this doctor was away," Burke continued. "He could not be called to sign the death certificate. An unknown doctor from the phone book or called by the nurse came who knew nothing about the case. Somebody had to sign a death certificate to get the body out of the room into the morgue. This doctor looked at his record and the chart and he saw 'radical surgery, carcinoma.' This new man wrote on the death certificate, 'Carcinoma, prostate.'

"When my doctor returned and I told him about this, he said 'This is not correct. I attended Hoxsey the day before he died and I was surprised he lived through the night. His heart was failing at that time and he died of heart failure and old age. Please have somebody send that to me, and that's what I want to write on it. I'm his doctor of record.' It's clear that Hoxsey did not have cancer when he died. Whether his own tonic together with surgery cured him, or whether the tonic cured him, or whether the surgery, who knows?" I verified Burke's assertions in a personal interview with Dr. Paul Peters, who confirmed that Hoxsey did not have cancer when he died.[35] But he never corrected the death certificate.

"While he was on his deathbed," Burke recollected philosophically, "I was tempted to tell him that his pills and his tonic were no good, that he was curing people with his own power and magnetism, making them cure themselves. I wanted to tell him how he cured them like Jesus Christ did.

"I never did tell him because I wanted to be sure myself. Now, as time goes on, looking back, maybe his medicine, his herbs and nostrums, maybe they did cure. He was only using derivatives of what Indians made cures from and what the ancient Greeks used. I'm glad now I didn't tell him, because just maybe Harry was way ahead of his time and he had a cure, or some part of a cure, for cancer. I can never be sure how he did it. One thing is certain from my viewpoint: He did make people well from cancer."

Burke paused, sighed, and recalled a rueful exchange he shared with his dying friend. "On his deathbed, I went to see him every other day or sometimes twice a day, and we'd talk about old friends and old times and good times and bad times. Harry would suddenly get a faraway look in his eye and he'd say 'Jimmy, we could have beat them sons of bitches!'"

As we filmed this poignant rememberance with James Burke, his wife, Angela, joined us. A stately, silver-haired woman in an azure dress, she too had a story.[36] "I first met Harry in May in 1955. My husband and our three-year-old son and I were returning from living in Germany for many years. Harry and his wife invited us to stay with them when we first came to Dallas, and we did for a time until Harry helped us find an apartment. He was most kind and gracious, and so was his wife. That fall after we got settled in, there came a call from my mother, who had just been diagnosed as having uterine cancer. She was very upset, very worried. She wanted to know what we thought about her coming down here and having the Hoxsey treatment.

"I didn't want to give her a recommendation to absolutely come or absolutely don't come. I felt she had to make up her own mind about that. What she didn't say was that the doctor had told my father and one of her sisters that he expected her to live only about six months, or at the very most a year. That part she didn't know. She did decide to come down here and have the Hoxsey treatment.

"She was here for about three weeks. She went home with her medication, and did come back some months later for a checkup. By that time she was well on her way to recovery, according to the doctors here at Hoxsey's clinic. She did not have any further serious health problems and certainly no recurrence of the cancer until 1980, twenty-five years later, when she then did develop a malignant brain tumor."

"Don't you think, Angela," Jim asked, turning to his wife, "that the irony, if not the tragedy, of our old friend Harry Hoxsey was that in his last days there was no Harry Hoxsey to minister to Harry Hoxsey?"

"Yes, he had been there for so many people throughout his lifetime. He certainly was there for my mother, and for hundreds and probably thousands of other people, but there was nobody there for him."

Largely forgotten, Harry Hoxsey was buried in Dallas by a small clutch of family and friends just before Christmas in 1974. He died without an obituary in the Dallas papers. Yet even in death, Harry Hoxsey was marked by a conflict of medical opinion.

The test that Harry Hoxsey sought never happened. It would be another several years after his burial before our film and other independent researchers would pick up the trail and precipitate for the first time a serious look into the medicines Hoxsey claimed could cure cancer. The findings would be startling.

PART TWO

A Conflict of Medical Opinion

The Hoxsey Remedies vs. Conventional Cancer Treatments

"What is a weed? A plant whose virtues have not yet been discovered."

Ralph Waldo Emerson

Tempest in a Tonic Bottle: A Bunch of Weeds?

For decades organized medicine ridiculed the Hoxsey remedies as a bunch of "weeds" and refused to look into them. Typifying this kind of cavalier dismissal was a classic 1940s archival medical film we located called *Fraud Fighters*.[1] Cast in much the same style as the heavy-handed antimarijuana propaganda film *Reefer Madness*, the melodramatic movie relates the parable of "Elixerex," an ersatz nostrum in a thinly disguised Hoxsey-like tonic bottle. Under the *Dragnet*-style narration, the movie follows Elixerex through the FDA's 1950s state-of-the-art labs, which today look as archaic as the era's Univac computer. Elixerex lands in the blocky hands of grim, square-jawed junior G-men intent on rounding up the unscrupulous crook behind the scam. The medical ideology is as black and white as the film footage.

"And now the Food and Drug people want to know," booms the narrator's voice over crescendos of music, "What is Elixerex? In every district station is a battery of crack chemists and microanalysts who fight the battle against filth and fraud. To one of these comes Elixerex. The magic formula to relieve sickness and pain turns out to be nothing more than a mixture of water and an alcoholic extract of certain herbaceous weeds that grow in profusion in the maker's backyard."

During Hoxsey's era, organized medicine took a uniformly contemptuous view of botanical medicine. Dr. Fishbein himself mocked herbs as "veritable vegetable soups."[2] It was in the unhappy wake of one of Hoxsey's court victories affirming the efficacy of his tonic that the AMA *Journal* echoed the FDA's frustration in its acerbically titled editorial "Cough Medicine for Cancer."[3] "It is fair to observe that the American Medical Association or any other association or individual has no need to go beyond the

Hoxsey label to be convinced. Any such person who would seriously contend that scientific medicine is under any obligation to investigate such a mixture or its promoter is either stupid or dishonest."

While sifting through the contentious terrain of the Hoxsey saga, I realized with consternation that no one seemed to have actually looked objectively at the ingredients of the Hoxsey tonic and salves. I decided to conduct an investigation for the film to ascertain what might be known about the herbs that caused this tempest in a tonic bottle.

In 1985 I set off for Washington, D.C., to meet with James Duke, Ph.D., a renowned botanist and author of twenty books and over two hundred scientific articles.[4] He has devoted his professional life to the study of pharmacognosy, the branch of pharmacy that develops medicines from natural sources. At the time, Dr. Duke worked for the U.S. Department of Agriculture (USDA), where he founded a world-class database on plant medicine. He also collaborated for many years with the National Cancer Institute as part of a modest government program for drug discovery from natural products including plants. Along with a small handful of other botanical explorers, Duke helped lead the way to plant medicines that have produced pharmaceutical drugs such as the cancer drug Taxol from the Pacific yew tree. During this period, the NCI reputedly screened about 10 percent of the plant species of the world, including all those in the Hoxsey formula.[5]

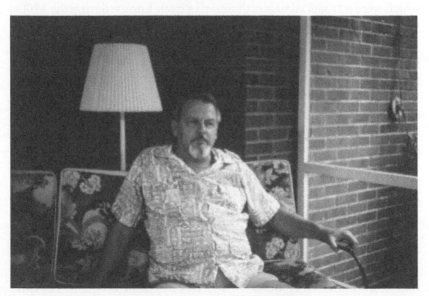

James Duke in his Maryland home.

I sent Duke the revised list of Hoxsey herbs published in the 1950s, which Mildred Nelson ostensibly continued to use. Duke decided to tap not only his own extensive USDA database, but also NAPRALERT, the Natural Products Alert computer database at the University of Illinois in Chicago. Founded by Dr. Norman Farnsworth, a globally revered pharmacognosist, NAPRALERT gathers data from scientific and medical studies all over the world on plants and other natural substances, and collates them into a comprehensive, centralized information source. It can sort the data into multiple categories of chemical properties and biological activities, a task ideally suited to computers working with gargantuan volumes of information.[6]

When I arrived at USDA headquarters in Beltsville, Maryland, Duke shuttled me to his nearby Herbal Vineyard, the small farm where he lives. A tall, gentlemanly figure sporting a trim goatee, he spoke in gentle, southern tones with understated authority. Guiding me around the lush Eastern deciduous forest, he delighted in pointing out a number of Hoxsey's "herbaceous weeds" growing in his own backyard. We inspected red clover, burdock, prickly ash, barberry, poke, and buckthorn, as well as bloodroot, the herb in one of the Hoxsey external formulas.

Duke noted that all the Hoxsey herbs have a long empirical tradition of Native American usage for cancer, several stretching back as far as three thousand years. Some of the herbs such as red clover and burdock, which were introduced to North America from Europe during the 1700s, were immediately adopted by the Indians.

Duke's first concern about the tonic was its safety, and he quickly pointed out that only one of the herbs, poke root, might be dangerous. A common plant throughout the Southeast, poke is a well-known herb and food to local residents, who like to parboil the leaves and add them to salads. The root, berry, and leaf are toxic in larger quantities. The amount in the Hoxsey tonic, however, is well below any threshold of danger. *[Warning: Do not even consider self-medicating with poke. Eating the leaves can also be toxic without proper preparation.]*

Back in Duke's study, stacked high with books, papers, and oversized reference works, he lifted a hefty three-pound volume called simply *Plants Used Against Cancer*. The encyclopedic tome was authored by Jonathan Hartwell, a chemist and virtual founder of the National Cancer Institute who went on to become an assistant chief of the NCI's new Cancer Chemotherapy National Service Center and head of the natural products section of the NCI's Drug Research and Development Program. Hartwell spent many years compiling a comprehensive cross-reference of information on the global folkloric traditions of anticancer plants. "The history of the herbal treatment of cancer," he wrote, is synonymous with "the history of medicine, indeed of civilization."[7] Covering more than three thousand species, Hartwell's compilation listed all the Hoxsey herbs. They ranged from having three to over thirty citations each—a very impressive score, Duke noted.[8]

A number of the plants, Duke pointed out, contained chemical compounds "of considerable interest" to the NCI. "At least three of the herbs—barberry, cascara sagrada, and buckthorn—contain compounds that have been studied by the Cancer Institute as effective in some tumor systems, though not studied in humans. So there are certainly biologically active compounds in these species."

The data Duke provided were sorted into several categories that indicate both the nature of the tests performed and their relevance to possible anticancer activities. One grouping was for *antioxidants*, which protect cells of the body against precancerous damage. Another was for *antimutagenic* properties, which shield against cellular mutations that can lead directly to cancer. A third was *cytotoxic* activity, which is a toxic action that can kill any cells, but is particularly effective at killing cancer cells since they are more sensitive by virtue of dividing so quickly. Another class of activity was *antimicrobial (antiseptic)*, consisting of both antibacterial and antiviral activity. Antibacterial properties are considered indicative of potential antitumor activity, while antiviral activity is important because some cancers are now believed to be caused by viruses (as Hoxsey asserted in the late 1950s).

Dr. Duke ultimately wrote a short article based on his Hoxsey research, published in 1988 in *HerbalGram*, the peer-reviewed journal of the respected American Botanical Council.[9] Eight of the nine herbs in the internal tonic showed antitumor activity in controlled laboratory animal tests. Five showed antioxidant properties as protectants against cancer. All showed antimicrobial properties with activity against viral or bacterial infections.

Duke's assessment was that the Hoxsey internal tonic ingredients showed very significant chemical and biological anticancer activity. The formulation might or might not actually work, but in principle it definitely merited serious investigation.*

---

*For readers interested in further technical aspects of the botanical information presented in this chapter, as well as a list of citations and sources of additional data, see the appendix along with the endnotes. Technical terms here are limited to a minimum, but those less interested in the specifics about the herbs and ingredients may want to skip to page 187.

In preparing this book, I revisited the initial 1985 herbal sleuthing begun by Jim Duke to learn what new data might have come on-line. I consulted again with Duke as well as with several other researchers who have conducted independent investigations into Hoxsey in what turned into a medical detective story. One of these was Francis Brinker, a naturopathic physician and scholar of botanical medicine who made his own visit to the Bio Medical Center in 1983. Brinker subsequently published a definitive article in the *Journal of Naturopathic Medicine* containing surprising conclusions about the Hoxsey tonic.[10]

Another was Patricia Spain Ward, Ph.D., an esteemed medical historian who prepared a contract report on Hoxsey for the federal Office of Technology Assessment, the former research arm of Congress. (The alarming episode of Ward's controversial report is told in chapter 17.) Finally, the American Botanical Council's executive director, Mark Blumenthal, supplied the most current update on the Hoxsey herbs from NAPRALERT, voluminous data filling 267 tightly spaced pages that Dennis McKenna, Ph.D., a prominent pharmacognosist, reviewed and appraised.

Before looking at these herbs, however, it is necessary to probe the mystery surrounding the secrecy of Hoxsey's formula. The list of ingredients I originally provided Jim Duke was the one published in Hoxsey's book in 1956.[11] That formula contained barberry, buckthorn bark, burdock root, cascara sagrada, licorice root, poke root, prickly ash, red clover blossoms, and stillingia root in a water base with potassium iodide.

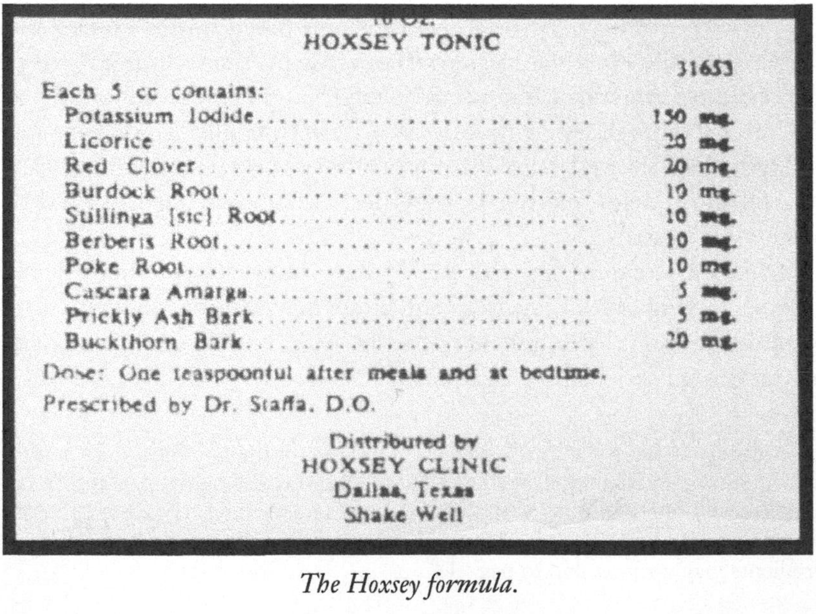

10 OZ.
HOXSEY TONIC

31653

Each 5 cc contains:

Potassium Iodide	150 mg.
Licorice	20 mg.
Red Clover	20 mg.
Burdock Root	10 mg.
Stillinga [sic] Root	10 mg.
Berberis Root	10 mg.
Poke Root	10 mg.
Cascara Amarga	5 mg.
Prickly Ash Bark	5 mg.
Buckthorn Bark	20 mg.

Dose: One teaspoonful after meals and at bedtime.

Prescribed by Dr. Staffa, D.O.

Distributed by
HOXSEY CLINIC
Dallas, Texas
Shake Well

The Hoxsey formula.

However, Hoxsey had previously given two different versions. After keeping its composition secret for twenty-five years, he first released it only under court order during the 1949 Hearst trial.[12] Several years later Hoxsey listed on his labels yet another recipe almost identical to the one published in his book.[13]

In court depositions Hoxsey admitted changing the formula over time, starting out with his original inheritance but significantly augmenting it under the direction of Dr. Joseph Durkee from 1946 to 1952.[14] Dr. Durkee saw himself as a serious researcher knowledgeable in traditional osteopathic and naturopathic medicines. Hoxsey readily admitted Dr. Durkee's contributions, but he never specified what they were.

Hoxsey remained cagey as to whether any of these was the true formula. Pharmaceutical companies have always been notoriously and justifiably secretive about their recipes and manufacturing techniques until they gain patents. Even then, such commercial interests remain evasive, like Coca-Cola and its famous secret formula. Because Hoxsey's herbal remedies were not patentable, he had reason to be cautious. Perhaps Hoxsey felt, as Winston Churchill once remarked, that the truth was so valuable that it had to be protected "by a bodyguard of lies." The MacGuffin might still be in play, after all.

So the question remains as to what exactly is in the Hoxsey tonic. Mildred Nelson has continued to hold the precise recipe close to the vest and never confirmed or denied its makeup. She gave a sly wink that Hoxsey might have admitted under court order only what the AMA believed to be in the tonic. However, botanical formulas containing multiple ingredients are famously complex, and the analytical methods of the day and understanding of plant chemistry were primitive. Mildred did hint to us that licorice may never have been in the formula at all, and has remained altogether opaque about the contents. In the last few years she elliptically stopped listing buckthorn and prickly ash bark on the label. She also maintains that the tonic formula may be customized according to the type of cancer and stage, as Hoxsey also claimed to do.[15]

As a naturopathic scholar, Francis Brinker delved deeply into the old literature of the Eclectic medical tradition. After attending the National College of Naturopathic Medicine in Portland, Oregon, his fascination with the rich heritage of the Eclectic physicians of the nineteenth century set him on an intensive review of their botanical remedies where he would eventually make a puzzling discovery about the Hoxsey tonic.

The name Eclectic originated with a group of doctors devoted to clinical research and the use of herbal preparations in treating disease. They flourished in the late nineteenth and early twentieth centuries, and between 1826 and 1939 had a string of medical schools that taught sophisticated methods of botanical prescribing, the mainstay of therapeutics of that era. Their work represented the apex of plant medicine in the United States and persists as a rich reservoir of practical knowledge, some of which has yet to be equaled.[16]

"The Eclectics were able to differentiate well the activities of various plants," the erudite researcher notes. "But most importantly, they were effective clinical observers. They could tell what worked and what didn't. Even though their results were positive, their explanations were very often wrong, based on the limitations and understanding of medicine and science at that time. They had an empirical approach to medicine in which it's clinical results that one looks for, not the absolute guarantee of understanding the process involved. They were willing to use anything that worked. In fact, conventional medicine eventually incorporated that philosophy of Eclecticism using clinical results and observations, which today are established through controlled, double-blind studies."[17]

In researching the Hoxsey formula, Brinker found that it bore a striking similarity to an old red clover–based Eclectic formula. He traced the origins of the Trifolium (red clover) extract back to the nineteenth century, when Parke, Davis, and Co. produced a Syrup Trifolium Compound approximating the modern Hoxsey formulas, except that in 1890 it did not contain buckthorn or licorice. "Several decades later," Brinker noted, "in advertisements appearing in medical journals, Parke, Davis, and Co. identified the Syrup Trifolium Compound as a long-established success prescribed in every civilized country in the world."[18] Credited to an obscure Dr. Rush, about whom nothing more is known, the formula was also described in an official American Pharmaceutical Association listing of drugs called the *National Formulary* in 1926 and 1936.

Yet another Extract of Trifolium Compound was listed in the 1898 *King's American Dispensatory*, the preeminent compilation of medicines used by Eclectic doctors. Produced by the W. S. Merrell Co. of Cincinnati, it was celebrated for "the alterative, tonic, and eliminative properties of the recently expressed juices of extracts from fresh or green plants with potassium iodide." It was prescribed for syphilis, scrofula, rheumatism, and glandular and skin conditions. This "Compound Fluidextract of Trifolium" contained all the Hoxsey ingredients except buckthorn, and also had mayapple root, *Podophyllum peltatum*.[19] However, Brinker adds, there is no evidence that anyone ever applied the Trifolium compound to cancer before Hoxsey did, an innovation for which Brinker gives him formidable credit.

Why might Hoxsey apply it to cancer? Brinker points out that the Trifolium compound was essential to the very fabric of the Eclectic and naturopathic view of disease. It was used for its *tonic*, *alterative*, and *eliminative* properties. He explains these important concepts.

"*Tonics*, often bitter, were employed to increase the appetite and enhance the processes of digestion and assimilation. They improved the quality of the blood and the nutrition of the entire system.

"*Alteratives*, known in folk medicine as 'blood cleansers,' were seen as assisting organs that remove metabolic waste and toxins from the circulation. Alteratives were believed to improve the quality of the blood by assisting digestion, improving circulation, and accelerating the processes of elimination, thereby correcting faulty metabolism. The knowledge concerning their action was wholly empirical. Health was seen as a product of the quality of the blood, since the blood brings nourishment to tissues and cells and must remove the cellular waste." In the Eclectic view, an alterative favorably *alters* the course of an illness. It is used for chronic conditions in small amounts over prolonged periods. Dr. Durkee explicitly characterized the tonic as an alterative.

The *eliminative* function is also essential. "Cleansing the blood," Brinker continues, "occurs as it is filtered through the organs which excrete cellular waste products. When these organs of elimination do not function adequately, it becomes increasingly difficult to maintain a healthy ecology of the cells. This makes them more susceptible to carcinogens.[20]

"Attempting to enhance elimination and immune function can be done by utilizing a variety of methods and agents including herbs," Brinker observes. "This model for the action of alteratives was practically applied by the late-nineteenth-century Eclectic prescribers in the treatment of chronic and cancerous conditions. Such was their success that the alteratives were considered to have been among the most useful medicines in Eclectic therapeutics."

The Hoxsey formula's real purpose was not to kill cancer cells directly. Rather, it was to create an overall *terrain* unfavorable to the growth of cancer cells. Simultaneously its effect was the enhancement of the body's own immune response and capacity to eliminate toxins. From these perspectives, the Hoxsey tonic is a credible approach.

Independent scientific research has validated certain effects of the Hoxsey herbs on overall physiological function. "The tonic and alterative claims by Eclectics have been relatively substantiated," Brinker confirms.[21]

There is additional evidence that the tonic does also have a direct *cytotoxic* (cancer-killing) activity, according to Brinker. "All of the plants of the Hoxsey tonic or certain of their active constituents have shown some degree of antitumor activity in human cancer cell-culture laboratory studies or in living animal systems. Constituents of red clover, licorice, and burdock inhibit the effects of tumor promoters or mutagens." He cautions, however, that these results cannot necessarily be assumed to apply to human beings, but serve rather as a screening method useful for speculative hypothesis.[22]

When I met again with Jim Duke in 1998, he joked that the new data on the Hoxsey herbs were by now so abundant that I would need another briefcase to lug the papers home. He culled his own private plant database, one of the most extensive in the world (Duke retired from the USDA in 1997), and dug up even more contemporary evidence of compelling anticancer properties in the Hoxsey tonic herbs.[23] Several are of special interest. Duke as well as the other researchers were particularly enthusiastic about recent discoveries concerning red clover, burdock root, and poke root.

RED CLOVER

Red clover blossoms, *Trifolium pratense*, which are proportionally one of the largest ingredients in the tonic, "show up in all the 'quack' remedies," Duke told me.[24] Historically red clover blossoms have been used as a folk cancer remedy both internally as a "blood purifier" and externally as a plaster. But, he added, "now it turns out that it contains genistein, the same estrogenic isoflavone for which the soybean has been getting all the press lately. It also contains three other compounds which are estrogenic [mimic natural hormones]. I suspect those four are synergistic at preventing or slowing the development of cancer." These components have all been documented to produce anticancer effects.[25]

Duke further underscored the fact that these compounds are especially notable in light of recent findings about tumor growth. They are *antiangiogenic*, meaning that they prevent the formation of new blood vessels, thereby cutting off the ability of a tumor to grow.

Red clover contains many biologically active compounds, including *phytoestrogens*, plant compounds with hormonal estrogenic effects. These plant hormones may be responsible for the low incidence of breast and other female reproductive cancers among women in Japan, where soybean products are regularly consumed.[26] Further research continues to confirm that consumption of soy as a dietary source of these phytoestrogens is associated with a lowered risk of leukemia as well as cancers of the breast, lung, and prostate.[27] Among 150 herbs tested for such hormone activity, the top six included Hoxsey's red clover and licorice, along with soy.[28]

Science News in May 1990 reported that a compound was discovered in soybeans that resembles the conventional cancer drug Tamoxifen. Duke noted that this "Tamoxifen look-alike may block cancer at an early stage. They attributed the results to genistein, found also in red clover. By blocking a wayward cell's growth at this early stage, genistein might give the immune system a better shot at destroying the cells."[29]

Duke further highlights the fact that only recently have scientists acknowledged the data that phytoestrogens such as genistein regulate the immune system and appear to prevent the spread of breast cancer. The recent flurry of excitement around tests of the synthetic drug Tamoxifen, claiming it can prevent breast cancer in up to 50 percent of women, downplays the fact that it also can produce serious "side effects" such as uterine cancer and fatal blood clots.[30] The compounds in red clover, says Duke, are a much safer natural alternative to this toxic synthetic drug.

This angiogenic direction in cancer research has gained some currency in recent years, and became the object of a media feeding frenzy in May 1998 around the research of Dr. Judah Folkman. Celebrated on the front page of the Sunday New York Times as a potentially momentous cancer breakthrough, two new drugs devised by Dr. Folkman were designed to utilize angiogenesis in preventing tumor growth by cutting off the blood supply that feeds cancerous tumors.[31] Subsequent research has confirmed Dr. Folkman's experiments, and several angiogenesis inhibitors are now being tested for tumor suppression in clinical trials.[32] These new directions in cancer research, Jim Duke says, "make the Hoxsey formula seem even more credible."

Duke additionally points out that red clover's folk tradition against cancer was strongly cited in Hartwell's *Plants Used Against Cancer*, as well as in the foundational herbal book *Back to Eden* by Jethro Kloss, who devoted many pages to its anticancer properties. Duke also names it extensively in his own scholarly work, *CRC Handbook of Medicinal Herbs*.[33]

Francis Brinker adds that the Eclectics prized red clover as an excellent alterative. "It was said unquestionably to retard the growth of cancer when administered internally for a prolonged period and was given freely to those with a tendency toward getting cancer."[34]

BURDOCK ROOT

Duke considers burdock, *Arctium lappa*, an especially distinguished Hoxsey ingredient for its strong immune-boosting properties. It contains chemicals that have shown anticancer activity in laboratory tests on cancer cells, and has other compounds with potent immune-enhancing effects.[35] Duke notes that burdock has been long used as a folk cancer remedy in Chile, China, India, Canada, Russia, and the United States.

Patricia Spain Ward's medical research also turned up compelling evidence of burdock's anticancer properties. One Hungarian study found "considerable antitumor activity" in a purified part of burdock. The researchers first included the plant in the project because of its history as a folk remedy for new growths and ulcerations.[36] Another test demonstrated how burdock inhibits tumor growth.[37] A Japanese study discovered a new substance in burdock uniquely capable of reducing mutagenicity. "So important is this new property that these scientists named it the 'B-factor,' for 'burdock factor,'" Ward reported.[38]

Herbalists often recommend burdock as a blood purifier and alterative, and it is also famous for its inclusion in another herbal combination for cancer called Essiac. A formula widely used in Canada and the United States, Essiac originated in Canada in the 1930s with founder René Caisse (*Essiac* is *Caisse* spelled backwards), a nurse who attributed the formula to Ojibwa Indians as a traditional cancer remedy.[39] It is notable when the same plant recurs in independent formulas.

POKE ROOT

Duke believes that poke root, *Phytolacca americana*, is another star in the Hoxsey tonic and he underscores its folk tradition. Poke roots, leaves, and berries, all of which can be poisonous, have long been used as anticancer remedies. Indians used the powdered root for cancer and early settlers applied the berry juice to skin cancers. Traditionally the juice was believed to alleviate cancer. As an ointment or decoction, the root as well as the leaf have long been used to treat cancer and tumors.

Poke was widely celebrated by the early Eclectics for its anticancer properties. After forty years of use, Eli Jones, a famous Eclectic physician whom science writer Ralph Moss has called "one of the founders of modern oncology," considered poke the most valuable general remedy available for treating cancer.[40] Among its common names was cancer root.

Poke hit the headlines in 1998 when *Antimicrobial Agents and Chemotherapy*, the official journal of the American Society for Microbiology, published a study about a promising new drug that eradicates HIV infection (AIDS) in mice.[41] The new agent contains a potent antiviral protein from the pokeweed plant and was found to be 100 to 1,000 times more active than any other anti-HIV agent produced to date. The new medication works like a magic bullet, delivering the plant-derived inhibitor selectively to AIDS-infected cells. The mice in the study were cured of human AIDS without side effects. Therapeutic drug levels were achieved in monkeys without side effects. Based on these very promising results, the FDA granted permission to start clinical trials in HIV-infected patients at treatment centers in the United States. Additional testing has begun in South Africa using this derivation from the folk cancer remedy.[42]

Patricia Spain Ward also found significant citations on poke in her research. She noted that in multiple studies poke's activity helped trigger the immune system.[43] Brinker unearthed yet other references from old Eclectic medical journals.[44] "Phytolacca is so potent," Brinker suggests, "that I am surprised that conventional medicine doesn't make more use of it."[45] (*Again, do not self-medicate with poke.*)

BARBERRY AND PRICKLY ASH BARK

Barberry and prickly ash have shown activity against cancer. Jim Duke highlights barberry, *Berberis vulgaris*, as especially significant for its anticancer activity, attributable to the alkaloid berberine in particular. (Alkaloids are bitter, organic bases found in plants.) Barberry contains a wealth of anticancer, antitumor, antioxidant, and mutation-preventing compounds, as well as cancer-preventive properties.[46] Native Americans used the plant to cleanse the blood, among many other uses.

Duke emphasizes that prickly ash bark, *Zanthoxylum americanum* or *Z. clava herculis*, contains some of the same alkaloid compounds found in barberry, and he considers it another leading agent in the formula. Because the quantities in the tonic are relatively small, however, its possible effect should not be overstated.[47]

BUCKTHORN BARK, CASCARA SAGRADA, STILLINGIA ROOT, AND LICORICE ROOT

The rest of the Hoxsey herbs have all shown meaningful anticancer activity as well. Buckthorn bark, *Rhamnus frangula*, has traditionally been used for internal cancers.[48] It has long been a remedy for cleansing the blood, liver disorders, and constipation. It contains aloe-emodin, a laxative compound that has shown activity in animal tests against several tumor systems including leukemia.[49] Ward identified a study that isolates an antileukemic principle from buckthorn. This discovery prompted the scientists to recommend retesting other similar laxative plant components for antitumor activity.[50]

Cascara sagrada bark, *Rhamnus purshiana*, contains the same aloe-emodins as buckthorn in twice the amount.[51] It has traditionally been used as a purgative, laxative, tonic, and liver medicine. An extract of cascara inhibited the tumor growth of breast cancer transplanted in mice after ten days.[52]

Stillingia, *Stillingia sylvatica*, also known as queen's root, is a medicinal plant of the Southeast known for its unsurpassed alterative influence on lymphatic and secretory functions. Eli Jones listed stillingia as another long-standing Eclectic remedy for internal cancer.[53] An alcoholic extract of stillingia reduced tumor growth in mice with breast cancer transplants after nine days.[54] According to Ward, in 1980 two German scientists discovered two new members of a chemical group with known antitumor activity in stillingia's root, the part used by Hoxsey.[55]

Licorice root, *Glycyrrhiza glabra*, which may be used by Hoxsey, also exhibits many relevant activities. It has estrogen-like properties, enhances immune function, and further serves to assist elimination.[56] It has long been employed as a tonic and blood purifier, as well as for soothing internal inflammations. It contains compounds potent against certain bacteria.[57] A number of components isolated from licorice have shown antitumor activity in animal test systems.[58] Recent studies have also found that a licorice fraction and amino acids helped prevent liver cancer in patients with hepatitis C.[59] Licorice is highly prized in Chinese medicine for its synergistic effects in formulas with multiple ingredients.[60]

POTASSIUM IODIDE

The most overlooked factor in the tonic is its nonherbal ingredient, potassium iodide, the base in which the herbs are contained. It is a compound of potassium and iodine also known by its chemical symbols as KI. Potassium iodide has a long history of usage in Eclectic and folk medicine, as well as in veterinary medicine. The Eclectics used potassium iodide extensively, but not for cancer.[61] Conventional doctors also employed it earlier in the century for many diseases.[62]

In the AMA's own files I uncovered obscure but important articles showing anticancer properties for potassium iodide. They were published in *The North American Veterinarian* and in *Veterinary Medicine* respectively in 1926 and 1930 by Arthur Bryan, a Baltimore veterinarian.[63]

Bryan corresponded with the AMA in 1951 about his findings. Writing to the Bureau of Investigation, he noted that "Hoxsey's treatments admittedly came from a veterinary surgeon. Some twenty-seven years ago, my brother, Charles Bryan, M.D., and myself found that solutions of potassium or sodium iodide, when injected or crystals instilled into all kinds of neoplasms [cancers] in domestic animals, broke them down, presumably by escharotic action, so that they usually disappeared in a week or so. Tumors of horses and cattle larger than a pumpkin responded to the treatment dramatically."[64]

Dr. Fishbein's attorney, preparing for a Hoxsey trial, brought the publications to the attention of Oliver Field, who never acknowledged the studies.[65] At the time, the AMA officially held that potassium iodide might accelerate the growth of cancer.[66]

Potassium iodide was also an important element of the therapy of Dr. Max Gerson. A German physician who emigrated to the United States, he achieved dramatic results against cancer and other conditions using a rigorous diet of natural foods, fresh juices, liver injections, and coffee enemas. He was celebrated by Nobel laureate Dr. Albert Schweitzer as "one of the most eminent medical geniuses in the history of medicine."[67] Dr. Gerson believed that potassium iodide corrected important bodily defiencies and enhanced metabolism, which in turn retarded and inhibited tumor growth.[68]

Other physicians in the 1940s and 1950s experimented with potassium iodide for cancer with demonstrable results. Dr. Kleiner, a professor of biochemistry at the New York Medical College, and Dr. M. M. Black of the Brooklyn Cancer Institute treated advanced-cancer patients with KI with encouraging results.[69]

An interesting contemporary footnote is that U.S. public health officials dispensed potassium iodide pills to nearby residents after the Three Mile Island nuclear accident. The substance is believed to block ionizing radiation from damaging the thyroid gland. The FDA itself distributed KI liquid to the population around Three Mile Island.

The same method was used in the former Soviet Union following the Chernobyl nuclear disaster. The Nuclear Regulatory Commission's *Report on the Accident at the Chernobyl Nuclear Power Station* found, "The Russians were apparently well prepared for large-scale distribution of KI tablets to the general public. Thousands of measurements of I-131 (radioiodine) activity in the thyroids of the exposed population suggest that the observed levels were lower than those that would have been expected had this prophylactic measure not been taken. No serious side effects of KI use have been reported." Spurred by new research from Chernobyl, the Nuclear Regulatory Commission is today preparing to distribute potassium iodide to states with nuclear power plants.[70] Clearly potassium iodide is an intriguing therapeutic agent.

Despite this encouraging data for the individual ingredients, the Hoxsey tonic has not been tested as a whole entity, and nothing is known about the complex synergy of its components. "When you're talking about the contents of active constituents in a plant," comments Francis Brinker, "the variables are enormous. You've got not one active ingredient, but many. Then when you start combining nine different plants into this complex, you have no idea really how those various factors are interacting, and which is more important than another. Trying to develop drugs from plants by reducing crude extracts into their component parts in order to obtain an active isolated constituent never duplicates the effect of the whole plant. There are minor constituents that can have a very significant impact as part of the overall complex of components that work together to act therapeutically in a human system."

James Duke strongly concurs. "You'll find that these plants have several different types of activities that might contribute toward cancer cure or prevention. Several compounds contribute to each of those types of activities."

Duke portrays the situation as a clash of paradigms between the isolated, purified *magic bullet* favored by allopathic medicine and the *herbal shotgun shell* preferred in the natural medicine tradition. "The whole is better than the sum of its parts," he asserts. "The suite is what's most effective. But FDA regulations are such that, if you've got several active ingredients, you've got to prove not only that every one of them is safe and efficacious, but that *all* of them are safe and efficacious. All plants contain thousands of compounds, most of them biologically active. Are we going to have to prove all thousand of them safe and efficacious?"

The National Cancer Institute did perform laboratory tests on all the Hoxsey herbs using cancer cell lines in petri dishes. Almost all the results were negative, contrary to other data presented here.[71] Most of these testing methodologies have since been abandoned because they are unreliable, and many scientists find that the outcomes do not match actual results with human subjects. Both Duke and Brinker are not fazed by the preponderant failure of the Hoxsey herbs to show anticancer activity in the NCI screens because these experiments have been designed for one very narrow band of activity: the cytotoxic capability to kill cancer cells directly in a dish. "If it were tested against cell cultures and the tests came up negative, I wouldn't be surprised or bothered," Brinker states. "That's not what I'm expecting or looking for from that herb." While some of the plants may directly kill cancer cells to some degree, most work by indirectly interfering with malignant cell growth through other mechanisms.

Duke, who worked closely with the NCI, is critical of its protocols. "One of the major problems with the NCI screen is that they do not test the plants in the way humans use the plants. I don't know that they have ever given an oral extract of red clover to a human being, and that's how it's used in folklore. If you're going to test red clover tea, you've got to give it to a human being."

Dr. Richard Early, an Ohio physician with a family practice did conduct a modest laboratory experiment with the Hoxsey tonic as a whole entity. Not a sympathizer of alternative medicine, he decided to look into the herbal brew after his father unsuccessfully tried it as a last resort against his terminal cancer. In 1990 Dr. Early gave the leftover tonic to Dr. David Ho, a senior research associate in the Ohio State University College of Pharmacy, who tested it against cell lines for five types of cancer. "Surprisingly the mixture was active against all five of the lines," Dr. Early wrote. Dr. Ho verified the results by repeat testing.[72]

The overall evidence is that the Hoxsey tonic is a biologically active substance whose components have individually shown significant immunomodulating, anticancer, and antitumor properties. "You can make an educated guess," suggests Dennis McKenna from behind the thick glasses through which he daily pores over reams of scientific data, "that, yes, there is some potential here for anticancer activity. These are interesting leads. All this activity is indicative that these are biologically active plants. But it's a long way from being able to say it's effective."

McKenna further qualifies the data by pointing out that the compounds in the Hoxsey herbs are widely distributed in many plants. He notes the scarcity of human studies as a severe limitation preventing any definitive conclusions.

One admittedly preliminary review of Hoxsey patients did take place beginning in 1984 by a contemporary naturopathic doctor, Steve Austin of Oregon. The study tracked a small sampling of cancer patients from the Pacific Northwest over a five-year period who went to three Tijuana alternative cancer clinics offering, respectively, Hoxsey, Gerson, and laetrile (the extract of apricot pits).[73]

Published in the *Journal of Naturopathic Medicine*, the review found that six of sixteen Hoxsey patients survived for five years and were disease-free. These survivors included two cases of melanoma and two of lung cancer. In each category, one was very advanced, and both types of cancer are often fatal. There were no survivors from the other two therapies. Dr. Austin was entirely forthright in acknowledging the severe limitations of the modest study. "Our Hoxsey results are uncertain due to the preliminary nature of our investigation. Nevertheless, we note that several long-term survivors had very poor initial prognoses. Plausible explanations might include misdiagnoses, small sample size, and erroneous information from patients. However, we believe any apparently successful treatment of late-stage lung cancer and melanoma should provoke interest."

But Dr. Austin's report certainly did not stimulate the media outpouring greeting the 1998 reports of Dr. Judah Folkman's experimental work with angiogenic drugs. The excitement, upon closer examination, boiled down to laboratory tests showing only modest results on mice. It is well known that mouse systems often do not translate to human beings, and the NCI itself abandoned the mouse screening test several years ago. Nor was consideration paid to possible side effects. Given the well-documented antiangiogenic properties of Hoxsey's red clover and licorice, why has there not been comparable attention paid to these and other plants? Is a difference of medical philosophy creating a double standard for research?

In her report to Congress, Patricia Spain Ward summed up her perspective on the Hoxsey tonic herbs. "More recent literature leaves no doubt that Hoxsey's formula, however strangely concocted by modern scientific standards, does indeed contain many plant substances of marked therapeutic activity. In fact, orthodox scientific research has by now identified antitumor activity of one sort or another in all but three of Hoxsey's plants—and two of these three are purgatives, one of them containing the anthraquinone glycoside structure now recognized as predictive of antitumor properties. Whether there is therapeutic merit in Hoxsey's particular formula for internal use remains as much a question today as it was in 1925, despite provocative findings of antitumor properties in many of the individual herbs he used."[74]

The lack of human studies has not stopped thousands of desperate cancer patients from using the treatment. But only the scientific test that Harry Hoxsey sought can finally resolve the question of the tonic's efficacy. The controversy surrounding it, however, belies a much deeper conflict of medical opinion about the very nature of treating cancer. How did Hoxsey believe his tonic worked?

12

Hoxsey's Eclectic Approach to Cancer

Until the 1950s orthodox medicine viewed cancer purely as a *local* disease. Doctors sanctioned only surgery and radiation as effective treatments, both being localized approaches reflecting their belief that tumors were independent growths on an otherwise healthy organism. After decades of taking the position that "there is no known liquid medicine which cures internal cancer," orthodoxy acknowledged a systemic approach with the development of chemotherapy drugs in the 1950s.[1] Even then, the exclusive orientation was to kill cancer cells by using strong poisons.

To the contrary, Hoxsey and the lineage of natural medicine he espoused characterized cancer as a *systemic* illness. He described it as a "systemic disease which occurs only in the presence of a profound physiologic change in the constituents of body fluids and a consequent chemical imbalance of the organism. Its real cause must be sought in the basic body chemistry and cell metabolism. We believe that the organism's attempt to adapt itself to the new and abnormal environment causes certain mutations in newly born cells of the body. Eventually a viciously competent cell evolves which finds the new environment eminently suitable to survival and rapid self-reproduction. These cells are what are known as cancer."[2]

Hoxsey believed that a systemic approach could remedy the imbalance. "It follows that if the constitution of the body fluids can be normalized and the original chemical balance in the body restored, the environment again will become unfavorable for the survival and reproduction of these cells. They will cease to multiply and eventually they will die. Then if vital organs have not been too seriously damaged by the malignancy (or by surgery or irradiation), the entire organism will recover to normal health. We attempt to get at the roots of the disorder, rather than deal merely with its end result. Our primary effort is to restore the body to physiological normalcy."[3]

Hoxsey called his approach "nontoxic chemotherapy" and, like the Eclectics, saw the internal tonic serving several functions: to stimulate the elimination of toxins poisoning the system; to correct abnormal blood chemistry; and to normalize cell metabolism. In essence, he proposed, the tonic alters the metabolic terrain to discourage the cancer's growth.

"In assessing the potential value of the Hoxsey formula in cancer treatments," naturopath Francis Brinker observes, "the current conventional scientific method has been to look at its component plants individually or their isolated constituents in regard to cytotoxic or antitumor activity. While this may or may not help establish some degree of justification, it does not address the intended purpose of using the formula as a means of normalizing physiologic processes and thereby assisting the body in its own control of cancerous growth."

Rather than specifically aiming to kill the cancer, Hoxsey deliberately sought to support the body's ability to cure itself. The Hoxsey herbs do in fact present a strong profile for precisely that activity. The tonic is also harmless. Unlike toxic chemotherapy drugs, the worst it will do is nothing. The seminal Greek physician Hippocrates, whose famous Hippocratic Oath doctors take, is well known for his primary principle: "First do not harm." Clearly the Hoxsey tonic honors this credo.

Hippocrates's second, less quoted principle was to "revere the healing force of nature." This precept is at the heart of the Hoxsey tonic as well as virtually all the other unconventional cancer treatments. It hearkens back to a long-standing concept known as *vis medicatrix naturae*, the healing force of nature, which was central to Hoxsey's medical philosophy. He exalted the ability of nature to heal and the capacity of the body to right itself when given proper support.

This medical philosophy originates from a centuries-old tradition prominent in the United States in the 1800s and early 1900s among "irregular" physicians. The irregulars were represented by diverse schools including the Eclectics, Physiomedicalists, homeopaths, and the naturopathic profession, which evolved in stages from all these approaches. The renowned turn-of-the-century Eclectic physician Eli Jones stated, "The Eclectic school of medicine was the pioneer in the successful treatment of cancer by internal medication. By my method of treating cancer as a blood or constitutional disease (as I was taught in the Eclectic college over forty years ago), I have cured 80 percent of the cases of cancer which have come under my treatment. I honestly believe, from my own experience, that 95 percent of the cases of cancer in our country could be cured by medicine if treated before any operation or the use of X-ray."[4]

Whatever the real origin of the Hoxsey medicines, they mirrored this empirical Eclectic tradition. Following their reputed discovery by a horse, Hoxsey consistently claimed his father added other ingredients from popular home remedies of the day. Potassium iodide would likely have been among them, given its empirical veterinary tradition. Because 1840 Illinois was also Indian country at the western frontier of the nation, John Hoxsey most likely had contact with Native American healers who used herbs extensively and maintained wide-ranging continental trade routes that brought remote plants into general circulation.

The nonlocal herbs would have been familiar because the region was also a hotbed of irregular medical practice.[5] There were major Eclectic and Physiomedical medical schools in Cincinnati as well as in Illinois, Indiana, and throughout the Midwest and Southeast. The most popular form of American folk medicine, called Thompsonianism, was rooted in indigenous American herbs since importing medicines from the East Coast or Europe was too expensive. These various traditions converged to become a re-indigenized, botanically based medicine naturalized to North America.[6]

Epitomizing the tradition of empiricism, the Eclectic school developed essentially a native materia medica of indigenous American plants. The parallel school of Physiomedicalists eschewed chemical medicines of any kind along with toxic herbs, relying solely on "nature's medicines." Brinker concludes that "it made eminent good sense for a veterinarian or a doctor in the Midwest in the mid-nineteenth century to rely upon the local plants as medicine." Hoxsey's herbs and latter

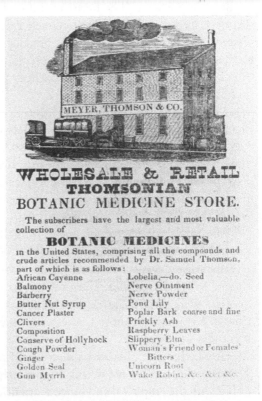

A nineteenth-century promotion for a Thompsonian drugstore offers herbs.

formulas were all cited in *King's American Dispensatory*, the Eclectic book of remedies first published in 1854. It incorporated the rich new discoveries of indigenous plants and Native knowledge with existing European traditions.[7]

The Hoxsey herbs were also listed in the *National Formulary*, which originated around 1888 in response to the mounting exclusion of many botanical formulas from the *United States Pharmacopoeia (U.S.P.)*, the official listing of the American Pharmaceutical Association. Even though the rise of the synthetic-drug industry began to displace many traditional plant medicines, both the *National Formulary* and the *U.S.P.* still contained a preponderance of botanical remedies well into the twentieth century. Their continued inclusion indicated not only their popularity but also their probable efficacy.

Apart from the herbs themselves, the special preparation of the tonic also owes much to naturopathic tradition. The tonic contains no alcohol, and no alcohol is used to make it, a fact that Mildred believes to be of primary importance. The herbs are infused or boiled in water to obtain extracts. Hoxsey was the first to concoct the formula strictly as a water extract, which is an old naturopathic practice. (Like Harry Hoxsey, Mildred Nelson has never fully revealed the precise method of making the tonic. She compares it to mixing paints, where the outcome depends on the precise order and sequence.)[8]

The twentieth-century naturopathic movement in which Hoxsey participated grew directly out of this Eclectic lineage. Originally called "drugless healing," naturopathy emphasized cleansing and detoxifying the body as the currency of good health. It added botanical medicine to its repertoire of nutrition, hydrotherapy, and other nature-based practices. The naturopaths relied exclusively on medicines from natural sources rather than on synthetic pharmaceuticals.[9]

The influential naturopath Dr. John Bastyr, after whom Seattle's naturopathic Bastyr University is named, agreed with Eli Jones about treating cancer systemically, and utilized Jones's seminal work, *Cancer: Its Causes, Symptoms and Treatments* (1911). As medical knowledge has progressed, the Eclectics and naturopaths have proved to be ahead of their time in recognizing cancer as a systemic or constitutional disease, which it is today known to be.

Hoxsey himself obtained a diploma from the Southwest College of Naturopathy, and his physicians, particularly Dr. Durkee, were quite familiar with the empirical and Eclectic traditions. In the 1949 trial against Hearst, Hoxsey made a strong case that all his remedies were listed in the homeopathic pharmacopoeia. Dr. Fishbein's medical experts took the stand to denounce the Hoxsey herbs as "absurd and ridiculous" for treating this "local disease."[10] Dr. Fishbein denigrated Eclecticism's plant remedies as "the apotheosis of the old grandmother and witch-doctor systems of treatment."[11]

"There is an empirical tradition in all cultures involving plants and their formulas," observes Brinker, "which have been utilized through the ages because they are effective. There is no definitive explanation or rational understanding at this point as to why and how these things work together to do what they can do. However, despite a very limited nineteenth-century knowledge of health and disease from a scientific stance, the empiricists obtained many positive results and were exceptional clinical observers unbound by philosophical strictures. Ironically, their very pragmatism of using whatever worked was later largely incorporated by orthodox medicine, if scientifically validated. For their day and age, the Eclectics were well in advance of conventional practice."

Even today, botany endures as the cornerstone of pharmacy. About 25 percent of prescription drugs contain at least one plant constituent, and another 25 percent are modeled on plants. Fully 40 percent of modern pharmaceuticals are directly derived from either plants or other natural products.[12] The heart medicine digitalis comes from foxglove, supposedly given to Dr. William Withering in 1775 by a Gypsy. Aspirin originated from willow bark, and to this day its action is not completely understood, though its efficacy is accepted. Quinine, a drug used against the scourge of malaria, came from a South American tree bark. The poppy flower yielded the painkiller morphine, and the Bayer corporation named its potent derivative "heroin" for its "heroic" anesthetic effects. The list of plant-based drugs is long and illustrious.

In fact, a high number of standard cancer chemotherapy drugs originate from plants. Vincristine and Vinblastine, used for acute childhood leukemia and Hodgkin's disease, are derived from the Madagascar periwinkle flower, *Vinca rosea*. The Pacific yew tree has yielded Taxol, whose sales are now approaching $1 billion. Etoposide, the chemotherapy drug of choice for testicular cancer, small-cell lung cancer, nonlymphocytic leukemias, and non-Hodgkin's lymphoma, comes from the mayapple, *Podophyllum peltatum*, an old Native American anticancer plant. It too was listed in the Extract Trifolium Compound.[13]

About 30 percent of anticancer compounds presently in clinical use originate from natural products or their derivatives. As Ralph Moss notes, "Of the thirty-two most common multidrug protocols used in cancer treatment today, only four do not contain some natural product ingredient. The majority contain either an herb-derived product, an agent derived from a microorganism, or, in one case, a drug derived from a sponge. Chemotherapy as we know it today would be inconceivable without the contributions of Vincristine, Vinblastine, Taxol, and Camptothecin [from the wood and bark of a Chinese tree]."[14]

"I would rather take the Hoxsey formula than Taxol or Etoposide," Jim Duke says bluntly. "That sounds heretical, but I do not believe that the pain endured with these hard-core semisynthetic chemotherapeutic drugs is worth the extra month or two they might add to your life. Is the herb as good as the synthetic? In many cases, it's as efficacious and in some cases probably more so. In almost all cases, it's cheaper. In almost all cases, it's gentler. I have good evolutionary reasons to suspect that in many cases the natural will be safer and as good, largely because my genes already know the natural chemicals. My genes do not know tomorrow's synthetic chemicals.

"Chemotherapy is really assaulting the immune system and assaulting cancer at the same time," Duke goes on. "But we have to strengthen ourselves as we weaken the enemy, and most of the NCI approaches have been weakening the patient while weakening the cancer. I would rather take something like Hoxsey that would boost my immune system at the same time it was fighting the cancer."

Throughout history, herbs have served as a primary tool for healing. Medicinal herbs have been found with the remains of Neanderthal humans dating back 60,000 years. Pollen from eight flowers and branches spread at their graves in a cave in Iraq was identified as originating from eight different species, seven of which are still used as traditional herbal medicines by the local residents.[15] The thrilling 1991 discovery of the "Iceman," a traveler whose 5,300-year-old mummified body was found frozen in the ice in the Alps of northern Italy, revealed that he carried two walnut-sized lumps tied to a leather thong probably attached to his clothing. Microbiologists have identified them as the fruit of the birch fungus, which contains a natural antibiotic he was apparently using against the parasite found in his colon.[16] Not unlike the Iceman, over 75 percent of the world's population still relies on plant-derived medicines for basic health-care needs, according to the World Health Organization.[17]

At the NCI's own Cancer Chemotherapy National Services Center, studies have found that the occurrence of drug activity is higher in plants reported in folk literature than in plants collected at random, "suggesting a correlation between plants used in folklore and those with anticancer activity."[18] When researchers compared the efficacy of drugs screened at random against those suggested by folk use, the folk tradition yielded a 20 to 50 percent "hit" rate in contrast with 10 percent from random screening.[19]

Dennis McKenna's greatest interest in the Hoxsey tonic emanates from its folk tradition rather than from any laboratory data. "The folk usage is another kind of screen. What it means is that somebody somewhere used it and found it useful, and was impressed enough with the results to continue using it. Herbalism in general and especially the way it was practiced in the nineteenth century and still today is a pretty empirical science. The real significance is that, if it does work from the standpoint of the person trying to cure the disease, that's good enough. They can let the molecular biologist worry about how it works. The Eclectic school and these others were pretty savvy and they didn't use things if they didn't feel that they were getting some results."

McKenna points out that even conventional cancer drugs derived from plants, such as Vincristine and Vinblastine, were missed in NCI screens until some researcher went back to look at them again on a hunch.[20] "There is no substitute for the human factor, the human intuition," McKenna smiles, tossing his beloved science to the winds for a philosophical moment. "That's where the tie to folk medicine comes, because the Eclectics were very astute observationists. That fact weighs more heavily than a simple screen or a petri dish. All it means is that somebody should take a very close look at these Hoxsey plants because they've been practically used, apparently with some success."

Nevertheless, hearkening back to the dictionary definition of an *empiric* as a "quack," the AMA's Oliver Field compared Hoxsey's tonic to "running cars on carrot juice" and stated flatly, "To go back to folk medicine is kind of foolish."[21] William Grigg of the FDA also took a derisive view of the empirical tradition. "The idea that the American Indians or a veterinarian would accidentally stumble upon some herb that would cure a large number of problems is rather far-fetched. It's like the idea that, if you put three billion monkeys in a room, one of them might write a Shakespearean sonnet."

And what about Hoxsey's horse? Francis Brinker is respectfully skeptical. A horse might possibly have nibbled on poke root, barberry, and burdock, while consuming substantial amounts of red clover. Prickly ash, however, is a decidedly aversive experience, inciting severe burning in the mouth. Animals seldom eat barks such as buckthorn, which causes sharp spastic contractions when taken fresh and must be aged for a year prior to human use.[22]

On the other hand, the field of zoopharmacognosy, the natural sources of veterinary medicines, is now a legitimate discipline, practiced at Harvard, among other places. Jane Goodall, who has studied chimpanzees in Africa for several decades, reported observing the creatures straying twenty minutes from their normal feeding grounds in search of the aspilia bush. They consumed only the leaves and swallowed them whole. Researchers later discovered the leaf to contain a potent antibiotic that the chimps sought out when they were ill. African folk healers have long used the same plant for treating stomach upset and wounds.[23]

Many indigenous peoples around the world maintain that they did not discover their rich tradition of botanical medicine by the perilous trial-and-error tasting of each plant. Rather, they observed the animals, a much surer and safer way to go. Though implausible, Hoxsey's horse story may well have had a kernel of truth to it. Hoxsey's horse also rides a symbolically rich heritage. According to ancient mythology, it was the Greek god Chiron, half man and half horse, who gave herbal knowledge to human beings from his cave.

Jonathan Hartwell, in the article "Plant Remedies for Cancer" published in *Cancer Chemotherapy Reports*, wrote, "Plants provide a fertile source of compounds with novel structures which are needed in cancer chemotherapy, but which are difficult for the chemist to synthesize. Higher plants are one of the great sources of compounds not yet tapped. The empirical application of plants to the ailing human body over thousands of years has resulted in certain observable effects interpreted as beneficial, and has culminated in the development of many useful drugs for a number of diseases. If there is any hope in a chemical treatment for cancer, it is reasonable to believe that such an agent is as likely to originate from a plant as well as from pure synthesis."[24]

In fact, Hartwell decided to write *Plants Used Against Cancer* after learning that the Penobscot Indians were the first to use the mayapple against cancer, eventually leading to the chemotherapy drug Etoposide.[25] Yet even today, about 90 percent of the world's flora remains uninvestigated by scientific medicine.[26]

Hartwell closed his discourse on botanical cancer remedies with words from the esteemed professor George Sarton, a scholar of medical history. "The remembrance of these astounding folk discoveries should sober our thoughts when we criticize too freely the old pharmacopoeias. It is easy to make fun of mediaeval recipes; it is more difficult and may be wiser to investigate them. Instead of assuming that the mediaeval pharmacist was a benighted fool, we might wonder whether there was not sometimes a justification for his strange procedure."[27]

Mildred Nelson situates herself firmly within this empirical tradition. "When you really get right down to the whole scope of medicine, the only stable drugs we have today are a product of the herbs. But scientifically we do not know all the interactions that take place. Not being scientifically minded, and being a nurse at heart, I have found that it is more important to have results than scientific proof."

At the Bio Medical Center, Francis Brinker witnessed Mildred Nelson's treatment of a melanoma in a patient's ear canal. Because the area was too sensitive for the caustic escharotics she otherwise might apply, Brinker watched the nurse prescribe solely the internal tonic, which had begun to reduce the tumor in size. As a result, he gained an added appreciation for the importance of the tonic. "I merely went to observe and try to get a sense of the value of this therapy. I left with great respect for Mildred as a person. Having been there, I am not at all reluctant in recommending it to people with cancer."

Mounting scientific data on the anticancer properties of the Hoxsey herbs certainly make it appear that Hoxsey's "bunch of weeds" have been the unjust victim of orthodox medicine's flowery rhetoric. As the American Botanical Council's Mark Blumenthal quipped, "The epithet of 'a bunch of weeds' is fine with me. As Ralph Waldo Emerson said in *The Future of the Republic*, 'What is a weed? A plant whose virtues have not yet been discovered.'"

The Hoxsey Escharotics: "Like a Pit from a Peach"

The earlier story of Mrs. Martha Bond's recovery from melanoma (chapter 2) is typical of Hoxsey successes removing external cancers. We heard numerous similar accounts of how external cancers dried up and fell out after application of the red paste or yellow powder. The Hoxsey method is justifiably famous for its escharotic remedies. In fact, since about 1950 organized medicine has not even contested their efficacy.

Mrs. Bond's case shows the standard procedure for the Hoxsey escharotics, which are usually applied topically. (*Escharotic* means "scar-forming.") They are always used in combination with the tonic. Whenever possible, patients start on the tonic before external treatment and continue on it for many years after. As a true escharotic, the red paste is used only externally. But as a selective agent, the yellow powder can also be used internally, as the following dramatic story describes.

While making the film in 1985, we traveled to California to meet Stephen Crutcher, a Hoxsey patient living in a suburb near the San Francisco Bay area. He was very soft-spoken, his eyes slightly masked behind lightly tinted glasses. Casually dressed in a sport shirt in his modest home, he exuded gentleness in contrast to the chilling events that shook his life beginning in 1975.

"I talked to a dentist who noticed a lump in the roof of my mouth," Stephen began softly. "He wanted to know if I'd had it checked out, but at the time I hadn't really thought about it. So I went to an ear, nose, and throat specialist who took a biopsy right there. He called me at work one day and said he had to talk to me.

"That's when he told me it was malignant—cancer of the mucous glands. They wanted to do surgery right away, and not knowing about other things, we set it up right off the bat. Then my wife was very reluctant about letting it go through and we started asking questions. The doctor said it had to be done right away, but we wanted to get some other opinions first. He gave us the names of some doctors and they generally all had the same opinion: It was either radiation or surgery. That's when my wife's sister, who had heard friends of hers who had gone to see Mildred at the clinic, started trying to talk me into going."

Stephen paused, revisiting the grim crossroads. We asked him exactly what kinds of treatment the doctors were recommending. "They wanted to start by removing the upper palate and then go to the jaw, then get at the upper gum by removing the teeth. And then 'whatever else they found' is what they told me—that's the term they used—which kind of scared me. One of the doctors had said something about removing most of the palate, and plating it in gold or putting a gold one in, so that they could do radiation in the rest of the areas of the mouth without affecting the lower skull or brain area. But they never really did say they could cure it. That was one of the first things Mildred did say to me. She said, 'Well, we can cure this.'"

Stephen Crutcher decided to make the trip to Bio Medical. He was understandably anxious. "When I first went to Hoxsey, I had the opinion that if it's so good, why isn't it here in the U.S.? Seeing the place for the first time in the old building was kind of a shock after seeing modern hospitals. My first impression was, 'What am I doing here?' But after talking to them, they put me at ease."

Mildred injected the roof of his mouth with a liquid preparation of the Hoxsey yellow powder. She also put him on the internal Hoxsey tonic for several years to follow.

"I was going back every couple of days during the first two weeks while they checked it to make sure there was no infection. All this time it was draining, and it felt like runners running down in my mouth and across the jaw. Mildred said it was probably from cancer trying to spread through the system. After that I went back regularly, every three or six months. Basically that's all the treatment I've had, and I feel pretty lucky that that's the only thing I did do." His cancer disappeared completely, and his mouth healed perfectly.

When I tracked down Stephen Crutcher more than twelve years later to check his standing, I found him alive and well. He has had no recurrence and continues to work at a large Air Force base and serve in the National Guard. His records confirmed his cancer. According to the Hildenbrands' epidemiological verification, it was clear from the physician's original notes that "something was still there" when he left for Hoxsey. Only after Mildred's treatment did it go away. Crutcher has now been cancer-free for twenty-four years. He had no conventional cancer treatment, only Hoxsey.

Let's look more deeply into these ancient medicines. As a "true" escharotic, the red paste is a corrosive substance that will burn or destroy any tissue in its path. It has a radiant effect that precipitates a chain reaction up to two inches from where it is applied. It is used mainly on large tumors. It does not so much cure the cancer as *kill* it, forming a dead, hard, black remnant, or *eschar*, which then sloughs off.

As an an indiscriminate killer of cells, the red paste can be extremely dangerous and disfiguring unless used by a skilled practitioner. Its main detriment is the intense pain it causes, though many patients are willing to tolerate it given the alternatives of radical surgery, radiation, or chemotherapy. Local anesthetics do not really work over a prolonged period. Mildred Nelson is opposed to morphine because of its addictive power and asks patients to withstand the pain.

The red paste contains the mineral-based antimony trisulfide and zinc chloride, as well as the herb bloodroot, known by its botanical name of *Sanguinaria canadensis*. Antimony trisulfide is a salt of the highly toxic heavy metal antimony, also known as stibnite. It is believed to act as a "permeant" to facilitate infiltration of the zinc chloride. Zinc chloride is a caustic chemical that opens the skin and permits the slough to form. It acts as a "fixative."[1]

Bloodroot is a red root that acts as a chemotherapeutic agent to kill the cancer cells. With a long history of widespread Native American usage, it was used by the Cherokee Indians for breast cancer, and both the Cherokee and Iroquois used it topically for cancers.[2]

Bloodroot contains important chemical compounds that have shown antitumor activity in laboratory tests with mice as well as in petri dish cell lines. It has also demonstrated action against disease-causing bacteria.[3] Jim Duke points out that it has been extensively studied by the National Cancer Institute, and that it got a formidable twenty-two citations for external cancer in Hartwell's *Plants Used Against Cancer.* According to Duke, bloodroot possesses strong chemical antitumor and anticancer properties.[4]

The old "quack" remedy of zinc chloride is also being validated scientifically. A recent study published in a dermatology journal concluded that its fixation of certain melanomas increased resistance to tumors by acting as an immune booster.[5]

The formula for the red paste has several historical antecedents. It is similar to Fell's Remedy, developed by Dr. J. Weldon Fell, an American physician who credited the Cherokee with showing him their use of bloodroot. Descended from a line of prominent physicians, Dr. Fell was among the founders of the New York Academy of Medicine and was a faculty member of the University of New York. After acquiring the root from the Indians, he added zinc chloride to amplify its activity and claimed to be able to eradicate large tumors in a matter of weeks. He published his formulas in 1857.

Dr. Fell soon ran afoul of the orthodox medical community and eventually expatriated to London. He conducted extensive work at Middlesex Hospital and freely published the formulas and results. The treatment was later endorsed by the hospital. Nevertheless, it was not adopted and disappeared from view. Another London physician, Dr. John Pattison, apparently took up the same formula. An outspoken critic of surgery, he incurred the opposition of orthodox medicine.[6]

Several other similar formulas were used and published in the early twentieth century, when escharotics were a common form of treatment used by medical doctors, empirics, and folk healers alike. Along with surgery, these caustics were the allopathic profession's principal tools against cancer. Regular doctors historically favored mineral-based treatments including arsenic and mercury. It is likely that the Eclectics appropriated escharotics from the allopaths. The use of escharotics actually dates back in India as far as 2,500 years to an arsenic paste, and the Greek physician Hippocrates also used one around 400 B.C.[7]

Bloodroot and zinc chloride were favored by the Eclectic physician Eli Jones in tandem with an internal tonic and other internal remedies. Like Hoxsey, Dr. Jones was adamant that caustics were to be employed only in conjunction with internal medicines because of the systemic nature of the disease. (He used another external paste made from poke root.) In his era around the turn of the century, escharotic pastes were commonly available in drugstores.[8]

The most startling parallel to Hoxsey's red paste, however, was an identical formula used by dermatologist Dr. Frederic Mohs at the University of Wisconsin medical school. Starting in the 1930s, Dr. Mohs conducted meticulous experimentation on hundreds and eventually thousands of cancer patients. He called his method *chemosurgery*, a microscopically controlled process he conducted with painstaking care. By the time he published his results in 1941 in the journal *Archives of Surgery*, he had already conducted eight years of laboratory work followed by four years of clinical practice on six hundred cancer patients.[9]

The kicker, however, was that Dr. Mohs published his ongoing research seven years later in 1948 in *JAMA*. "The term 'chemosurgery,'" wrote Dr. Mohs, "was coined to designate a newly developed method for the treatment of cancer. The most important feature is the technic by which thorough microscopic control of excision may be obtained. This microscopic control makes possible the selective destruction of cancer with the dual advantages of unprecedented reliability and conservatism."

In 814 cases, he achieved an "unusually high proportion of successful results," ranging from 96 percent on basal cell carcinoma to about 85 percent in squamous cell skin cancers.[10]

Dr. Mohs achieved these results despite treating many advanced cancers, over a third of which had recurred following surgery and radiation. "The unprecedented reliability of the chemosurgical treatment of cancer is indicated by comparison with statistical results from other centers for cancer treatment," he wrote. The curative success for Mohs's technique was 93.5 percent compared to the standard 88 percent rate. His success rate underscored the treatment's conservatism, since it harms very little healthy tissue. The method's other notable virtue was that it eliminated deaths from surgery.

Dr. Mohs combined the escharotic treatment with tedious microscopic surgical excisions, a factor that may have made his hybrid approach more palatable to the medical profession.[11] He acknowledged the long usage of zinc chloride by many "quacks and irregulars," but distinguished his own protocol by its microscopic control, able to avoid the wholesale destruction of tissue that escharotics can cause.

Dr. Mohs never did address the mystery of how he came to add bloodroot to his formula. As Ralph Moss has noted, "That out of thousands of agents Mohs just stumbled upon bloodroot by complete happenstance strains credulity."[12] When Dr. Andrew Ivy visited the Dallas clinic, he noted the similarity of Hoxsey's red paste to the "Wisconsin paste" used by Dr. Mohs. Dr. Durkee said it was the same.[13] Did Dr. Mohs actually learn about the red paste from Hoxsey?

Thus it was, when Hoxsey faced Dr. Morris Fishbein in court in 1949, that the AMA no longer disputed Hoxsey's external cures. The *Journal's* publication of Dr. Moh's procedure with a paste identical to Hoxsey's provided irrefutable proof of its efficacy. Fishbein's attorneys spent considerable energy preparing defensive strategies to explain away the undeniable success confirmed by Dr. Mohs's data. They advised Fishbein to say that the *Journal* often published pro and con opinions, and that publication of the article did not represent an endorsement.[14] However, the AMA never again challenged the effectiveness of the Hoxsey external treatments, though belittling them as archaic. The FDA also stopped attacking Hoxsey's external preparations.

Dr. Mohs continued to work and publish into the 1970s, refining his method amid a deafening silence from his peer medical community. Some proponents, including researchers at Harvard and the University of Wisconsin, did adopt the practice, which is now considered a "standard," though seldom used, treatment for certain skin cancers. The only acknowledged disadvantages are the pain and labor-intensive nature of the treatment. Apart from superficial skin cancers, Dr. Mohs also found it useful for melanomas, as well as otherwise sensitive or surgically hard-to-reach areas.[15] Toward the end of his career, he relied increasingly on his microsurgery, perhaps in frustration over the lack of recognition his work received.

The Hoxsey yellow powder is yet another matter. It is the substance that the AMA charged "ate into patients' blood vessels" and caused death by arsenic poisoning. To the contrary, Hoxsey contended—as does Mildred Nelson—that it is nontoxic and selective of malignant tissue only. It is used for the "fine detail work" of tumor eradication, while the red paste is reserved for large tumors that need to be attacked quickly. Hoxsey theatrically swallowed it in front of audiences or bathed his eye in it to demonstrate its harmlessness. While filming, we watched Mildred Nelson nibble a taste of it, and she was obviously unconcerned about getting it on her skin.

The yellow powder contains arsenic sulfide, yellow precipitate (powdered sulfur), sulfur, and talc. Arsenic trisulfide is also an old form of escharotic, but a notorious one considered generally very destructive, dangerous, and indiscriminate in its action against tissues. However, Hoxsey claimed to have rendered the compound nonpoisonous, which appears to be true. It is not entirely clear when or how he accomplished this. According to my own research, it appears to have occurred by 1930, because subsequent experience by other practitioners including Dr. Ira Drew confirmed the nontoxic quality of the medication. Previously Hoxsey may or may not have been using a toxic form of arsenic.[16]

The use of arsenic against cancer, which goes back to ancient Egypt and India, has been revived today in China, where complete responses are being achieved against leukemia. Memorial Sloan-Kettering Cancer Center is now experimenting with it as well.[17] As Ralph Moss points out, "Essentially, this is the same prescription an Egyptian doctor would have made 5,000 years ago."[18]

According to Mildred Nelson, tumors slough off "like a pit from a peach" within seven to fourteen days after starting escharotic treatment. The scar left by the red paste is readily identifiable, leaving a smooth depression. "The scar isn't as pretty as the surgical scar," she concedes, "but there are fewer metastases than with surgery." She generally starts external cases on the tonic for one to six months prior to using the escharotics.

Francis Brinker offered an intriguing conjecture about the possible combined actions of the ingredients in the Hoxsey remedies. "Given the presence of potassium iodide in the tonic, it is probable that the major direct antitumor activity for both the tonic and the escharotics is due in large part to the destructive effects of the mineral elements. On the other hand, the herbs indirectly make these mineral agents much more effective by the ways they provide the foundational healing and enhanced elimination to overcome the proclivity toward cancer. In balance, it seems more apparent to me that it is the integration of the toxic chemicals, representative of allopathy, and herbs, representative of natural healing, that empowers the death-defying Eclectic approach."

The use of escharotics in cancer has several benefits, according to Mildred. "The end result is where the advantage comes. There's less possibility of spread or recurrence in the same area. When I am in doubt if I got all the cancer, I put the yellow powder back on the good skin. If nothing happens, that tells me I have no problem left. They can't do this with surgery, and they have to wait until the tumor recurs, and then another surgery. The healing process is very rapid. Once the tumor comes out, it isn't sore and doesn't hurt."

While organized medicine charged that Hoxsey's escharotics were disfiguring, it failed to mention that surgery is too. As evidenced by Dr. Mohs's data, the disfigurement using the red paste is often milder than with surgery. In fact, the father of the famous "Halsted radical mastectomy," legendary turn-of-the-century surgeon William Stuart Halsted, wrote glowingly of his encounters with escharotics. "I have several times had occasion to operate on cancer which had been vigorously and repeatedly treated with caustics [escharotics] and to note the comparatively admirable conditions, the freedom from cancer permeation of the surrounding tissues of the axilla; whereas, after incomplete operation with the knife, the local manifestations of recurrence were almost invariably deplorable, and the prognosis, of course, invariably hopeless."[19]

Francis Brinker spent seven days at the Bio Medical Center observing Mildred Nelson treat external cases. He concluded that no two were treated exactly the same, and that she had a surprisingly broad repertoire of ways of applying the yellow powder. "I thought that Mildred had a lot of very practical skills, and her experience had taught her a lot in terms of being creative in variable approaches to applying the escharotics. With the powder, I saw her variously dip cotton balls on the end of a hemostat [a medical clamp] into the powder and then tap it over an area to sprinkle it on lightly. I saw her use an insufflator—a little bulb syringe device—over a larger area covering most of the half of a side of a face with really extensive lesions, where the powder was blown over the area. There were cases where she took a little K-Y jelly and mixed the powder and applied it with a cotton swab. She would modify her techniques specifically for whatever requirement that case had. She has a very homespun approach to clinical practice. She certainly was not embarrassed to appear simple, and at the same time she obviously had profound practical knowledge and didn't show it off. She was very genuine."

Why aren't these escharotics used more widely? "Frankly, I think the basic part is money," Mildred speculated. "Second, the doctors don't want to spend that much time taking care of patients when they could surgically remove it, send them home, and not worry about it. It is time-consuming. But the end makes it well worth it." External treatments can require weeks or even months of frequent care. Dr. Mohs also indicated that using escharotics takes more time and attention.

The domination of conventional cancer treatment by surgeons has greatly depressed any interest in escharotics. Even the exceptional results achieved by Dr. Mohs combining surgery with escharotics made little impact on conventional practices, although, as mentioned earlier, the Mohs method is accepted and even listed in the orthodox *Taber's Cyclopedic Medical Dictionary*.[20]

Still, in the United States today, there is a large underground of people using several forms of escharotics. They come variously from Native American healers on Indian lands and from assorted folk traditions that have maintained them covertly. In a comprehensive and unique book, *Cancer Salves*, author Ingrid Naiman explores a multitude of escharotics, including many still in active use around the country today. Naiman has begun reconstructing and refashioning many old empirical formulas for treating external cancer with these salves and their adjunctive tonics.[21]

"There are reasons to accept the validity of this escharotic application to cancer based on empirical evidence," concludes Brinker, whose own grandfather was successfully treated with escharotics at the famous Nichols Sanitorium in Missouri, which treated almost 20,000 patients into the 1940s and claimed an overall success rate of around 75 percent.[22] "There shouldn't be any controversy regarding their use. The question is whether there is significant risk that doesn't exist with an equally effective conventional technique. The simplicity of these escharotic formulas would allow for some fairly easy studies and animal tests."

These escharotic treatments today occupy a nebulous legal standing. The basic practice has been validated scientifically and published in the medical literature, yet the use of these salves has been largely neglected, marginalized, or driven underground. This situation fosters the danger of their use in unskilled hands, where there have been cases of serious injury and disfigurement reported.

In light of their significant merits, it seems unfortunate that doctors and patients alike are not more familiar with escharotics. Today the incidence of skin cancer in Caucasians is skyrocketing, doubling since the 1980s in women and rising 25 percent in men.[23] It is likely that damage to the ozone layer resulting in increased exposure to harmful ultraviolet radiation will continue to cause the incidence of external cancers to balloon. Clearly escharotics represent a potentially important option for skin cancer and melanoma patients.

14

Nutrition with Attitude

A trip to Hoxsey has always provided patients with considerably more than a bottle of tonic. From early on, the Hoxsey method has offered substantial "supportive treatment" including a diet, vitamins, nutritional supplements, and other miscellaneous therapies. The approaches are both physical and spiritual.

The Hoxsey diet is relatively simple compared with many anticancer diets. Much of it is founded in excluding foods that are believed to counteract the activity of the tonic, based on empirical experience. Patients are barred from eating pork, vinegar, tomatoes, lard, carbonated beverages, processed white sugar, white flour, and alcohol. Fried and highly spiced foods are also eliminated. Overall it is a basic, reasonably healthy menu emphasizing fresh fruits and vegetables.

The clinic also offers extensive supportive treatments that are continually evolving with current knowledge. Mildred employs a special diet aimed at candida (yeast) infections, which she believes often precede cancer. She uses the BCG (Bacillus Calmette-Guerin) vaccine, an immune-stimulating serum widely used in Europe, which also combats tuberculosis. She dispenses vitamin C, yeast for B vitamins, and other vitamin and mineral supplements. "All I want is for that person to get well," Mildred declares. "If something else is going to help, more power to them." She has continued to experiment widely with other contemporary alternative practices, though the tonic remains the perennial.

"No study into the cause of cancer would be complete without weighing the nutritional factor," Hoxsey wrote in 1955. "Wrong eating habits unquestionably contribute to the origin and growth of many of the so-called incurable ailments. Pastries, colas, alcohol, pork, bread made from bleached flour, fluorinated water, and other abnormal foods and liquids create inhibitors to health in the human body. Vegetables grown in chemically treated soil depleted of the proper mineral content have a similar effect."[1]

Hoxsey saw himself as "born and raised as a naturopath and dietitian."[2] He vehemently opposed the advent of chemical additives to foods that flooded the market in the 1950s, and attacked the FDA for not upholding its mission of protecting the safety of the food supply while "throwing money away like drunken sailors at a carnival" in its assault against his natural medicine practices.[3]

Throughout Hoxsey's era, organized medicine denied any link between diet and cancer. As Dr. Morris Fishbein contended, "There is no scientific evidence whatsoever to indicate that modification in the dietary intake of food or any other nutritional essentials are of any specific value in the control of cancer."[4] Science has since contradicted him.

In general terms, contemporary research has shown that the Hoxsey diet does directly serve important anticancer functions. Reducing overall caloric intake, as this diet does, suppresses and retards tumor growth. Most tumors are also promoted by the kind of high-fat diet Hoxsey excludes.[5] Today this diet would surprise few health-conscious eaters, but in Harry Hoxsey's era the regimen was quite radical, especially in a place like Texas, where fried foods, meat at every meal, sodas and white sugar and white flour were standard fare. In many places in the United States today, patients still complain about the lack of availability of fresh, healthful foods to comply with the Hoxsey diet.

As is now commonly known, substantial data indicate that diet can both cause and alleviate cancer. Much contemporary research confirms that certain foods, as well as the plethora of synthetic additives present in most foods, can contribute to the onset of cancer.[6] Research has further shown that people who eat abundant fruits and vegetables have about half the risk of cancer and a lower death rate than those who don't. The National Institutes of Health now recommends a diet rich in vegetables and fruits and lean in fat. Of 156 dietary studies recently reviewed, 82 percent showed that fruit and vegetable consumption provided significant protection against many kinds of cancers.[7]

A Finnish study found an inverse relationship between lung cancer incidence and the consumption of dietary flavonoids found in fruits and vegetables.[8] A study in the Netherlands has shown that allium vegetables such as onions, garlic, and leeks reduce the risk of stomach and colon cancer.[9] A diet rich in antioxidants from fruits and vegetables has been found to be a factor in protecting against nonmclanoma skin cancer.[10]

A 1988 study by Dr. Harold Foster at the University of Victoria, British Columbia, reviewing two hundred cases of "spontaneous regression" from cancer discovered that almost 90 percent had made changes in their diet preceding their recoveries. Most involved shifting to a vegetarian menu and eliminating white flour, sugar, and heavily processed foods. Many also used vitamin and mineral supplements, as well as herbal teas.[11]

Orthodox medicine now increasingly acknowledges these connections. In fact, a great body of this knowledge already existed by the 1930s and 1940s, and Dr. Fishbein did much to obstruct it. Most prominent among his targets was Dr. Max Gerson, whose appearance at the 1946 congressional hearings on cancer conducted by Senator Claude Pepper brought forth provocative testimony on the ability of diet to palliate or even cure cancer.[12]

Dr. Gerson used an elaborate program of natural foods and fresh juices grown without synthetic chemicals, along with liver injections, potassium iodide, and a sophisticated course of vitamins and mineral supplements. The diet was low in salt, fat, and animal protein and high in carbohydrates and fresh organic fruits and vegetables. (Dr. Gerson adamantly opposed the use of chemical fertilizers.) It eliminated meat, milk, alcohol, and canned or bottled foods, and forbade smoking. Dr. Gerson claimed a documented success rate of around 30 percent with terminal cancer patients.

Numerous Gerson patients offered their testimonials at the hearing, followed by Dr. George Miley of New York's Gotham Hospital, who, as discussed earlier, would later land in hot water for his testimony on the failures of surgery and radiation. "We do know experimentally that diet definitely does influence cancer," Dr. Miley told the Senate committee. He called the Gerson method "the first promising method which treats cancer as a systemic disease, that is, a disease of abnormal chemistry of the whole body."[13] The basic elements of the diet Gerson recommended are today widely acknowledged for their general health virtues. Yet, like Hoxsey, Dr. Gerson was blackballed and harassed for the rest of his professional career.

Vitamin and mineral supplements such as those prescribed by Hoxsey are also being proved today to influence the onset and treatment of cancer. Research from Finland has shown a 32 percent reduction in prostate cancer incidence among patients using vitamin E, which may provide protections against colorectal and lung cancer as well.[14] (Even by the 1950s, Canadian doctors had scientifically established vitamin E as effective in preventing heart disease, although conventional medicine denied the connection.)[15]

In a 1994 study on the effects of vitamin megadoses on the recurrence of bladder cancer, patients with cancer who received only the recommended daily allowance of vitamins and minerals experienced a tumor recurrence rate of 91 percent. Those who got the megadoses had a recurrence rate of just 41 percent.[16]

Dr. William Fair, an eminent surgeon and former chairman of the urology department at Memorial Sloan-Kettering Cancer Center, began a nutritional, Chinese herbal and holistic approach to his own colon cancer after four surgeries and chemotherapy failed. His cancer shrank and he has survived to launch nutritional research focused principally on vitamins C, D, and E, as well as the soybean, Chinese herbs, and the mineral selenium.[17] Meditation, yoga, and other stress-relieving techniques were an important part of his therapy. A 1998 study by Harvard researchers published in the *Journal of the National Cancer Institute* found that "higher selenium levels were associated with a reduced risk of advanced prostate cancer."[18]

In regard to diet and nutrition, clearly Harry Hoxsey was ahead of his time. But what if the Hoxsey tonic and diet really were worthless against cancer? Could they merely be placebos, "lies that heal" that work only because patients believe they will? (A placebo is an inert, inactive substance with no actual physical therapeutic activity. *Placebo* is Latin for "I shall please.")

"Don't Give Up Hope," Hoxsey proclaimed on the cover of the 1936 brochure for the Spann Sanitarium. As he wrote in *You Don't Have to Die*, "Cancer is not only a disease, it is also a psychosis. Tell a victim he is 'hopeless' (or let him discover it from his family), and the will to live becomes paralyzed. Show him a way out, strip him of fear and hysteria, give him even a forlorn hope, and the will to live is stimulated. It becomes a powerful ally in the battle against death."[19]

In his film Hoxsey elaborated on his view of attitudinal healing. "These people have one simple thing in common: They were frightened, confused. They did not know which way to turn for help. Fear is like a bullet fired into the mind. It can kill with deadly accuracy. Sentence a patient to death, remove all hope, and he will obediently roll over to wither away. Their tissues, their bones, their blood may be diseased, but their will to live is sound and healthy. That is why they are here. When the horror of this ugly scavenger casts its shadow, each one of these people has asked, 'What do you do? Where do you go?' This place is their beacon of hope, the ray of light that might lead the way."[20]

Jim Burke remembered watching how Hoxsey mingled with his patients. "Dr. Hoxsey introduced me to the few patients around, and he would put his arm around them, these old women with cancer, and say, 'Mother, I ain't going to let you die. You're going to get well. Them doctors are going to cut you up and kill you. But I'm here and I'm going to see that you get well.' They believed him.

"When Harry would come into that clinic, it was filled with people who had come from all over the world. The doctors had given up on them. Pitiful sight. But the man had something. He would come in and he'd put his arm around those old people and somehow he had the ability to inspire them to get well. He must have triggered something in their psyche or in their physical makeup that perhaps triggered something in them that made them cure themselves."

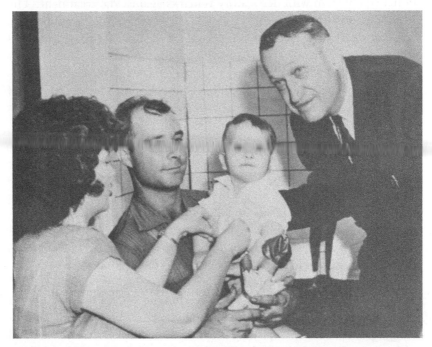

Observers noted that Hoxsey seemed able to talk patients into getting well.

Mildred Nelson agrees. "Harry felt that the patients' attitudes played a very, very big part in their getting well. If he could say anything or show them anything or convince them of anything that would lead them to believe they could do this, he would do it. 'Know that you're going to get well.' They believed him and would do it for him, along with the medication and everything."

Was Hoxsey just pitching an ephemeral "castle in the air where sick folks get well," as Norman Baker's hospital advertised? Organized medicine thought so. "There is a kind of hope that is useful and even therapeutic to some patients if it is based on reality, or even a small percentage of cures," the FDA's William Grigg remarked. "But to raise a person's hope in this way and then have it crash down, as you read in all these stories of these poor people, have them spend the money their families needed, and then discover that they had been duped in this way, you couldn't find anything crueler. Even cancer itself was not as cruel as the horrible realization by these people that they had been duped."

A poignant 1950s internal FDA memorandum described a Hoxsey patient's complaint about how agents came and disturbed her fragile emotional equilibrium with derogatory remarks against the treatment. The FDA Commissioner himself responded. "We are not unmindful of the well-known medical fact that sick people often show improvement from any new treatment. In many cases the psychosomatic response is sufficient justification for using the treatment even though its pharmacological activity may be questionable. This is not so, however, in the case of cancer, where early and competent treatment is of the utmost importance to the welfare of the patient."[21]

Although Dallas physician Harry Spence believed that Hoxsey's medicines were useless, he acknowledged their possible psychological benefits. "I think that hope is the greatest thing he had to offer. True, it was a misguided hope, a false hope. There was no hope. But still, from the patient's point of view, it was hope." Oliver Field of the AMA went further. "People who think they've been treated, it's up here in their minds and in their hopes, and their unwillingness to face reality. The hope has to be false if they do have the fact of cancer in their bodies."

"When you can define false hope, let me know, because there isn't any," countered Dr. Bernie Siegel as we filmed him in 1985 in his New Haven office near Yale University, where he taught and operated his private cancer surgery practice.[22] A spirited, radiant presence with shaved head and white doctor's smock, he spoke in swirling gusts of ideas. "What I think doctors call false hope are statistics. You take a disease, and it kills nine out of ten people. So you go down the line telling ten people they're supposed to die. You probably will kill ten out of ten by taking hope away. I see that in reverse. I say, 'Oh, 10 percent survive. That's good.' Then I go into every room and I say, 'You have a chance of getting well, and I'll tell you how the 10 percent who get well do it.' I might get 30 or 40 percent well. At least I have an option then. There is no false hope in the individual who has an illness. It is real, it is physiologic, and I have no difficulty giving it to people"—Dr. Siegel then echoed Harry Hoxsey—"because I know people today who are alive because I said, 'You don't have to die.'"

Dr. Siegel, who has authored several bestselling books on the subject of attitudinal healing, including *Love, Medicine and Miracles*, began to grope in his own practice for a profile of cancer survivors. "People do get well when they're not supposed to. I met a lot of people who didn't die when they were supposed to, and there are charts in this office of those people. The key factor was that, if you tell somebody they'll be dead in six months and they're feeling better than ever in six months, they don't come back for a checkup. So most physicians do not know who didn't die when they were supposed to.

"I read *Cancer Ward* many times before the words came off the page, where Solzhenitsyn uses the term *self-induced healing*—not *spontaneous* or *miraculous*. If we want to make medicine success-oriented, we would take the patients who get well or do better than they're supposed to, identify it as something they had something to do with, and then teach that to other patients who are willing to undertake it. That's what I started doing. Now, most patients don't want the added work. That's why we have so many doctors. It's more difficult to change your life than it is to have an operation. The submissive eight out of ten patients come in and lie down, but the two out of ten say, 'Hey, I want to participate.'"

Dr. Siegel illustrated the medical profession's own attitude toward people who get well when they aren't supposed to. "These are quotes from doctors: 'That case is a lie'; 'That's an error in diagnosis'; 'That's a slow-growing tumor'; 'Oh, that's a well-behaved cancer.' Never do they say the patient had anything to do with the outcome. That's the point I keep trying to make: People have something to say about what happens to them."

Dr. Siegel began to see a distinct portrait emerge of the "Exceptional Cancer Patient." "They're all the people that doctors and nurses don't like. When the nurse comes up to you and says, 'Your patient's a real nuisance. He won't take his clothes off, and I can never find him in his room, and he keeps questioning every blood test,' you say, 'Good, he's going to live longer.' In studies that are done at Yale with patients with melanoma, the woman who did it, a psychologist, said it got to be a joke because there was a 100 percent correlation between the opinion of the head nurse of the patient and immune-system activity. If the nurse said he's a real SOB and won't let you draw the blood for the test, no trouble with the immune system. If he was a wonderful, submissive, gentle patient who will not question anything, he was in trouble.

"In the study at Johns Hopkins, patients with breast cancer—all long-term survivors—were identified by the doctors as having a poor relationship with their doctors. So that's one piece of advice I give everybody. Want to live longer? Develop a poor relationship with your doctor. The so-called 'bad' patient is a good patient from the standpoint of survival, and you can train people to be a good/bad patient."

Although it is dangerously simplistic to generalize about a "cancer personality," studies of patients experiencing remarkable remissions do generally affirm that survivors display a fighting spirit.[23] Mildred Nelson sees the same profile in her clinic. "They're all free-thinking people, or they wouldn't even be here. The majority of them make up their mind before they get here. This is what they're going to do, and they are going to win it. There are some people, who are practically dying, telling you what they are going to do tomorrow, next week, and next year. For some it's a front. Others believe that they will win the battle. They're that determined. Some of them do win it. Everyone's told them that they cannot, and they say, 'I will show you.' But those people have a totally different mental attitude toward life and the value of life, what's important to them, as far as their religion, their faith in God."

In some sense, patients seeking out Hoxsey and other alternative cancer treatments are self-selecting. They are taking charge of their lives and making a willful decision to live. They are sufficiently adventurous to journey across an international border to a "quack" clinic. As such, they are already distinguishing themselves as possible survivors by sheer force of will and intention. It is difficult to know how much impact this personality profile affects the healing process.

The atmosphere at the Bio Medical Center is decidedly upbeat. When we filmed with Florence and Frank Gibson, a couple there to check up on Florence's breast cancer, they described their experience. "Just coming to this clinic," Florence confided in a warm voice, soaking in the Mexican sunshine, "you get an entirely different sense than when you go to a cold, sterile hospital, where nobody talks to anybody and everybody is afraid."

"That's the thing that impressed me," chuckled husband Frank. "I thought this was a psychiatric place, all these people laughing and talking, and they're supposed to be sick!" "Because we have hope," Florence added. "We know cancer doesn't have to be a death sentence."

When Rex Major came from New Zealand, he was unprepared for what he found. "The thing that I was intrigued about was the attitude of most of the people in the waiting room. There's an awful lot of sick people there, usually the first-timers. But the laughing and the jokes and the friendly camaraderie created in that place is something to behold.

"I was only supposed to be there for one day, but I decided to stay for three days. I kept going back, hopped on the shuttle bus with Raul from the International Motor Inn and went back across the border, my wife and I, just to be there. Just to chat with other people. I didn't have to be there. I was sort of looking for excuses to be there, because I got so much motivation and confidence from just being in the building and watching and talking and listening to what was going on around me. I had to really tear myself away from that place."

Dr. Bernie Siegel finds Rex Major's experience common among patients using alternative cancer therapies. "Something that you see as you travel around the world and visit alternative cancer clinics is that there are some people who got better. Maybe it's only 10 percent. My comment generally is it's those people who have done it. I'm not sure that any of those therapies mean anything, but it has given them hope and instant group therapy, because a lot of people come together with those beliefs and you see something happen.

"A placebo is a hope-giver," Dr. Siegel underscored with conviction. "You have to remember the power within that word. We tend to label things we don't want to understand, like 'spontaneous remission.' You don't have to study that: That's a word. 'Placebo.' Oh yeah, placebo. But for somebody to get a shot of water and have his hair fall out because he thinks it's chemotherapy, or the other side of the coin—to get a shot of water and be told it's an anticancer agent and have your cancer melt away— is incredible! That means within the body is this incredible power that the mind and body communicate, so why not stimulate that?"

Dr. Herbert Benson of Harvard, an early pioneer since the late 1960s in the nascent field of mind-body medicine, has extensively studied the "placebo effect" among people who exhibit actual medical effects after using the inactive decoy. A cardiologist, he successfully treated his own high blood pressure in the late 1960s through meditation. He was appalled to find that there was not one citation describing this mind-body interaction in the *Index Medicus* by the 1930s, when such phenomena were discounted as impossible.[24] Even by 1985, a famous editorial in the *New England Journal of Medicine* derided the ability of emotions to contribute to disease outcomes as "folklore . . . a myth [that] serves as a form of mastery."[25] As Dr. Norman Sartorius of the United Nations World Health Organization wrote, "The healing process has been relegated to the position of a disturbing effect, summed up under the name 'placebo,' equated to some kind of noise in the system."[26]

Yet what does the placebo trigger in a person to be able to accomplish such "miraculous" results as significantly lengthening survival time or even dispatching a supposedly incurable cancer? How is it that people exhibiting multiple personality disorder have real physical diseases come and go with shifts in persona? Are there other interactions among the body, mind, and spirit that compose what Norman Cousins called a "healing system" capable of self-diagnosis, self-repair, and self-regeneration, "a grand orchestration of all the body's systems enabling human beings to meet a serious challenge"?[27]

In fact, very startling data on placebos emerged in 1998 in what the *New York Times* billed as "The Brain's Triumph over Reality." Several studies have shown that placebos often work as well as actual treatments. Doctors in Texas performing arthroscopic knee surgery found that a placebo group given only anesthesia and three little cuts in a sham operation where surgical instruments were not used reported the same amount of relief from pain and swelling two years later as those who had the real surgery. Another review of placebo-controlled studies of antidepressant drugs showed that placebos and drugs worked about the same. Dr. Irving Kirsch, a psychiatrist at the University of Connecticut who conducted the review, concluded that placebos are about 55 to 60 percent as effective for controlling pain as most active medications.[28]

"Explanations of why placebos work," reported the *New York Times*, "can be found in a new field of cognitive neuropsychology called *expectancy theory*—what the brain believes about the immediate future. The expectations that result are internally generated brain states that can be as real as anything resulting purely from the outside world. 'We are misled by dualism or the idea that mind and body are separate,' said Dr. Howard Fields, a neuroscientist at the University of California at San Francisco who studies placebo effects."

Dr. David Spiegel, a specialist in hypnosis and dissociative disorders at Stanford University, conducted a study of breast cancer patients to determine whether "psychosocial intervention" could affect their degree of pain and disposition. He structured the experiment with two groups, one that offered mutual support and social contact from the families and a control group without these factors. The subjective experience of pain in members of the support group was decidedly less and their ability to cope was enhanced.[29]

Several years later, skeptical of the results he himself observed, Dr. Spiegel returned to the group to see what had happened to the women. Although eighty-three of eighty-six ultimately died, the physician was amazed to learn that, where all the members of the control group died within four years, a third of the intervention group was still living after the same time frame. The intervention group lived an overall average of twice the length of the control group. He also saw a "dose response" indicating that the more support sessions the women attended, the longer they survived.[30] A follow-up study looking at actual survival time among breast and prostate cancer patients using psychosocial intervention found that the intervention group did live "significantly longer."[31]

Evidence is now accumulating that demonstrates the general health benefits of a positive outlook. "People who look on the bright side have reason to be optimistic," wrote Susan Gilbert in the *New York Times* in 1998. "Evidence suggests that they have healthier, longer lives than their gloom-and-doom counterparts. For years, research has shown that optimists weather coronary bypass surgery better and live longer with H.I.V. Now a new study suggests that positive thoughts are also good for healthy people." A study of first-term law school students found that those who were optimistic about doing well had more T-cells and natural killer immune cell activity than they had before the semester started. The study further showed that the greater the optimism, the higher the immune measurements.[32] These findings clearly illustrate that thoughts and feelings affect the immune system.

As a consequence of these and other definitive studies, the medical profession is increasingly embracing attitudinal healing as a valuable adjunct in cancer therapy. As a nonsurgical and nondrug treatment, attitudinal healing in a certain sense represents less of a material threat to conventional medicine than, say, an herbal tonic. It does pose a philosophical challenge, however, as evidenced by the fact that cases of remarkable remissions have seldom been studied until fairly recently.

Today, mounting evidence shows that mind and body are not separate entities, but blend in a fluid plasticity of fantastically complex interactions. Dr. Bernie Siegel, citing a physicist noting important advances in our understanding of quantum physics, oberserves simply, "Desire and intention alter the physical world. They can thus cause things to occur which would not normally occur if they were not desired. From my experience determination is necessary too."[33] Hypnosis is well documented as a practical technique for speeding the healing of wounds and altering basic physiologic processes. Emotional and mental states have been shown to increase the neuropeptides and endorphins that seem to mirror or regulate moods and which have a direct relationship with immune cells. Dr. Candace Pert, former chief of the Brain Biochemistry Section of the National Institute of Mental Health and codiscoverer of endorphins, suggests, "It's not far-fetched to think of cancer treatment based partly on emotional intervention. Maybe that's the reason emotional catharsis seems often to precede healing; it's like kicking an old TV set stuck on vertical hold."[34]

In the comprehensive book *Remarkable Recovery*, authors Marc Barasch and Caryle Hirshberg roved the scientific literature and scanned numerous cases of improbable remissions from many afflictions, including cancer. In their exhaustive "search of the miraculous," they found a biology of belief, a chemistry of caring, and a physiology of feeling all weaving into an altered state called healing. "If we have learned one thing from the extraordinary and inspiring people we have met on our journey," they wrote, "it is that healing is as much wild as domesticated, as much raw as cooked. It requires a certain daring, a willingness to explore many dimensions of wholeness. Only a handful who got well did so without coloring outside the lines. A new medicine, too, must learn to color outside the lines; lines that sometimes artificially divide doctor from patient, fact from feeling, surgery from synergy, chemo from caring. A medical system sensitive to the genuine needs of patients would base health care as much on the individual's intangible values and beliefs as on tangible pharmaceuticals and operations."[35]

Barasch and Hirshberg found several key commonalities across the profiles of these survivors. Many described a profound emotional release often resulting in a spiritual catharsis preceding their recovery. They took the opportunity to redirect their lives and choose a more satisfying path. Most had close personal loving relationships and an emotional support system. Many experienced a deep faith and surrendered their troubles to a higher power.

Barasch and Hirshberg raise the fascinating conundrum of what role these spiritual factors may play across the entire spectrum of remissions, including those attributed to conventional therapy. "Can we ever be certain whether 'real' treatment does not owe an unknown portion of its curative power to these 'nonmedical' factors? For that matter, how can we know the extent to which mind-body factors might account for the successes of even ostensibly well-proven treatments? In 1994, at a meeting convened by the National Institutes of Health Office of Alternative Medicine, a paper was presented analyzing responses of various disease conditions to 'nonspecific effects'—that is, placebos—using both alternative and standard therapies. It is reported that for either approach 'when both healers and patients believe that a treatment is likely to be effective, one can commonly expect improvements in up to 70 percent of the patients treated, even when the treatment is entirely nonspecific.'"[36]

Part of the power behind placebos is the enthusiasm of the physician as an "agent for optimism and hope and a great inducer of beliefs."[37] As Dr. Bernie Siegel relates, "When Cisplatinum [the chemotherapy drug] first came out at Sloan-Kettering and they gave it with great enthusiasm, 70 percent of the people were free of cancer six months later. Then the drug gets dispensed and the rate dropped to 30 percent, because the enthusiasm didn't go with the drug. So, yeah, I deliver surgery and drugs with enthusiasm and hope." As a droll French doctor once quipped, "Use the new therapies as quickly as possible before they lose the power to heal."

From their perspective using standard cancer treatments, conventional doctors report the danger of another kind of false hope: Many terminal patients want to believe that their odds for survival are better than the prognosis offered by their physician. One study of terminal cancer patients demonstrates that this kind of belief can lead patients to insist on "aggressive therapies that are useless and increase suffering," such as certain chemotherapy regimens.[38]

At the same time that conventional medicine has ignored the potential value of the placebo, it has been casual in applying its opposite. When doctors "give a cancer patient six months to live," they are delivering a *nocebo*. The shadow side of a placebo, a nocebo has the potential to be equally powerful as a kind of hex whose underlying message to the patient is to die. The beliefs of patient and doctor, as well as their shared projection, fashion a double-edged sword that can cut decisively to either life or death.

"You always have to be realistic, but hope is not unrealistic," said Dr. Larry Norton, head of the solid tumor division at Memorial Sloan-Kettering Cancer Center. "I can't necessarily tell you how to guarantee victory but I can tell you how to guarantee defeat: Be pessimistic. People who do well with the disease are those who know they will do well and will do anything to accomplish that. They have an irrational confidence in the future."[39]

"The history of [allopathic] medicine before one hundred fifty years ago is the history of the placebo effect," Dr. Benson points out. Only with relatively recent discoveries did scientific medicine enjoy tangible therapeutic successes. The proof by Robert Koch and Louis Pasteur of bacterial causes of disease resulted in effective antibiotics. Deadly tetanus was effectively ended by an antitoxin, just as streptomycin cured most strains of tuberculosis. Penicillin finally defeated syphilis and gonorrhea, and sulfa drugs proved effective against meningitis and scarlet fever. Significant contemporary allopathic technologies, Dr. Benson notes, include artificial heart valves, aortic pacemakers and defibrillators, blood and plasma transfusions, and organ transplants.[40]

Yet Dr. Benson warns that an overemphasis on these mechanistic advances has eclipsed the undeniable wholeness of the human being. He finds that 60 to 90 percent of visits paid to doctors should appropriately be treated in the mind-body realm, and from 10 to 40 percent of conditions are fitting for conventional physiological medical approaches. He envisions a new style of medicine reconstituted as a three-legged stool consisting of drugs, surgical procedures, and self-care founded in belief systems. Only around 1910 did the word *placebo* become a pejorative term in medicine. He suggests that "placebo" be rephrased as "remembered wellness" and celebrated again as an invaluable therapeutic tool.

The first national conference on spontaneous remission was launched in 1998 under the auspices of the Institute for Noetic Sciences, a non-profit California group founded by astronaut Edgar Mitchell that was among the first to bring scientific rigor to this crucial area. Under the direction of the late Brendan O'Regan, the Noetic Sciences remissions database began collating many of these astonishing cases in the 1980s, starting with the sixty-five "miracle" cures certified by the Catholic Church at the sacred shrine of Lourdes in France.

For the first time in its sixty-year history, the National Cancer Institute has started an Office of Survivorship to begin to look at spontaneous remissions. The startling work of Dr. Larry Dossey documenting the positive effects of prayer and other seemingly "miraculous" forms of spiritual healing has gained wide interest and credibility.[41] The best-selling book *Spontaneous Healing* by acclaimed physician and author Dr. Andrew Weil has also focused attention on the subject.[42]

Journalist Ron Rosenbaum witnessed the profound healing power of hope during his visits to several Mexican alternative cancer clinics, including Hoxsey, around 1980.[43] "As long as orthodox medicine continues to fail with its fearsome and destructive therapies, there's a role for the deluded dreamers, the biomystic visionaries, the masked microbe detectors, apricot pit alchemists, mind cure mesmerists—all who keep supplying us with theory after elaborate theory about the elusive malignant plague. Somehow the periodic transfusions of false hope the cancer cure cults supply us with serve a purpose. We need a Tijuana of the mind, a place we can retreat to to smuggle back some illicit hope when our own world doesn't offer much. We need a fertile poetics of fraud to fool ourselves into fighting for our lives. I don't know what's in that Hoxsey tonic, don't want to know, in fact, but having immersed myself in the mystique and made a pilgrimage to the shrine, I have a feeling—yes, a false hope, the American Cancer Society would call it—that the old-fashioned elixir might do me some good someday."

While disparaging any cancer treatment using a therapeutic mix of herbs, diet, and attitude for the better part of a century, conventional medicine has instead promoted the exclusive use of surgery, radiation, and chemotherapy. One would expect that this sole reliance on these techniques stems from a strong record of proven efficacy. The truth, however, may be one of the better-kept secrets of conventional medicine.

Conventional Cancer Treatment: "Heroic" Medicine

Doctors use surgery, radiation, and chemotherapy as the standard treatments for cancer. Even if one accepts the National Cancer Institute's widely disputed statistics, at least half of cancer patients still die within five years of diagnosis, some 560,000 Americans in 1999.[1] If we are winning the war against cancer, as the NCI asserts, why has the U.S. cancer death rate increased by over 10 percent since 1950?[2] What proof really is there to justify the use of these "proven" methods?

It must be unequivocally stated at the outset that *there is no question that conventional treatments are effective in certain cases and cancers*. Patients reviewing their options would certainly be wise to avail themselves of these choices before considering other avenues, especially for those cancers that have been documented respond successfully to these treatments.

Even by today's science, cancer remains vaguely described as a broad group of diseases characterized by the uncontrolled growth and spread of abnormal cells. It is an unusual disease because it afflicts vegetable, animal, and human life. It is a very ancient killer, first recorded more than four thousand years ago in Egypt and India. Hippocrates first characterized tumors as *karkinos* or *karninoma*, giving rise to the word *carcinoma*. The physician Galen (A.D. 131–200) first gave it the term *cancer*, likening it to a crab's feet.[3]

There are hundreds of kinds of cancer, and its etiology remains mysterious. Causal theories abound ranging from chronic irritation to environmental factors, genetic inheritance, and viruses or microbial hosts. Each theory has valid data to support it in certain instances. Chronic irritation is certainly a factor in cigarette smoking. Environmental and industrial pollutants have been widely documented to cause cancer.

Genetic predisposition is accepted as an important factor in some cases, yet it is seldom deterministic.

Conventional medicine currently sees cancer as a disease of damaged genes. One viewpoint suggests causality by carcinogenic chemicals that induce genes to mutate and stimulate uncontrolled growth. Another proposes a viral origin in the creation of tumors. Both factors produce cancer genes called oncogenes, from the Greek *onkos*, meaning a lump or mass. Although organized medicine rejected any viral theory of cancer for the better part of this century, there is now credible data to indicate viral involvement in certain cancers. Some scientists go so far as to suggest that cancer may turn out to be a virally transmitted infectious disease like smallpox, bubonic plague, and others that were the primary cause of death in 1900.[4]

Whatever the theoretical disagreements, the medical profession's overall failure treating cancer is evident in its very terminology. Orthodoxy long ago ceased using the word *cure* in favor of *five-year survival rate*. A patient living five years after diagnosis is statistically counted as cured, even if the person still has cancer or later dies of the disease. According to credible critics, seeming improvements in survival rates are often the result of statistical manipulations such as earlier diagnosis. Called "lead-time bias," this numerical sleight-of-hand misleadingly only appears to extend the life span of the patient.

Since the 1950s evidence has steadily accumulated that surgery, radiation, and chemotherapy are far less effective than the public is being led to believe. Investigative journalist Daniel Greenberg, writing in the *Columbia Journalism Review* in 1975, produced the first widely reported exposé showing that cancer survival rates since the 1950s have not progressed, and that improvements from 1930 to 1950 were mainly a consequence of improved hospital nursing care and support systems. The existing body of data came from a scant four "tumor registries" around the country representing only a fraction of the cancer population. He further warned against statistical misrepresentations stemming from wrong diagnoses, as well as the fact that cancer surgeons frequently rejected cases of advanced cancer to make their track record appear better.[5] The potential margin of error and possibilities for distortion were great.

Greenberg stated that even the valid improvements were very, very small, and that there had been no significant advancements in treating any of the major forms of cancer. Certain kinds of the disease such as lung and pancreatic cancer remained essentially incurable by conventional means. Greenberg found that after the introduction of chemotherapy, the survival rate for people with certain cancers actually appeared to decline.[6]

This anomaly raises serious questions as to whether these highly toxic drugs might actually be harming patients more than helping them.

Years before, in 1969, Dr. Hardin Jones had already released a shocking report on this issue at the Science Writers Convention sponsored by the American Cancer Society. Dr. Jones, a respected professor of medical physics from the University of California at Berkeley and an expert on statistics and the effects of radiation and drugs, essentially concluded that "the common malignancies show a remarkably similar rate of demise, whether treated or untreated." He went on to identify fundamental flaws in methods of medical measurement, and stated, "The possibility exists that treatment makes the average situation worse."[7]

Since 1956, when Dr. Jones initially made this kind of assertion, the scant three studies testing his devastating thesis have supported it.[8] Joining the fray, Nobel laureate James Watson charged that the American public had been sold a "nasty bill of goods about cancer."[9] This eminent codiscoverer of the DNA double helix remarked seathingly that the war on cancer was "a bunch of shit."[10]

Surgery is the oldest and most successful of conventional cancer therapies. When the tumor is localized, surgery can be a life-saving procedure, and the scalpel accounts for the majority of successes. One limitation is that surgery is a purely local application that is helpless when the cancer has spread through the system.

Surgery, which dates to ancient times, has always been controversial. Hippocrates, writing around 400 B.C., considered cutting into tumors below the surface dangerous and likely to shorten the life of the patient. He viewed cancer as a systemic disease, as did many early physicians, whose consensus was to leave it alone beyond the early stages.

By the twelfth century, doctors were closely tied to the church, which officially deflected the then barbaric practice of surgery from doctors to the disreputable class of "barbers." Their practice was gruesome and filthy, and filled the population with dread. Prior to the discovery of anesthesia, surgery was an agonizingly painful procedure, and few were willing to endure it. Before the recognition of asepsis (infection control), patients were as likely to die from infection as from the disease. Ironically, for hundreds of years the medical profession shunned surgery as quackery.

The first statistical analysis of the value of cancer surgery was conducted in 1844 by Dr. Leroy d'Etoilles and published by the French Academy of Science. Spanning a thirty-year time frame, the study looked at case histories of 2,781 patients from 174 doctors. It compared survival after using either surgery, escharotics, or no treatment. "The net value of surgery or caustics was, in prolonging life, two months for men and six months for women. But that was only in the first few years after the initial diagnosis. After that period, those who had not accepted treatment had the greater survival potential by about 50 percent."[11]

In the mid-nineteenth century the discovery of anesthesia and asepsis suddenly made surgery viable on a large scale. Now able to control pain and infection, surgeons began to flourish. Their new power coincided with the spike in cancer incidence synchronous with the Industrial Revolution. What had been a relatively rare disease commenced its long ascendancy to a pandemic.

The figurehead of infatuation with the scalpel was J. Marion Sims, infamous as a "woman's doctor" in the South during the latter part of the nineteenth century.[12] Practicing on black slave women, he began a set of grotesque experiments that his biographer characterized as "little short of murderous."[13] Sims started his practice even before anesthesia and asepsis, doping his captive subjects on opium. Relocating to New York City, he cofounded the Women's Hospital and amplified his activities with a coterie of other surgeons. Among his special interests was cancer.

The "Lady Managers" of the hospital dismissed Sims in horror over his practices, although he later regained his position. When the wealthy Astor family, several of whose members were stricken with cancer, offered a large grant to the Women's Hospital to build a cancer wing, Sims convinced them in 1884 instead to fund the New York Cancer Hospital, the first in the country exclusively devoted to the disease. Later to become Memorial Hospital and then Memorial Sloan-Kettering Cancer Center, it was destined to be the flagship of conventional cancer treatment, seeding a new medical terrain.[14]

Cancer surgeons now had a vast theater of operations to advance their craft. Excesses were common, operations such as the hemicorporectomy to remove the entire lower half of the body below the pelvis for bladder or pelvic cancers, and the "commando" to remove the jaw in its entirety. (Also especially popular were women's operations, including the routine procedure of a hysterectomy—removing uterus, ovaries, and fallopian tubes—for "emotional problems.") Surgeons thrived on "heroic" acts, the more radical the better. Most prominent among these was the "Halsted procedure," a radical mastectomy for breast cancer pioneered by and named for its originator, the previously mentioned Dr. William Halsted of Johns Hopkins University in Baltimore. Halsted and other surgeons became the rock stars of American medicine. Physicians and surgeons who objected to the excesses of heroic surgery were censured or ignored.

Surgery became standard practice, an assembly line of cancer treatment. Its dangers have since been only superficially acknowledged or studied. Dr. Hardin Jones suggested the likelihood that "radical surgery does more harm than good."[15] By the 1970s it was clearly determined that massive amputations such as the Halsted procedure were generally unnecessary. Far more conservative "lumpectomies" eventually proved at least as effective, as well as far less disfiguring and traumatic to the patient.[16] There is disturbing evidence that surgery may release cancer cells into the blood and lymph systems to spread.[17] Further studies have shown that cutting a tumor may increase its subsequent growth if it is not entirely removed.[18] In addition, ample documentation exists showing that the physical trauma of surgery depresses the immune system immediately afterward, just when metastasis is most likely to occur. Even needle biopsies may spread cancer.[19] There is also concern that tumors may actually secrete factors that control metastasis, and that removing them can disrupt a subtle balance in the body preventing the cancer's spread.[20] Physically and emotionally traumatic, surgery is the treatment most feared by patients.[21]

"Surgery is not really a 'cure,'" says Ralph Moss, whose rigorous research on conventional cancer treatments and the exclusion of alternatives led him to write several eye-opening books including *The Cancer Industry* (originally titled *The Cancer Syndrome*) and *Questioning Chemotherapy*. "Rather it's an amputation of the problem. It doesn't say anything about solving it, but simply eliminates the symptom."[22]

It must also be said that cancer surgery has saved innumerable lives and is the best option under certain circumstances. Surgery has produced more remissions than radiation and chemotherapy combined. Yet its limitations are also evident, and it does not fundamentally address the underlying causes and mechanisms of this systemic illness.

Surgeons came to dominate and define cancer treatment for the first thirty years of the twentieth century until radiation treatment began to emerge as a serious competitor in the 1920s. Ironically, surgeons vehemently opposed radiation as quackery, and it was not until 1937 that the American College of Surgeons finally endorsed it.[23] Throughout its tenure, radiation has remained fiercely controversial, among other reasons because radiation causes cancer.

Radiation is a modern version of another very old form of treating cancer: burning the tumor. Cautery, or burning, was a prevalent technique as long ago as ancient Egypt and Greece—Hippocrates used a sizzling iron—but even then it was controversial and believed by many to do more harm than good. Like surgery, radiation is a local treatment. It is used on about half of cancer patients, despite the fact that it can definitively be said to "cure" only a scant number of types of the disease such as early Hodgkin's disease (lymphatic cancer), and at times testicular, cervical, and prostate cancer. Its principal role is to keep tumors from recurring, but it does not seem to affect the remission rate or long-term survival significantly.[24]

Radiation is frequently used as a palliative treatment to alleviate pain, especially in lung, esophageal, pancreatic, breast, and colon cancer. It is often combined with surgery despite the fact that tests have generally shown it made no apparent favorable difference.[25]

Radiation can, however, cause temporary remissions, a fact that induced "radium fever" around the turn of the century and led to its widespread medical use by the 1920s. Because it was already well known several years after the discovery of X-rays in 1895 that the invisible beams caused severe burns, radium pioneer Dr. Emil Grubbé surmised it might be medically applied to cancerous tumors.[26]

Serendipitously, Dr. Antoine-Henri Becquerel, a noted French physicist and early radium researcher, discovered that the uranium ore called pitchblende emitted comparable rays, and Marie Curie and her husband isolated radium from it. When Becquerel carried a tube of radium in his vest pocket to a lecture in London for a few weeks, he noticed a consequent irritation on his abdomen growing worse and harming the tissue. Experiments were soon conducted putting radium inside screens and focusing the beam on skin cancer. It did kill the cancer, but exposure to the radioactive element also caused leukemia, cancer of the blood. Both Marie Curie, the discoverer of radium who coined the word *radioactivity*, and her daughter died as a result of their exposure to the seemingly magic element that glowed in the dark.[27] Fully half the cases of cancer from exposure to radioactive materials at that time occurred among doctors and technicians. Radiologists began to die from cancer in large numbers by the 1920s. The AMA attributed the deaths to an epidemic of communicable diseases.[28]

But by now industry had caught radium fever. Popular radium products included doll's eyes, fish bait, gunsights, and the lids and handles of chamber pots.[29] Radioactive fluoroscopes were the rage in shoe stores for measuring feet with X-ray vision, and doctors bathed the faces of teenagers with acne in the magic rays.[30] Companies produced chocolate bars infused with radium, along with radioactive "tonics" and milk sugar.[31] Companies manufactured watches and instruments brushed with radium paint. About 4,000 "luminizers," mostly women, applied the novelty in factories by "lip-pointing," using their lips and tongues to shape the brushes to a fine point. By the 1920s, many became ill with "radium jaw" and started to die, often from cancer.[32] The radium companies at first denied any link.

Scientists and doctors applied X-rays as a wonder cure for removing facial hair and for depression in women. X-rays were used to test eggs for freshness and to scan human fetuses for possible complications in delivery.[33]

By 1920 the first "radium bombs" were inserted in long hollow needles into cancers of the breast, womb, and other organs. Radium pellets were propelled through needles into the tumors and left there for as long as thirty hours at a single stretch.[34]

At $150,000 a gram, radium quickly attracted ferocious exploitation.[35] The chairman of Phelps-Dodge mining corporation, James Douglas, founded the National Radium Institute in

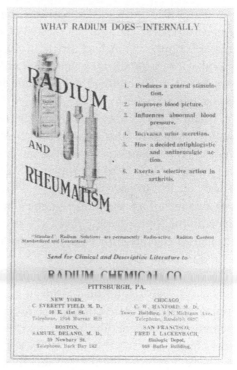

Radium fever overcomes medicine, ad c. 1900

1913 in concert with the U.S. Bureau of Mines to develop this newly precious resource. Douglas made a financial donation to Memorial Hospital with stipulations that the financially strapped institution treat nothing but cancer and use radium as a standard protocol. He insisted on installing his friend and physician Dr. James Ewing as chief pathologist. (Dr. Ewing later became medical director.) He linked with other business partners and allies including a close doctor associate at prestigious Johns Hopkins Hospital to emulate the scenario and spread the technology.[36]

Douglas succeeded in establishing radiation treatment for cancer as standard practice. A true believer, he watched his own daughter die of cancer using radiation therapy, and administered it to himself and his wife for minor medical complaints. He died of aplastic anemia, most likely the result of his radium folly.[37]

As radium enraptured the country and the press, Dr. Ewing aggressively innovated full-body irradiation at Memorial Hospital with virtually no safety precautions for either patient or practitioner. By 1937 the use of radiation surpassed surgery as the treatment of choice, despite "American characterizations of the 1937 Congress of Radiology as a 'congress of cripples.'"[38] A lead article in the *Dallas Morning News* in 1940 typical of the era proclaimed, "Diet of Radioactive Particles Possible Soon, Says Scientist," heralding the imminent day "when hospital patients eat radioactive particles for health."[39]

When Harry Hoxsey likely read that item in the Dallas papers, he was already intimately familiar with the effects of radiation on the patients landing on his doorstep. One of them was Mr. H. J. Myser, whose case was described in a 1954 FDA memo. "Mr. Myser is a victim of multiple cancer. He had to have almost one half of his nose removed and also an area two inches square on his forehead at the Mayo Clinic. Myser was given all the X-ray therapy that Dr. Ernst thought he could survive. He was nauseated constantly [and] lost considerable weight, which may have been due to the X-ray therapy."[40]

Another graphic example was Mrs. Ludie Johnson, who suffered uterine cancer. "Mrs. Johnson was given a series of radium treatments by implantation. She stated that the hemorrhages stopped completely after the radium treatment. She had another series of hemorrhages [about two weeks later]. She was then placed back in the hospital where the womb was packed [with radium]." She was then given a series of X-ray treat-

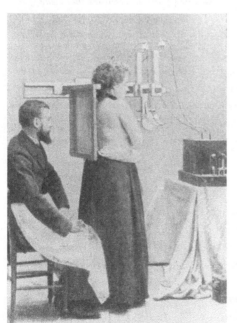

ments and suffered severe radium burns in her uterus before going to Hoxsey.[41]

By the 1930s the indiscriminate spree of irradiation was yielding a dark harvest of harm. It was already known by some scientists that even at low levels radiation caused cancer, and the ensuing debate engendered a sharp polarization of opinion within the medical profession exemplified by the words of one prominent critic, Sir Leonard

Doctors are enthralled by the magic of X-rays, but know nothing of precautions, c. 1900.

Hill, a renowned British physiologist. "The world would, I think, be little the worse off if all the radium in the country now buried in deep holes for security in bombings were to remain there."[42]

For years skeptics denied that X-rays were capable of causing cancer, until long-term surveys finally confirmed the connection. By 1946 a *New England Journal of Medicine* study found that radiologists died of leukemia eight times more frequently than other physicians. Studies published in the 1970s showed that children given X-rays for ringworm (a scalp disease) developed six times as many cancers as nonirradiated children.[43]

But in 1945 destiny held other designs. The horror of the dropping of the atomic bombs on Hiroshima and Nagasaki created a massive public relations problem for atomic energy. The result was a spirited campaign by the military to give radiation a positive image, and "our friend, the atom" presently donned a benign medical face. As the AMA claimed in 1947, "Medically applied atomic science has already saved more lives than were lost in the explosions at Hiroshima and Nagasaki."[44] The chairman of the Atomic Energy Commission was also a trustee of Memorial Sloan-Kettering Hospital, and promoted an aggressive strategy to hype the virtues and hide the perils of nuclear energy.[45]

In the 1950s President Eisenhower directed the Atomic Energy Commission to "keep them [the public] confused" about radiation, while Cornelius P. "Dusty" Rhoads, director of Memorial Hospital, publicly proclaimed the harmlessness of aboveground nuclear testing, minimized the hazards of radiation exposure, and celebrated its newfound medical marvels.[46]

The subsequent cover-up of the dangers of radiation by government and military officials has been well documented decades after the fact. The medical cover-up has taken longer to leak out.[47]

For most of its short life, nuclear medicine has been considered by the medical mainstream as harmless at worst.[48] The same negative information withheld from the public was also to some degree cloaked from the profession, which was often ignorant, though sometimes willfully so, of the data on the harmful health impacts of irradiation. A casual attitude toward radiation's dangers has prevailed, and those doctors and scientists who have spoken out against it have often been professionally stunted through the denial of grants or penalized with the loss of their positions.[49]

According to some estimates, around 78,000 people a year get cancer from medical and dental X-rays. In just one generation, the number of cancers caused in this way is estimated around 2.3 million.[50] John Gofman, M.D., professor emeritus of molecular and cell biology at the University of California at Berkeley, who worked on the atomic bomb and at the

Atomic Energy Commission, concluded in his 1995 book *Preventing Breast Cancer* that "our estimate is that about three-quarters of the current annual incidence of breast cancer in the United States is being caused by earlier ionizing radiation, primarily from medical sources."[51]

One Canadian study found a 52 percent increase in breast cancer mortality in young women given annual mammograms, a procedure whose stated purpose is to prevent cancer.[52] Despite evidence of the link between cancer and radiation exposure to women from mammography, the American Cancer Society has promoted the practice without reservation. Five radiologists have served as ACS presidents.[53]

Like surgery, radiation therapy has essentially been grandfathered in without being rigorously tested against a baseline measurement of no treatment. In the few tests comparing radiation treatment against no treatment, according to Dr. Hardin Jones, "Most of the time, it makes not the slightest difference if the machine is turned on or not."[54] Dr. Jones went even further, saying, "My studies have proved conclusively that *untreated cancer victims actually live up to four times longer.*"[55]

A recent study with patients with the most common form of lung cancer found that postoperative radiation therapy, which is routinely given, actually raises the relative risk of death by 21 percent, with its most detrimental effects on those in the early stages of illness.[56]

As Dr. Irwin Bross, the highly respected director of biostatistics at Roswell Memorial Park Institute, told Ralph Moss, "It is almost impossible to get 'peer review' that will accept a study of iatrogenic [doctor- or treatment-induced] disease. You just can't get people associated with the medical profession to accept a study that is frankly dealing with doctor-caused cancer. For thirty years radiologists in this country have been engaged in massive malpractice—which is something that a doctor will not say about another doctor."[57] Dr. Bross had his research funding dropped by the National Cancer Institute following the publication of his Tri-State Leukemia Survey in the *American Journal of Public Health*, which found medical radiation to be the principal cause of rising rates of leukemia, mainly from diagnostic X-rays.[58]

Nevertheless, although radiation has been found to be effective in only a very small number of cancers, it is administered today to about half of American cancer patients.

It was into this disappointing setting that chemotherapy entered as the next great hope of cancer treatment. Chemotherapy drugs are poisons that are indiscriminate killers of cells, both healthy and malignant. The strategy is quite literally to kill the cancer without killing the patient.

As early as the 1800s in the United States, doctors were injecting lead into women's breasts for cancer.[59] The word *chemotherapy* came from Paul Ehrlich, who also coined the term *magic bullet*. Ehrlich injected an arsenic compound into syphilis patients. Although most of them died horribly, a few extraordinary cures occurred, spurring a major boost for chemical medicine. Ehrlich's enthusiasm for chemotherapy spread, and the nascent chemotherapists brought a near fervor to their mission, despite a series of gruesome failures. Through the 1930s, within organized medicine chemotherapy was synonymous with quackery.[60]

The terrain was permanently altered in the 1940s by a twist of fate. After an Allied ship carrying the chemical warfare agent nitrogen mustard gas exploded in a remote Italian harbor, sailors who survived the catastrophe experienced a dramatic reduction of their bone marrow, and some perished from a severe drop in white blood cells. A Navy doctor recorded the mishap, but did not realize that covert government wartime experiments were already under way at Yale University on the effects of mustard gas on the blood.[61]

This government project created a soluble compound of nitrogen mustard and tested it on living tissues. One scientist proposed injecting it into mice with tumors. After two doses, the first mouse tumor shrank. Although the tumor returned a month later, another injection staved it off for eighty-four more days before the mouse died. Despite repeated attempts, the researchers failed to replicate the temporary remission in other mice, but this did not discourage them from commencing a clinical trial with a human subject in late 1942. The patient received "Compound X" for his lymphosarcoma, and the response was "as dramatic as the first mouse." Tumors softened and some even disappeared. Unfortunately, within a month that patient's white blood cell count dropped sharply and the tumor reappeared in the bone marrow. After several more courses of treatment, the patient died.

Investigators concluded that nitrogen mustard had potent antitumor activity, even though it failed to save the patient. Despite the fact that the next 160 subjects receiving the experimental drug all died, it did not slow the progression of this new "heroic" vector in cancer therapy.

As it happened, the chief of the U.S. Army Chemical Warfare Service was the aforementioned Cornelius P. "Dusty" Rhoads, a prominent figure in cancer research who had worked at Memorial Hospital before the war. When the war ended, Rhoads took over the leadership of the newly constituted Memorial Sloan-Kettering Institute for Cancer Research, the research arm of the burgeoning Memorial Sloan-Kettering Cancer

Center. Rhoads was a committed advocate of the new science of chemo-therapy, eager to discover a cancer cure in his own domain. He heralded a golden age of chemotherapy on the cover of *Time* magazine in 1949 from his leading-edge cancer hospital.[62]

Rhoads was riding the medical successes of penicillin and antibiotics in the 1930s, the first medical magic bullets that actually seemed to reach their target without destroying the host. It was also the carefree era of "better living through chemistry," a profound conviction in the human ability to rearrange nature molecule by molecule for precise human ends. This epoch trailed in the high-water mark of national unity caused by World War II, which generated Big Science and its pinnacle of mobiliza-tion: the Manhattan Project to produce the atomic bomb. The huge can-cer research effort adopted this Big Science model. The prestigious prov-ing ground of Memorial Sloan-Kettering Cancer Center started to ex-amine thousands of chemicals for their utility against cancer. It was a medical mobilization of unprecedented proportions against any disease.

Rhoads initiated the testing of over 1,500 different types of nitrogen mustard at Memorial Sloan-Kettering in the late 1940s. By 1955, the National Cancer Institute's Cancer Chemotherapy National Service Cen-ter started looking at 20,000 chemicals a year.[63]

Enthusiasm ruled the day as chemotherapeutic proclamations read like Hollywood press releases. The traditional conservatism of medical speculation was consumed in a frenzy of expectant optimism. The cure was on the horizon, year after mercurial year. The giddy anticipation drummed up formidable funding, climaxing in President Nixon's 1971 National Cancer Act: the "War on Cancer," with the biggest budget in history allotted for medical research. Entirely consonant with its desig-nation as a "war," cancer therapy marched forward armed with tumor-destroying weapons in a relentless campaign to conquer the disease.

Powered by massive funding, a new cancer industry was rapidly taking shape. A set of interlocking interests coalesced, ranging from giant corpo-rations to the government's National Cancer Institute and Food and Drug Administration, research hospitals and universities, and public nonprofits such as the American Cancer Society, the largest private charity in the country. The national press acted as hardly more than a credulous booster for the chemotherapy bandwagon. When David Dietz, president of the nascent National Association of Science Writers, addressed a science con-vention, he applauded the "fine and friendly relations which now *exist* between scientists and the press."[64] A subsequent study published in *JAMA* pointed out a troubling psychological factor in the emerging dynamic.

Given both positive and negative stories on a new drug, about half of reporters wrote solely about the positive conclusions, while none wrote exclusively about the negative.[65] In the decades to come, the press would consistently fail to shine light on the dark side of chemotherapy.

As Ralph Moss has pointed out in his critique *Questioning Chemotherapy*, "In the decades between 1960 and 1980, chemotherapists generally enjoyed a grace period during which the public ardently believed that a cure for cancer was around the corner. It was during this period that chemotherapy was shown to cause long-term remissions in relatively rare, but certainly tragic forms of cancer in children, such as acute lymphocytic leukemia, as well as in a disease of young adults, Hodgkin's disease. In addition, chemotherapy also contributed to the successful treatment of almost a dozen other rare kinds of cancer."[66]

Although these successes with children must not be belittled, what was unspoken was the fact that only 2 percent of patients who die are under thirty, as documented by John Cairns, M.D., an eminent biostatistician and professor of microbiology at the Harvard School of Public Health. Although chemotherapy's successful treatment of certain rare forms of cancer has been a life-saving contribution, Cairns continued, "For the vast majority of cancers, which arise in older patients, the results of chemotherapy are much more controversial."[67]

By the mid-1970s, the real numbers behind chemotherapy's alleged victories began to appear, like invisible ink held over a flame. Survival rates for 78 percent of cancers had not improved. There was an actual *decline* in survival in about 13 percent of cancers.[68] By the mid-1980s, prominent members of orthodoxy published unsettling assessments that could no longer be dismissed. Writing in *Scientific American*, John Cairns documented the failure of conventional treatments by examining the overall cancer death rates, which had risen. In other words, higher percentages of people were dying of cancer than ever before. According to Dr. Cairns, chemotherapy was able to save the lives of just 2 to 3 percent of cancer patients, mostly those with the rarest kinds of the disease.[69]

Yet another illusion faded with data provided by Dr. Ulrich Abel, a biostatistician at the Institute for Epidemiology and Biometry at the University of Heidelberg in Germany. A member in good standing of the cancer establishment, like many others he had believed that chemotherapy, even when it did not cure, did at least extend life. Instead, found Dr. Abel, "A sober and unprejudiced analysis of the literature has rarely revealed any therapeutic successes . . . There is no evidence for the vast majority of cancers that treatment with these drugs exerts any positive influence on survival or quality of life."[70] Abel called chemotherapy for the vast majority of cancers a "scientific wasteland," summing up his findings with one word: "Appalling."

In an arena theoretically based on meticulous clinical testing, chemotherapy has surprisingly meager proof to justify its widespread use. The standard of medical investigation is the randomized clinical trial (RCT). It is a carefully designed long-term study to determine the efficacy of a drug or treatment. Two groups of similar human subjects with the same condition are respectively given no treatment versus a new drug or regimen, and then compared against one another. The structure of the RCT is designed to eliminate bias and nullify expectation, while giving a large enough sampling to provide meaningful data.[71]

The RCT was initially proposed in the 1930s in England, and was first conducted there between 1946 and 1948. Only a handful of RCTs were conducted during the 1950s. Previously, there was little "objective" data in medicine, which relied on the same patient testimonials as Hoxsey used.[72]

A 1962 change in the U.S. Food, Drugs and Cosmetics Act requiring proof of efficacy as well as safety precipitated the widespread use of RCTs. It birthed a substantial and costly medical research infrastructure, weaving a web of close ties among universities, research hospitals, drug companies, and the government.[73]

The rising use of RCTs for cancer therapies paralleled the expansive burst of chemotherapy. But the abstract purity of the scientific method soon became fundamentally compromised by other exigencies. The gold standard of RCTs is the placebo-controlled, double-blind, randomized clinical trial in which a control group given a placebo is compared against the "arm" (branch group) receiving the real drug. In principle, neither subject nor doctor knows which arm is getting the real medicine, and the control group serves as a baseline for comparison. According to Ralph Moss, "In fact, true placebo controls have been almost abandoned in the testing of chemotherapy. Drug regimen is tested against drug regimen, and doctors hardly ever look at whether the drugs do better than simple good nursing care. The value of chemotherapy is a given."[74]

In fact, Moss asserts, oncologists have come to regard it as "unethical" not to give the drugs to all subjects. Consequently, there is no baseline marker of a no-treatment group against which to measure their actual effect. Critics say chemotherapy may actually be dispatching patients sooner and in greater numbers, but there are scant comparison data to verify the real scope of this possibility.[75] According to Moss, only about 1 percent of patients in clinical trials develop complete remissions.[76]

There are other reasons that make it virtually impossible to perform a blinded RCT with chemotherapy. The drugs have a kick like a mule, cause hair loss, nausea, vomiting, and many other obvious "side effects" such as turning urine blue, so that both subject and doctor will surely know who is getting the actual drug.

In fact, even the five-year survival rate is not applied to various measurements of chemotherapy "cures." For certain types of cancer, a one- or three-year surival may constitute a cure. As Moss suggests, this "rubber ruler" confuses any meaningful statistical analysis and provides a lot of wiggle room as to what "cure" means.[77]

But chemotherapy does exhibit undeniably dramatic results. "When a person is confronted with so-called terminal cancer," Ralph Moss told me, "you want to do something. The family wants to do something, and oftentimes the patient wants to do something. More often it's the family and the doctor who will want to do something rather than the patient. But in that situation, chemotherapy is the only thing they know to do. They don't know about or believe in any nontoxic or less toxic treatments. So they reach for the chemo bottle. Chemo produces a big effect. Everybody's thinks it's strong medicine. They realize the doctor is a powerful medicine man. This drug makes you really sick, so this must be really good. You don't have that feeling of just sitting around hopelessly waiting for the cancer to claim its next victim."[78]

While interviewing Ralph Moss at his Brooklyn office, I began to probe him on his extensive research on the efficacy of chemotherapy. Having recently completed his book on the subject, Moss went right into the weeds, citing highly specific data for each individual cytotoxic drug.

As he spoke, Moss rose and disappeared mysteriously into a back room stacked high with voluminous files. Reemerging, his curly-headed, rosy-cheeked appearance belied the fierce gravity and razor honesty he brings to his grim study of the dry medical records that mask the flesh-and-blood tragedy of real human suffering. He handed me the printout of a cancer case history from Memorial Sloan-Kettering. The eight single-spaced pages recorded the unimaginably massive regimen of experimental chemotherapy drugs administered to the patient over an eleven-month period before she died. Each line recorded a course of drug treatment. It seemed a miracle she survived the toxic assault as long as she did.

Researchers today are having an increasingly difficult time getting patients to participate in experimental clinical trials using the drugs Hubert Humphrey called "bottled death" before he died painfully under experimental chemotherapy.[79] Many doctors are now refusing to recommend such protocols to their patients, excepting the small percentage of physicians who are professionally associated with major research programs. The potential lack of subjects is a dire threat to the medical testing infrastructure, which is foundational to proving the efficacy of new drugs in order to bring the products to market.

The response of even oncologists themselves to chemotherapy is darkly instructive. In 1986 the McGill Cancer Center conducted a survey among doctors treating non-small-cell lung cancer. Over three-quarters of them actively recruited patients for clinical trials. The oncologists were asked what they would do if they themselves had non-small-cell lung cancer, a form of the disease for which standard treatment is the toxic drugs used in experimental trials. They were given six regimens from which to choose.

The survey concluded that "most specialists who treat lung cancer would not consent to participate as subjects in many of these trials." About three-quarters declined to take part in any of the trials because of the inefficacy of the treatment and the extreme toxicity of the drugs.[80] A comparable German study by Dr. Ulrich Abel came to the same conclusion, that "the personal views of many oncologists seem to be in striking contrast to communications intended for the public."[81]

Patients can easily be confused by misleading technical language about their chances using a chemotherapy regimen. One basic medical marker called the "tumor response rate" sounds to most patients like a positive regression. However, all that "tumor response rate" means is a 50 percent tumor shrinkage for just one month. In no way does it signify an actual remission or cure. Like the mouse whose tumor briefly receded before returning with a vengeance, cancer and death may well still result despite the statistically favorable short-term "tumor response rate."[82]

Nor does tumor response rate speak to the quality of life a person experiences. Many cancer patients receiving chemotherapy find the treatment worse than the disease. Considering the "side effects" of the drugs, it's hardly surprising that patients are increasingly loath to surrender their bodies on the cancer war's experimental chemotherapy battlefield.

Chemotherapy drugs are outright poisons, many of which are carcinogenic. One study among women surviving ovarian cancer after chemotherapy treatment showed a one-hundred-fold greater subsequent incidence of leukemia over those not receiving chemotherapy.[83] "Chemotherapy combinations can significantly raise the risk of secondary tumors," according to *Cancer Principles and Practice of Oncology*, the standard text written by the former director of the NCI himself.[84] In some studies, when chemotherapy and radiation were combined, the incidence of secondary tumors was about twenty-five times the expected rate.[85] It is common for chemotherapy patients not only to have virulent relapses, but their chances for recovery diminish even further if the cancer does recur.

Trials of one drug called ICE found 8 percent of the recipients dying from the drug itself in so-called "treatment deaths."[86] In another clinical trial with leukemia patients, the cancer drug killed 42 percent of the participants.[87] To add to the probem, the trend in chemotherapy has been toward "polypharmacy," a "cocktail" of mixed drugs. The very acronyms of these powerful, poisonous drugs highlight the mentality of the "War on Cancer" and inspire dread: BOLD, CHOP, COP-BLAM, and ProMACE.[88]

One of the biological "side effects" of chemotherapy is the destruction of bone marrow, the very basis of the immune system. The resulting weakening of the body's immunity makes patients subject to a plethora of secondary diseases and infections. They can easily die from minor maladies as a consequence. Because radiation and chemotherapy in particular lower or damage the patient's immune system, their early use can radically limit other options. Since Hoxsey and most other alternative therapies are based on stimulating the patient's immune system, conventional treatments can leave them little to work with.[89]

It is not only the patients who are in jeopardy. As Moss drily points out, "An oncology nurse's manual warns that cytotoxic agents pose a 'significant risk' of damage to the skin, reproductive abnormalities, hematologic problems, and of liver and chromosomal lesions. And this is just to the health-care workers preparing the drugs!"[90] Nurses are instructed to wear heavy protective gloves when administering them since an undiluted drop on the skin can burn a hole in the flesh. They are further advised to don face masks and long-sleeved gowns, and scrupulously avoid breathing in the agents. Disposal is accomplished in shielded containers labeled CAUTION: BIOHAZARD. Because of medical cost cutting, increasing numbers of patients take these dangerous drugs at home, and even bodily excretions saturated with the drugs are a toxic waste.[91]

Chemotherapy has presented a macabre set of new challenges for undertakers. As Jerome D. Frederick, director of chemical research for the Dodge Chemical Company, wrote in the *Dodge Institute for Advanced Mortuary Studies*, "Today's embalmer must cope with problems unknown to the morticians of earlier generations. For now, as in no other era in the history of the profession, chemotherapeutic agents (drugs) are used extensively by the medical men. Such changes may be comparatively minor in nature—limited to causing slight discolorations which respond readily to cosmetic treatment. But when they assume major proportions such as acute jaundice or saturate the body tissues with uremic poisons, the fixative action of the preservative chemicals contained in the arterials used become seriously impaired."[92] The study goes on to present a grisly taxonomy of anatomical deformities associated with each cytotoxic agent, advising morticians to work closely with doctors to ascertain which drugs were used.

While making the film, we searched out considerable footage ranging from old medical propaganda movies to contemporary treatment scenes. The only footage we couldn't locate was a documentary depiction of patients undergoing chemotherapy. Apparently it is considered so off-putting that medical institutions are resistant to release the depressing images. We finally got the film through another independent crew working on a show called *The Cancer War*.[93]

As far back as 1973, the head of the NCI Cytochemistry Division, Dr. Dean Burk, wrote to the NCI chief in dismay over the failed promise of chemotherapy. "Virtually all the chemotherapeutic anticancer agents now approved by the Food and Drug Administration for use or testing in human cancer patients are (1) highly or variously toxic at applied dosages; (2) markedly immunosuppressive, that is, destructive of the patient's native resistance to a variety of diseases, including cancer; and (3) carcinogenic. I submit that a program and series of the FDA-approved compounds that yield only 5–10 percent 'effectiveness' can scarcely be described as 'excellent,' the more so since it represents the total production of a thirty-year effort on the part of all of us in the cancer field."[94]

As Ralph Moss and others have documented, at best chemotherapy is *unproved* against 90 percent of adult solid tumors, the huge majority of common cancers resulting in death.[95] Nevertheless, *chemotherapy is given to about four of five U.S. cancer patients today, around a million people a year*.[96] "There's tremendous overmedication going on," says Moss. "It becomes an outrage when chemo is given in the vast majority of cases where they *know* that it's not likely to do anything."[97]

Again, however, it must be made clear that chemotherapy drugs do work for certain cancers. Lives have been saved or prolonged as a result of using specific chemotherapy regimens under the right circumstances, and patients should seriously review these options. Moss has cataloged these drugs in great detail in *Questioning Chemotherapy* and cited which drugs are documented to have life-saving results for particular cancers. (He also produces *The Moss Reports*, customized analyses for patients showing which treatments, including alternative ones, have shown valid data for specific cancers.)[98]

Putting a human face on these conventional cancer therapies is a harrowing experience. While making the film, we interviewed Bob DeBragga, a cancer patient who began his journey using conventional treatments. A passionate, graying man with a charismatic presence, DeBragga worked as a high-powered marketing representative for a large defense corporation when he learned he had a usually fatal lung cancer. His doctor gave him ten months to live.[99]

"I, like so many millions before me, started down the road of orthodox therapy. I knew of no other options that were available. I, like the average person, believed everything my doctor told me. I took six thousand rads of radiation, which is the most you can take—any more and you run the risk of total paralysis, since the electron beam has to be focused on the spinal column. And then I started the most feared part of cancer management: cytotoxic chemotherapy.

"You get the feeling, even before you take it, that if it would work, then you could deal with it. It's not a matter of cytotoxic drugs making you ill or that your hair falls out, because you don't care about that. When somebody has told you already to get your affairs in order, you don't care about things like that. All you want to do is live. And if Cytoxin and Adriomycin and Methotrexate and Procarbyzene, which were the four drugs that I took, can give you even some extra months, at a reasonable quality, you'll settle for that. But I had the book from the Mayo Clinic, and I knew that the median survival for my exact cell type under my exact conditions was thirty-six weeks with the best of orthodox treatment.

"I'll never forget what it was like the first time, the first moment the intravenous solution is shot into your veins, because I took Cytoxin as the first drug and it works instantaneously. The plunger is moved a sixteenth of an inch from the great big syringe and *you turn on like that!*" DeBragga shouted, snapping his fingers loudly and pounding on the table at the same time. "It was absolutely mind-blowing. It was like somebody hit me with a sledgehammer in the middle of the head and I got sick to my stomach all at the same time.

"But I want to make this very clear. If you really believed that these things worked, and if the data supported Cytoxin or Cisplatinum or any of the chemotherapeutic drugs—all of which are cytotoxic, all of which are indiscriminate killers of cells, all of which are carcinogenic, which is philosophically extraordinary—if you really thought it would help you, you'd go with it."

DeBragga paused to sip some water, breathe deeply, and regain his composure. "One of the things that was so extraordinarily terrifying in the course of treatment during the radiation phase would be to watch the patients come in. We'd all sit together waiting to go into the room with the linear accelerator, where we were the only one in the room and everybody else was outside the room looking at the patients that had already started to receive chemotherapy. The women had wigs. The complexions of the men and women were like a piece of white paper. Most of them had already lost weight. I know there are people that have done well with chemotherapy—a very small minority of people—but I never saw any-body in the entire four weeks of radiation treatment look remotely healthy at all. And it terrifies you because you know, as the days of the radiation go by, that you count the days till you begin the chemotherapeutic pro-gram. It's terrifying. It really is. Because not only are you worried about dying, now you begin to worry about how it's going to be to die."

Bob DeBragga became a cancer activist, founding a group called Project Cure, which continues today to inform patients about alternative options and to support their medical civil rights of access to them.[100] Us-ing nutrition and a variety of alternative therapies, he greatly outlived his prognosis.

Where has this state of affairs left the war on cancer? In a landmark study of cancer survival published in the *New England Journal of Medicine* in 1986, John Bailar, M.D., former editor of the *Journal of the National Cancer Institute*, reported disturbing findings that continue to prevail to-day. "Age-adjusted mortality rates have shown a slow and steady increase over several decades, and there is no evidence of a recent downward trend. In this clinical sense, we are losing the war against cancer." He tagged the cancer mobilization a "qualified failure." He was attacked by the Na-tional Cancer Institute for his public criticism, but the war on cancer was visibly becoming a war of attrition.[101]

Even the federal government's General Accounting Office has had little positive spin for the NCI's war on cancer in its review covering 1950 to 1982. It found that "actual improvements" in patient survival "have been small or have been overestimated by the [NCI's] published rates."[102]

By and large, however, the rigorous clinical testing that could reveal the objective facts about conventional cancer treatments has not taken place. Ironically, one of orthodox medicine's central rationales for reject-ing alternative therapies is that they are unproved, which turns out to be largely the case with its own approaches. Medicine is operating by a double standard, professing rigor but practicing elasticity.

Clearly, conventional cancer treatments can and do save lives, and have a rightful place. Yet they also have serious shortcomings and have not been sufficiently proved to justify their use in many cases. Overall, their limitations and destructive effects highlight the urgent need for fresh directions in research and treatment, as even mainstream oncologists are advocating today.

But why then is chemotherapy given to the huge majority of patients even when it is known not to work for most kinds of cancer? According to Dr. Victor Richards, a prominent oncologist, "Chemotherapy serves an extremely valuable role in keeping patients oriented toward proper medical therapy. Judicious employment and screening of potentially useful drugs may also prevent the spread of cancer quackery. Properly based chemotherapy can serve a useful purpose in preventing improper orientation of the patient."[103]

This "improper orientation" of the patient is a subtle code signifying a much deeper rift within medicine, a long-standing conflict of medical philosophy. Today's allopathic cancer treatments come from an unbroken therapeutic lineage called "heroic medicine" which is entirely consistent with present practices. What is this heritage?

The Hidden Roots of "Heroic" Cancer Treatment

The conflict of opinion between Hoxsey and the doctors is actually a very old story in medicine. Reflecting the long-standing therapeutic disagreement between allopathic and irregular practitioners, the conventional treatments of surgery, radiation, and chemotherapy bear an unmistakable philosophical birthmark placing them soundly within the genealogy of allopathic practices.

The word *allopath* was actually coined by Samuel Hahnemann, the founder of homeopathy. Where homeopathy is conceptually anchored in the law of similars, the precept that like cures like, allopathy uses "other" ("allo") approaches with no direct pathological relationship to the disease. Hahnemann intended the word as a slur since he believed the allopathic approach bore no meaningful connection to the specific illness and constituted the blind use of brute force.[1]

In broad terms, the two schools of medicine have been classified as the Rationalist and Empirical traditions.[2] While the diverse sects of empiric medicine were united around the belief in *vis medicatrix naturae*, the Rationalist or allopathic school placed no stock in nature's healing power. Instead, allopathy championed "heroic medicine," the need for aggressive intervention by the physician to vanquish disease with powerfully invasive treatments. Among its early leaders was Dr. Benjamin Rush, who lived in the late 1700s and early 1800s, and whose overarching influence extended for at least another hundred years. Thus did Rush comment on nature: "I would treat it in the sick-chamber as I would a squalling cat— open the door and drive it out."[3]

A prominent and prosperous physician and a signatory of the Declaration of Independence, Dr. Rush created an enduring legacy through his teachings as professor of medicine at Pennsylvania University, which then trained three-quarters of the doctors in the young nation. Like most allopaths of the era, he was adamant that theory must precede practice, a direct contrast with the empirics, who relied on experience and observation. He posited elaborate theories such as the "unity of all disease," the idea that all illness emanated from but one source: "irregular arterial action" resulting from a state of "debility" that first laid the basis for its appearance. He was further convinced that the cause of disease is fully knowable. His principal "weapons" were bloodletting and the administration of mercurous chloride, the form of mercury called calomel.[4]

Where the empirics favored gentle vegetable remedies, Dr. Rush and the doctors considered plant remedies to be "inert" and viewed the botanical knowledge of the Indians as contemptible. Dr. Rush's allopaths opted for toxic minerals including lead, arsenic, antimony, and, above all, mercury. They celebrated mercury and its derivative calomel as "the Sampson of the materia medica" and pronounced it "a safe and nearly universal medicine."[5] Doctors enlisted it for almost all maladies, even the most trifling of ailments.

Perhaps the quintessential prototype of allopathic therapeutics was the infamous treatment of George Washington, the aging founding father of the United States. On Friday the 13th of December 1799, the former president awakened in the middle of the night with a sore throat and fever. He proposed to his staff that perhaps a bleeding was in order. A local bleeder arrived who promptly relieved Washington of about fourteen ounces of blood.[6]

Still ill in the morning, Washington sent for his doctor, who soon summoned two other physicians. As the *Reformed Medical Journal*, an empiric publication, later recorded, "Think of a man being, within the brief space of little more than twelve hours, deprived of eighty or ninety ounces of blood; afterward swallowing two 'moderate' American doses of calomel, which were accompanied by an injection; then five grains of calomel and five or six grains of emetic tartar [antimony]; vapours of water and vinegar frequently inhaled; blisters applied to the extremities; a cataplasm of bran and vinegar applied to his throat, upon which a blister had already been fixed, is it surprising that when thus treated, the afflicted general, after various ineffectual struggles for utterance, at length articulated a desire that he might be allowed to die without interruption!"[7]

Scholars have estimated that Washington was drained of about half the blood in his body, a condition that would today be considered a medical emergency. The heroic doses of mercurous calomel he received— probably about 650 milligrams—constituted fatal heavy metal poisoning. Hardly twenty-four hours after waking up with a sore throat, Washington expired at the hands of his doctors.

The treatment afforded Washington was entirely commonplace. As Oliver Wendell Holmes, professor of anatomy at Harvard, commented on the wild west of heroic medicine in the United States, "How could a people which has a revolution once in four years, which has contrived the Bowie knife and the revolver . . . which insists on sending out yachts and horses and boys to outsail, outrun, outfight and checkmate all the rest of creation; how could such a people be content with any but 'heroic' practice? What wonder that the stars and stripes wave over doses of ninety grams of sulphate of quinine and that the American eagle screams with delight to see three drachms [180 grains] of calomel given at a single mouthful?"[8]

Dr. Rush and his contemporaries theorized that calomel worked by purging disease from the body or by displacing it and transforming it into a 'mercurial fever' that would get better by itself. As Barbara Griggs described the actual effects of mercury: "Following salivation, extensive areas of the facial flesh and bone sometimes became blackened and mortified, then sloughed away, eye, cheek, and all. Sometimes whole portions of the jaw rotted and fell out; occasionally the diseased jawbones fused together as in lockjaw, dooming the victim to a silent death from starvation unless the condition was corrected by painful surgery."[9]

Mercury also resulted in the invariable loss of mouthfuls of teeth and the destruction of jaw muscles. It severely impaired the salivary system, causing the tongue to swell to three times its normal size and discharge a stream of malodorous mucus over the lips. As heroic medicine journeyed across the continent farther away from Eastern medical institutions, heroic doses became "Herculean" ones.[10]

Bloodletting, which became widely popular among doctors after Harvey's proof in 1628 of the circulation of the blood, was administered to sick and healthy alike. Bloodletting by the lancet or leeches was considered to have "vast remedial powers." It was administered as readily to children and infants as to adults. Dr. Rush recommended it for any malady, draining up to four fifths of the blood from the body. "Among American physicians there is no one remedy of greater importance in the

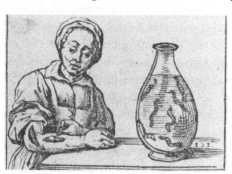

Allopathic medicine celebrated leeches and the knife to bleed away disease, and as much as 80 percent of the patient's blood.

treatment of diseases than the lancet," the preeminent doctor enthused, despite the fact that it engendered debility, fainting, and convulsions.[11]

Surgery was also exalted among heroic allopathic practices even in the absence of anesthesia and infection control. Doctors competed with one another to amputate the most body parts without dispatching the patient. As medical historian Harris Coulter sanguinely noted, "No life insurance company would insure a surgeon's wife."[12]

This was "heroic medicine," extreme measures for serious or mild conditions that produced undeniably dramatic results. As a highly organized professional class that began the 1800s as a virtual medical

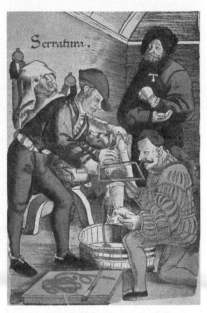

The horrors of early surgery.

monopoly, doctors were exceedingly confident they could know the source of illness and intervene boldly against nature to cure.

The widespread medical use of toxic minerals and chemicals dates back to at least 1500 in Europe. When the scourge of syphilis ravaged the continent, the only practitioners having any apparent measure of success were the surgeons. They had adopted the use of mercury from Arab physicians who were enthralled with alchemy, the mystical marriage of chemistry and philosophy. Alchemy began captivating Europe in the thirteenth century, and for three centuries it would preoccupy those seeking to unlock nature's great mysteries.

The European surgeons made pastes containing mercury, which would temporarily alleviate symptoms of syphilis because of its antibacterial action. The surgeons triumphantly heralded their apparent cures, claiming to transform poisons into medicines by their alchemical magic. Any therapy for syphilis other than mercury was promptly outlawed, and the commerce of apothecaries prospered greatly off the new business.

When the legendary sixteenth-century Swiss-German doctor Paracelsus came on the scene, he forever changed medical practice with his passionate embrace of the mineral remedies. He ridiculed mild vegetable medicines while celebrating the new mineral poisons of mercury and antimony. Known as the "founder of chemical pharmacology," Paracelsus is characterized by

Barbara Griggs as "the patron saint of the drug companies."[13] Allopathic medicine would mine his legacy in one form or another for five hundred years to come.

Before long, however, the hideous aftermath of mercury poisoning surfaced. As Griggs observed, "Since toxic substances were readily absorbed into the bloodstream through the open wounds to which they were applied, many of these apparently innocent and wonder-working cures must have left a trail of deadly side effects in the form of systemic poisoning. The new generation of progressive surgeons were probably blissfully ignorant of the damage they were doing. By the end of the sixteenth century, medical chemists all over Europe were feverishly experimenting with every metal or mineral known to man, reacting it with other chemicals, turning it into salts or oils, and then administering it to a patient."[14]

The excruciating effects of the chemical medicines performed an odd double duty. Since syphilis in particular and disease in general were widely believed to be manifestations of sin, the horrific effects of the mineral therapies served as both remedy and retribution. Many doctors were reluctant even to treat the immoral affliction of syphilis, though prominent aristocratic families such as Italy's Borgias begged for relief. "In Rome this kind of illness is very partial to the priests, and especially to the richest of them," Benvenuto Cellini coyly wrote.[15]

The advent of the controversial chemical medicines, which were already deepening the schism with plant medicines, further ruptured the medical profession itself. The derivation of the word *quack* originated with herbalists who described doctors using mercury and mineral poisons as "Quacksalvers" for their affinity for quicksilver.[16] Even other physicians held these mineral medicines to be the most odious expression of quackery, and dragged fellow doctors into star chambers—secretive tribunals acting as kangaroo courts—to seek censure against their brethren's mercury madness.

Nonetheless, by the late 1500s most surgeons were enthusiastically adopting the mineral poisons. They added arsenic, lead, and copper to their armamentarium of mercury and antimony. Although they still relied heavily on plants as well, the minerals brought irrefutably bold results, and the early adopters energetically used them to induce the vomiting, purging, and intense diuretic expulsion that they believed were curative. Patients, awed by the raw power of the new remedies, eagerly sought them out.

By 1600 clever tinkerers transmuted mercury into its modified form of calomel and applied it with abandon. The four classes of popular therapies were vomitives, purgatives, diuretics, and diaphoretics (to increase perspiration), and their effects were vomiting, sweating, raging bowels, intense salivation, and convulsions. By the end of the century, royalty was being treated with heroic doses of mercury and with pills made of gold leaf and turpentine. Mercury was the treatment of choice for syphilis, as well as for eczema. Calomel quickly became the standard prescription for purges and launched a frenzy of mineral medicines that would persist for three centuries among allopathic doctors.

Paracelsus himself had been conservative in his use of the deadly silvery metal, whose very mining the ancient Romans had feared enough to forbid. Even the father of chemical medicine would most likely have been appalled at its gleeful proliferation, a trend that would continue unabated in their journey from Europe to the therapeutic repertoire of the distant British colonies soon to become the United States.

Armed with heavy metals and the knife, doctors in the United States discounted the body's ability to cure itself and intervened aggressively. Dr. Benjamin Rush described his heroic stance as "that bold humanity which dictates the use of powerful but painful remedies in violent diseases. The conscientious, or bold physician who by the use of a remedy of doubtful efficacy turns the scale in favor of life, performs an act that borders on divine benevolence." [17]

The dire consequences of "regular" therapeutics exhibited a manifest destiny of their own. As Coulter observed, "An intriguing question is the responsibility of the medical profession for the generally recognized bad health of Americans in the period 1830 to 1860. *Harper's Monthly* stated in 1856 that the youth of this country were a 'pale, pasty-faced, narrow-chested, spindle-shanked, dwarfed race.' In 1856 the War Department published the results of its examination of recruits during the Mexican War: American volunteers weighed less than European or English recruits, and there were nearly twice as many rejections of Americans for being 'too slender, and not sufficiently robust' or for 'malformed and contracted chests.'

"Worst off, however, were the women," Coulter elaborated. "Thomas Wentworth Higginson wrote in 1861, 'In this country it is scarcely an exaggeration to say that every man grows to maturity surrounded by a circle of invalid relatives, that he later finds himself the husband of an invalid wife and the parent of invalid daughters, and that he comes at last to regard invalidism [as] the normal condition of that sex—as if almighty God did not know how to create a woman.'"[18] Higginson went on to record the horrid condition of American teeth, an unmistakable consequence of mercury poisoning: "One seldom talks to a dentist who did not despair of the Republic."[19]

An empiric critic of the period wryly cited allopathic treatments as "one of those great discoveries which are made from time to time for the depopulation of the earth."[20] The public seemed to agree and was by now considerably less than enthusiastic about these "heroic" procedures. People migrated in droves to the diversity of empiric healers by the 1830s. For the balance of the century, allopaths struggled to survive, suffering a humiliating nadir of unpopularity and poverty. As a droll observer of the period remarked, "With allopathic treatment, the patient dies from the cure. With empiric treatment, the patient dies from the disease."

These heroic practices of allopathic medicine evolved seamlessly into the twentieth-century expressions of radiation and chemotherapy. Radiation relies on yet another toxic mineral, radium, used in heroic doses to "kill" the disease. Nor does it beg a philosophical leap to trace the arc from mercury to chemotherapy drugs. They bear the same allopathic disdain for the healing power of nature. Only late in the twentieth century did allopathic medicine in effect acknowledge the existence of the Empiric *vis medicatrix naturae* by its recognition of the immune system, the therapeutic principle underlying Hoxsey's herbs as well as virtually all the nontoxic alternative cancer regimens.

In the twentieth century the renewed allopathic contempt for herbal medicine partly stemmed from its failure to cure syphilis or produce a dependable remedy for acute infection. Dr. Morris Fishbein expressed this aversion to botanicals in *Fads and Quackery* in 1936 when he observed with satisfaction the steady removal of plants from the U.S. Pharmacopoeia. "All the signs and portents indicate that the great deluge of modern scientific chemotherapy is about to wash away the plant and vegetable debris."[21]

This same conflict of medical opinion is playing out again today in the recurring cancer wars. As in the nineteenth century, however, the allopaths are experiencing waning public confidence in their practices. Their heroic cancer therapeutics do not sufficiently cure and often bring the same fearsome effects. By the mid-1980s, the "plant and vegetable debris" was beginning to wash back on the shores of medicine in a rising tide of popular favor and scientific validation. The allopaths had good reason to be anxious about once again losing their patients to the new generation of empirics, including the heirs of Hoxsey.

PART THREE

Money, Power,
and Cancer

Healing the Politics of Medicine

*"We must admit that we have never fought the homeopath
on matters of principle. We fought him because he came into
our community and got the business."*
Dr. J. N. McCormack, AMA, 1903

17

Cancer Scandals in the Capital: The *Hoxsey* Film Goes to Washington

As we raced to edit the *Hoxsey* movie in 1986, then in its third arduous year of production, a flash flood of events swept over us, dumping alarming new footage on the flatbed editing table and requiring maddening revisions in the narration. Echoes of Hoxsey's charge of conspiracy were thundering through the nation's capital. The scenario resembled a rerun of the divisive drama we were viewing every day in a darkened room in Santa Fe.[1]

In 1985 a group of cancer patients receiving Lawrence Burton's unorthodox Immuno-Augmentative Therapy (IAT) met in Washington, D.C., with Congressman Guy Molinari. The Bahamian government had recently closed Burton's controversial Freeport clinic, in exile in the Bahamas, based on reports from the United States that its blood supplies were contaminated with antibodies to the AIDS virus. The patients, mortified at being deprived of what they saw as their only lifeline, told Molinari they doubted the contamination reports. They believed the entire incident was simply the latest skirmish in the U.S. medical establishment's long war against Burton and other practitioners of unconventional cancer therapies. Molinari, having lost a parent to cancer, was sympathetic to the patients' plight. He flew to Freeport to inspect Burton's clinic personally, then held a congressional hearing on the matter.

The unfolding events implicated the usual suspects. The contamination reports, which had been widely disseminated by a top official at the National Cancer Institute, later proved to be wrong—the result of a false positive result on a preliminary screening test. Also involved was the American Medical Association, which had published the NCI contamination report in its *Journal*.[2]

Like many others, Lawrence Burton began his travails with what seemed like good news. A credible Ph.D. medical researcher in good standing, he and his associates were working along immunological lines under grants from the NCI, among other establishment institutions. They devised a serum extracted from a tumor-inhibiting factor found in fruit flies and later in mouse blood. Working at St. Vincent's Hospital in New York, where Burton was a senior investigator in the Hodgkin's Disease Research Laboratory, he was eager to show his astonishing laboratory results dissolving mouse tumors in a matter of hours. The cancer would return later, so Burton was not claiming to have found a cure, but he was demonstrating a dramatic force for inhibiting tumors that merited serious attention.[3]

Memorial Sloan-Kettering dispatched an investigator who coauthored a paper several months later and appropriately put his own name last on the list of authors.[4] Apparently his boss chastised him for diminishing the reputation of Memorial Sloan-Kettering's elite status by this association with an inferior research lab. Before long, Burton was offered a contract by Sloan-Kettering, which he rejected. His grants immediately evaporated.

Undaunted, Burton went back to work at St. Vincent's, where he continued experimenting on animal tumors and achieved the same astonishing results. Serendipitously, the same Pat McGrady Sr. of the American Cancer Society who once visited Hoxsey's Dallas clinic was a patient at the hospital and witnessed one of Burton's demonstrations. He invited the researcher to show his stuff.

Burton unveiled his method at a meeting of the American Cancer Society Science Writers Seminar, where he injected cancerous mice with his Immuno-Augmentative Therapy. The outsized mouse tumors literally shrank before the eyes of the assembled press, who reported the next day with rapturous headlines in their newspapers such as "15-Minute Cancer Cure for Mice; Humans Next?"[5] But the clamorous event marked the beginning of Burton's blues.

Burton and his associates soon saw their research defamed, their funding short-circuited, and credentials attacked. After a false start attempting to institute clinical trials with the NCI, Burton found the FDA blocking him. The director of the FDA Bureau of Drugs subsequently acknowledged that these kinds of stalling tactics were intended to "hinder research" on unconventional cancer therapies.[6] The researcher disgustedly pulled up stakes in 1977 and expatriated to the Bahamas, where he maintained a low profile, quietly treating cancer patients with the full permission of the autonomous island government. He refused to disclose or publish any further research, fearing theft and also registering his disdain for the medical establishment.

It became clear that the NCI started working along similar lines soon after an associate of Burton's left for Sloan-Kettering and took the work with him. There he developed TNF, Tumor Necrosis Factor, drawn from animal blood. The work surfaced in 1987 with the release of the next greatest hope of cancer drug treatment: Interleukin-II, a pharmaceutical analogue similar in concept to Burton's "de-blocking" agent.[7] But now the NCI was itself claiming the discovery.[8] "Dr. Burton's heresy," asserted science writer Robert Houston, "is to have brought such techniques to clinical realization long before Sloan-Kettering or NCI."[9]

Independent studies of Burton's work confirmed positive results. After a researcher at Columbia University's College of Physicians and Surgeons referred twenty advanced cancer patients to Burton, he validated tumor regression in half of them.[10] Other researchers at the University of Pennsylvania found markedly increased survival time among seventy-nine IAT patients, including 63 percent still alive after five years, about twice as long as those treated conventionally.[11] The research team, apparently embarrassed by the findings, balked at publishing them and began qualifying them. Throughout, Burton had never claimed to "cure" but rather to "control" cancer.[12]

Another high-profile case of alleged suppression simultaneously ensnared Dr. Stanislaw Burzynski. Having fled his native Poland to escape the communists, he relocated to Houston, Texas, only to run up against even more rabid foes at the Texas Medical Society and FDA. The M.D. and Ph.D. who had graduated first in his medical class of 250 and published over one hundred peer-reviewed papers was working on "antineoplastons," tumor-inhibiting peptides, chains of amino acids extracted from the urine of cancer patients. Dr. Burzynski maintained that he had identified chemicals in the human body capable not only of treating some forms of cancer but also of diagnosing and preventing the disease. Rather than destroying cancer cells, he believed, these antineoplastons could reprogram and correct them without negative side effects.[13]

Dr. Burzynski set up a Houston research institute in 1977 to treat terminal cancer patients under an explicit understanding with the state medical society that his drugs were not yet approved by the FDA, yet would be considered legal. In 1983 the FDA filed suit against the clinic to stop any further research, development, manufacture, and administration of antineoplastons. The judge forbade any interstate commerce, but allowed the doctor to continue his research in Texas. Dr. Burzynski immediately applied in good faith to the FDA for Investigational New Drug (IND) status to pursue his testing, but the agency denied it. By 1985 the

State of Texas passed a law barring non-FDA-approved drugs altogether, and he came under siege. Three months later, on the same day Burton's Bahamian clinic was ordered to close, the FDA raided Dr. Burzynski's institute using an improper search warrant, seizing 20,000 files and patients' records.[14]

Three and a half years after the raid, the FDA still had not returned the files, and Dr. Burzynski's staff was forced to install a copy machine at the local FDA office to obtain its own clinic records, by appointment only. Insurance companies ceased making payments, and the institute had to curtail its production of the medicine, stranding its terminal cancer patients. Ten years later, the FDA still had not filed charges.

Dr. Burzynski endured an unending series of trials and tribulations. At the same time that he was being prosecuted in the United States, Japanese researchers started clinical trials of antineoplastons, finding "anticancer activity." Four other independent groups of distinguished scientists verified the efficacy of antineoplastons in the United States, England, Italy, and China. His work was highlighted in a special session at the International Congress of Chemotherapy in Europe in 1987, and he spoke at the 14th International Cancer Congress, the most respected global gathering in cancer research.[15] The paper he presented there documented a 60 percent remission rate, including complete recoveries in almost half his subjects.[16] Nevertheless, the Houston doctor was embroiled in an ongoing legal battle that was rapidly draining his resources and preventing the clinical investigation he vainly sought.

Nor were Lawrence Burton and Dr. Stanislaw Burzynski isolated cases. Numerous other prominent scientific and medical researchers watched their careers be destroyed and their work waylaid when, like Hoxsey, they dared treat cancer by unorthodox means.

Congressman Molinari's research convinced him that the subject of alternative cancer treatments deserved more study. He and thirty-nine other concerned members of Congress requested that their own research arm, the Office of Technology Assessment (OTA), do the work.[17] The OTA was generally regarded as an evenhanded agency. Subject only to Congress, it tended to be relatively free of political pressures and had produced assessments considered by many to be among the most scrupulously objective done by the government.

Congress instructed the OTA to prepare a report not only on Burton's operation but on the full range of controversial alternative cancer therapies. The government's first evaluation of unconventional cancer treatments was under way at last.

The subtext was that by 1987 an estimated 40 percent of cancer patients were experimenting with one or more alternatives to conventional cancer care. Yet, despite their popularity, most alternative cancer therapies had never been thoroughly tested. There was very little objective data on them, let alone the voluminous research needed to "prove" their efficacy in a way that would satisfy the mainstream medical community. Despite the lack of hard evidence, however, a national poll (which is never lost on Congress) found that the majority of the American public favored allowing unorthodox cancer clinics to operate freely in the United States.[18]

Although mainstream medicine's war on cancer had little to show for itself, cancer treatment had become a huge industry. Given the high-stakes competition—getting a new drug tested and approved, for example, required on average an investment of $230 million—it seemed unlikely that the medical-industrial complex would cheer the outsider who came up with the enviable prize of a cancer cure.[19] Commented Dean Burk, one of the NCI's own most respected researchers, "It's the NIH syndrome—Not Invented Here."[20] Nor would the cancer establishment likely take much interest in promoting someone else's proprietary formula, much less in studying an herbal compound, diet, or vitamin that cannot be patented. As a result, cancer patients were caught in a life-threatening medical crossfire.

Outsiders thus faced a Catch-22: Without research dollars, they could not conduct tests to gather data; without data, they could not publish; without published articles, they could not get research funding. If they somehow managed to operate outside of the system, their work was almost always discounted.

That's why the alternative medical community was watching the OTA so closely: If this authoritative and widely respected research agency concluded in its final report that at least some unconventional cancer treatments were worthy of further investigation, it could pave the way for Congress to demand that the NCI fund such studies. And that's also why alternative therapy advocates were so concerned about what they said was disturbing evidence of bias and suppression at the OTA. I began to follow the story closely as an investigative reporter.[21]

In 1986 the OTA started to gear up for the massive task of designing procedures for evaluating and testing Burton's therapy in particular and for reviewing the broad spectrum of alternative cancer therapies in general. The study was designed to examine everything from the scientific to the mystical, the promising to the fantastical: laboratory therapies designed by doctors; techniques involving acupuncture, herbs, and diet; even metaphysical therapies using shamanism and crystals.

The OTA, which was accustomed to processing vast quantities of complex technical information, routinely relied on advisory panels of outside experts in close consultation. For its cancer report, the agency selected a well-balanced panel reflecting both sides of the highly polarized medical landscape. It also contracted with numerous specialists to provide information and data. Among them was Patricia Spain Ward, a medical historian at the University of Illinois at Chicago, asked by the OTA to write historical summaries of three major proponents of alternative cancer therapies. The daughter of a South Dakota eye, ear, nose, and throat specialist, Ward had planned on becoming a doctor until she took her first medical history course and fell in love with the subject. Since then, her work, which focused almost entirely on orthodox medicine, had been widely read and praised.

Only once in her career had Ward written about the history of an "alternative" therapy, in a paper on Krebiozen, Dr. Andrew Ivy's hotly debated immunological method from the 1950s and 1960s. Her well-known article, which was skeptical of its subject, was almost certainly instrumental in her selection for the OTA assignment.[22]

Ward said she knew from the start that trying to compose "objective" histories of such provocative treatments would mean entering "the thorniest brier patch in American medicine," as she put it.[23] "I didn't believe anyone could be objective on this controversial and difficult subject."[24] However, she had always been impressed with the OTA's impartiality, and, after reassurance from the agency that it would seek the truth—whatever the political cost—Ward agreed to take the job. Soon she was painstakingly researching the herbs of Harry Hoxsey, the nutritional regimen of Dr. Max Gerson, and the BCG vaccine, which related to the turn-of-the-century immunological formulation of William Coley, a famous New York surgeon and cancer researcher.

Ward was particularly fascinated by the work on Hoxsey and his clash with the powerful AMA and its primary spokesman, Morris Fishbein. When the medical historian began her research, she acknowledged, everything she knew about Harry Hoxsey painted him as "the original flim-flam man, the premier quack."[25] Soon, however, she too began to believe that the forces opposing him were far from blameless. Rhetoric such as Fishbein's, she wrote, "has done much to set the low level of discourse and the emotional—rather than analytical—tone that has characterized the American medical profession's response to unorthodox remedies."[26] She went on to note that the AMA had simply refused to investigate the Hoxsey medicines, disregarding science's most fundamental question: What is the evidence?

As her project progressed, Ward inadvertently discovered that the OTA had not bothered to look into whether Hoxsey's herbs had ever been tested for their pharmacological effects (though the agency had asked a researcher to look in the medical literature for citations about their dangers). "I should have known right then," Ward recalled, "that something was terribly wrong."[27] She agreed to do some detective work. After a preliminary search of the literature, she went to Norman Farnsworth, the world-renowned professor of pharmacognosy at her own University of Illinois at Chicago. With Farnsworth's help using the NAPRALERT botanical database, Ward found that six of the nine Hoxsey herbs had shown immune-enhancing or antitumor activity, corroborating what we had learned earlier from James Duke.

Ward was excited. For the first time, there were questions in her mind about her "flim-flam man." Nevertheless, she was "flawlessly circumspect" in her final presentation to the OTA. But word soon reached Ward that her reports had been selectively edited. "I was sick to my stomach," she told me. "I knew I'd been had."[28]

Ward turned in her Hoxsey paper on April 19, 1988, three months prior to the target release date of the OTA's preliminary draft report and about three months later than she had promised. She continued to work under deadline pressure on her histories of the Gerson and Coley therapies. Those she submitted in May and June. A task originally designed to take two weeks had consumed six months.

The OTA issued a preliminary draft report to its advisory panel in July 1988, just days before the panel's meeting to discuss it. But Ward's contributions were not readily identifiable in its four hundred pages, a result, the OTA said at first, of the late submission. "It was not an official complete draft," demurred OTA Project Director Hellen Gelband. "A lot of things were left out."[29] The report did incorporate selected parts of her research (attributed to her sources), as well as a number of reports critical of unconventional therapies, some of them marginally anecdotal. In the Hoxsey section, Ward's data supporting the herbs' anticancer properties were absent, while another researcher's negative data about them were cited, such as one patient's freakish overdose on licorice and poisoning from contaminated burdock.[30]

Knowing that Ward had written a Gerson paper, Gar Hildenbrand, an OTA panel member and then director of the Gerson Institute, was puzzled not to find a copy or reference to it in the draft. The day after the panel met, Hildenbrand went to the OTA and asked to see the report. He said that, after initial resistance, Gelband gave him one to read but told him that it could not leave the office.[31]

As Hildenbrand perused the paper, he began to see why the OTA might have been so guarded. In her report on Gerson, Ward described the low-fat, low-sodium diet the doctor had developed in 1928, a regimen similar to the one now endorsed by the NCI, the American Cancer Society, and the American Heart Association. But during Fishbein's tenure, the AMA had stated flatly that clinical successes with the Gerson diet "were apparently not susceptible to duplication by most other observers." The AMA Council on Pharmacy, Ward noted, had claimed that it was a "false notion that diet has any specific influence on the origin or progress of cancer." (Ward also observed that, ironically, it may have been Gerson's opposition to tobacco that made it so difficult for the AMA to swallow, noting that at the time cigarette giant Philip Morris was *JAMA*'s major source of advertising revenue.)[32]

Ward's paper closed by citing the favorable results of a European clinical trial of Gerson's therapy. Fearing that Ward's research may have been suppressed, Hildenbrand blew the whistle. He drafted a letter of protest to the OTA and immediately contacted the other advisers. Three advisory panel members co-signed the protest, while two others also wrote letters and two more spoke with the OTA directly. In total, eight of the eighteen panel members objected to the omissions and other problems with the draft. "The product was unacceptable," Hildenbrand explained. "The advisory panel had been totally excommunicated from the process."[33]

Ward quickly learned that her reports had been selectively edited and that the originals had not been circulated to panelists. Like the practitioners she wrote about, a disoriented Ward found herself charging that the "OTA had actually tried to suppress my reports."[34]

Once-hopeful members of the alternative medical community began to complain that the draft report seemed to perpetuate the very process it was commissioned to rectify—condemnation without investigation. When Burton's Iowa-based IAT Patients' Association contacted its senator, OTA board member Charles Grassley, the lawmaker's query found the OTA explanation shifting. Ward's submissions were now not merely late but "selectively positive," "biased," and "nonobjective."[35] Said Gelband, "We're not saying it was an intentional bias, but a biased package of information."[36] In backing up its charge that Ward was selectively positive, the OTA pointed to controversial NCI tests on the Hoxsey herbs that indicated they had no anticancer activity.[37] However, these reports had never even been published.

In response, Ward protested to OTA Director John Gibbons. Why hadn't the negative NCI data been supplied to her? Had that information been obtained only after she had turned in her favorable findings? Why couldn't the NCI data simply have been included with her data? "This tendency to read any positive data at all as a full endorsement of an unconventional therapy is a major problem which the OTA must address," she wrote.[38]

Apart from the dispute over Ward's herbal data, the OTA charged further bias in her historical presentations, noting that the papers were perceived as "favorable" to alternatives.[39] In support of its position, the OTA cited the comments of two informal reviewers. One of them, sociologist Barrie Cassileth, criticized the findings for a lack of balance and accused Ward of portraying conventional science and medicine as "a collection of obtuse fools who are blind to the truth."[40] Having spent her adult life chronicling orthodox medicine, Ward was particularly outraged by these charges. "Exposing the mistakes of conventional medicine and the retrograde leadership that misled the profession during the more than three decades that Morris Fishbein served as *JAMA* editor hardly constitutes hostility to conventional medicine. . . . [Fishbein] was essentially a journalist and a propagandist. Although he held a medical degree, he never practiced medicine, did no research, and was not a medical scholar. He was instrumental in laying down the faulty machinery for evaluating cancer therapies which we have unhappily inherited," she wrote to the OTA. "These old ways of evaluation do not work well, but they entangle us still. Should not the OTA be studying them in an effort to suggest to the Congress some means by which we might break free of procedural snarls that tend to stifle or retard innovation?"[41]

"There were no grounds for withholding Pat's work," protested the fiery Hildenbrand. "The OTA avoided the entire socioeconomic environment and the historical pattern of the AMA and the government agencies that are supposed to regulate but don't. Without Ward, the OTA is not likely to be able to look critically at the AMA and understand leadership trends today. If you exclude Ward, you exclude that whole picture."[42]

The OTA continued to deny any suppression of Ward's work and subsequently distributed the missing papers. Gelband characterized the flap as simply a series of misunderstandings. "We have not been conspiring with anybody," she asserted. "Everything gets out eventually, and all these people have permission to publish independently."[43]

OTA advisory panel member Michael Lerner, a MacArthur fellow and author on alternative cancer therapies generally regarded as a neutral observer, agreed that the OTA's critics overstated the problem. "I believe the people at OTA are well intentioned and serious," he said. "There has not been a conspiracy or suppression."[44]

Only the OTA's final document could confirm or deny Ward's allegations. Gelband insisted that the report would include Ward's herbal data, tempered with the OTA's own findings. She noted the biggest problem as the lack of available information on the therapies. Meanwhile, the agency continued to explore how it could "flip the perfect coin" to design randomized scientific protocols for generating the data needed to evaluate the treatments. The Burton protocol, then under construction, represented the emerging model.[45]

Meanwhile groundbreaking court cases involving alternative cancer therapies and insurance companies took an unexpected turn. Christina Hanks, a Wyoming woman given six months to live when doctors discovered a brain tumor, went into complete remission after treatment by Dr. Burzynski. Her insurance company stopped payment, claiming that Burzynski's antineoplaston therapy did not constitute "usual and customary" treatment approved by the Food and Drug Administration. The judge ruled otherwise, determining that Burzynski had indeed cured Hanks and ordering her insurance company to pay her medical bill, $120,000 in attorney's fees, and, if her policy was not reinstated, an additional $650,000 in damages. Based on very strong medical documentation, other Burzynski patients who ostensibly recovered from "incurable" brain tumors won similar court suits soon after.[46]

Catherine Salveson and I boarded a plane for this hornet's nest of Washington, D.C., in 1988 at the invitation of Project Cure and Mike Torrusio, chief of staff of Congressman Molinari, to hold a special congressional screening of our finally completed feature-length *Hoxsey* documentary. Clutching the precious film print in my lap at 25,000 feet, I found it hard to grasp how four years of obsessive effort and voluminous research could possibly fit into this small metal can. Looking down at the solid ground far below, I anguished over whether we had dotted all the "i's" and crossed every "t" as fastidiously as we believed.

The film had been released only months earlier to standing ovations at international film festivals in New York City and Europe. When it premiered at a Manhattan movie theater, Vincent Canby in the *New York Times* called it "first-rate reportage". Later in 1988 the film was scheduled for a national TV premiere on HBO/Cinemax, which does not shy away from provocative programming. There it would garner the highest viewer response of any documentary ever shown till that time. Along with the investigative reportage I was writing about the brewing chicanery at the OTA, the film would go on to win the Best Censored Stories Award, a national journalistic honor associated with Bill Moyers.[47] While we were gratified at the response the film was receiving, our purpose was to use it to bring as much attention as possible to the life-and-death issues it portrayed. At that moment the curtain was about to rise at the center of political theater among key players whose decisions mattered the most.

The Washington screening was set for the Kennedy Center, and when we reached the nation's capital, it was abuzz with cancer patients and health activists from all over the country.[48] Catherine and I accompanied patient advocacy groups as they visited congressional offices all over Capitol Hill. It was a distressing experience to watch terminally ill cancer patients plaintively plead for access to the treatments they believed were prolonging and saving their tenuous lives. Congress was listening.

The morning of the screening, National Public Radio broadcast a feature story on the film and related issues. As Catherine and I sat in a hotel room tuning in to *Morning Edition*, the voice of Harry Hoxsey, resurrected from our film, boomed across the airwaves, demanding a fair investigation from the federal government.[49]

That night, the Kennedy Center filled with over seven hundred people, including two hundred representatives of congressional offices plus a fistful of OTA staff. Congressional screenings of this nature are rare events and the atmosphere was charged.[50] Cancer activists intently watched policy makers watching the movie, searching their impassive faces for any clues. After the film, activists deftly cornered congressional representatives and staff to lobby them in the lobby. There was no doubt that this movement represented a widespread constituency and the volatile issues were becoming irrepressibly public.

Harry Hoxsey's cinematic charge of conspiracy was all too relevant to current events to dismiss out of hand. Synchronous newspaper headlines were once again exposing the AMA at the center of a web of unlawful activities, including monopolistic practices and antitrust violations. In purely legal terms, it was called *conspiracy*.

18

Patented Medicine: A Way of Business

Just as the movie was about to be released in late 1987, we had to scramble at the eleventh hour to add a title card at the film lab with late-breaking news: The American Medical Association had just been convicted in federal court of a "conspiracy to destroy and eliminate" the chiropractic profession." The court judgment was unequivocal. "For over twelve years and with the full knowledge and support of their executive officers, the AMA paid the salaries and expenses for a team of more than a dozen medical doctors, lawyers, and support staff for the expressed purpose of conspiring (overtly and covertly) with others in medicine to first contain, and eventually, destroy the profession of chiropractic in the United States and elsewhere." Also convicted with the AMA were the American College of Surgeons and the American College of Radiologists.[1]

Many years earlier, Dr. Fishbein had once labeled the chiropractic profession "a malignant tumor" and clearly the legacy was unbroken. Part of the AMA's strategy, the trial disclosed, was to deprive chiropractors of any association with medical doctors. In practical terms, this exclusionary stance barred chiropractors from hospitals and from getting physicians' referrals because the AMA deemed it "unethical" for a doctor to associate with a chiropractor. The AMA strategy sought to brand chiropractors as "unscientific cultists." Judge Susan Getzendanner said that the function of the AMA's Committee on Quackery formed in 1963 as a successor to the expired Bureau of Investigation was specifically to destroy the chiropractic profession, which had grown to sizable proportions and overtaken osteopathy in popularity.[2]

Secret files on the campaign against the chiropractors were first leaked to the national press by a mysterious source known as Sore Throat. The mole turned out to be a member of the Church of Scientology angered at the AMA's attack against the group as a "menace to mental health" in

1968. The Scientology church retaliated with a "doom program" against the AMA. Releasing a wealth of damning evidence that soon saturated the mass media, the irate Scientologist, who had worked at the AMA, had a U.S. representative on his mailing list who then forwarded some of the documents relating to the AMA's war on chiropractic to the Federal Trade Commission for antitrust action.[3]

The case centered on restraint of trade, a violation of the Sherman Antitrust Act. The four chiropractors who brought the suit decided against seeking money damages because they didn't want to divert attention from the true issues of monopolistic practices and impairments to patient care. Fully 18 percent of hospital admissions, a very sizable market share, are for orthopedic and musculoskeletal disorders, precisely the conditions that chiropractors treat. Evidence in the case documented the fact that the AMA was fully aware of studies showing chiropractic care to be twice as effective as standard medical care in relieving some painful conditions of the neck, back, and musculoskeletal system.

Judge Getzendanner ruled, "I conclude that an injunction is necessary in this case. There are lingering effects of this conspiracy; the AMA has never acknowledged the lawlessness of its past conduct and in fact to this day maintains that it has always been in compliance with the antitrust laws."[4] The AMA was forced to circulate the contrite Order of Injunction through medical journals, hospitals, and many other outlets, and to cease and desist from obstructing the professional rights of the chiropractic profession.

The conviction marked the third time in the century that the AMA was found guilty of antitrust violations for conspiracy and restraint of trade. The medical association was first convicted in 1937 under Dr. Fishbein for trying to destroy an autonomous doctors' group applying cost-cutting health delivery and insurance in Washington, D.C. It was again found guilty in 1982 by the Federal Trade Commission—a decision upheld by the Supreme Court, just as the earlier conviction was. This time the verdict confirmed the AMA's decades-long, systematic violation of antitrust statutes. Clearly Judge Getzendanner agreed with the chiropractors that the AMA was engaged in an ongoing conspiracy.

With measured anger, Project Cure's Bob DeBragga framed the dilemma when we filmed him. "Now the question arises: Is there a premeditated, conspiratorial activity under way to maintain the status quo—to prevent, if you will, a cure for cancer? I say no. But there is a system that we have, which has evolved over the years, which includes the National Cancer Institute, the Food and Drug Administration, the federal government, parts of Congress that oversee these groups, pharmaceutical companies who

peddle the drugs, who do the basic toxicity testing of almost all the drugs—
a way of business has been established. And they're not going to let anybody from outside break into the inner club."[5]

At over $110 billion a year just in the United States, cancer is big
business.[6] The typical cancer patient spends upward of $100,000 on treat-
ment.[7] It is estimated that each hospital admission for cancer produces
two to three times the billings of a typical noncancer admission.[8] More
people work in the field than die from the disease each year.[9]

Dr. Samuel Epstein's explosive 1978 book *The Politics of Cancer* (recently updated) served as an early exposé of how large vested interests
have colored cancer research, prevention, and treatment. According to
Dr. Epstein, "For decades, the war on cancer has been dominated by
powerful groups of interlocking professional and financial interests, with
the highly profitable drug development system at its hub."[10]

"Cancer treatment," Ralph Moss adds, "is the essence of hope for the
future of the pharmaceutical industry."[11] Global sales of chemotherapy
drugs in 1997 were $30.9 billion, about $12 billion of it in the United
States.[12] Moss, who has documented the scope of the cancer industry in
his books, notes that chemotherapy drugs are the "leading edge because
that's the area where the big corporations monopolize that portion of the
marketplace. Obviously they exert a greater power than a thousand different hospitals gathered around a thousand different cities which don't
have the same clout in the marketplace that a few corporations do. The
chemotherapy marketplace is a highly monopolized situation. You've got
one company, Bristol-Myers Squibb, that controls 50 percent of worldwide sales of chemotherapy. They're highly aggressive and ingenious,
and they really are the company that for a long time has gone after the
cancer market with both hands. They give grants and make awards, and
they're everywhere."[13]

Bristol-Meyers Squibb, Moss adds, has had a long "incestuous" relationship with Memorial Sloan-Kettering Cancer Center through interlocking boards of directors. In fact, according to Epstein and other researchers,
a virtual revolving door has existed among large pharmaceutical companies, the NCI, FDA, and cancer research and treatment centers. The 1998
chairman of the hospital's Board of Overseers and Managers is a company
director of Bristol-Myers Squibb, as is the vice chairman, who is the
company's chairman of the board. Another example is the former director
of the NCI's Division of Cancer Treatment who went on to Bristol-Myers
Squibb to become head of drug research and development.[14]

Among those companies heavily engaged in producing chemotherapy
drugs are giant pharmaceutical concerns including Merck, Upjohn, Eli

Lilly, Burroughs-Wellcome, Miles, and Lederle. These industry corner-stones have been characterized by ever more relentless corporate central-ization. An example of the result of such vertical integration is the fact that the AstraZeneca corporation actually owns a chain of eleven hospitals and cancer clinics that dispense the company's own chemotherapy drugs.[15]

Despite chemotherapy's lack of proof of efficacy in at least 90 per-cent of cases, these drugs are administered to 80 percent of U.S. cancer patients. Moss points out that chemotherapy sales are increasing at double-digit rates with astronomical price tags.[16] He documented the not uncommon case of one patient who was charged $750,000 solely for chemotherapy drugs.[17] Since the 1980s, the number of such cancer drugs in development has doubled from 65 to 126.[18]

When I asked Moss about the bottom-line implications of the grow-ing awareness of chemotherapy's overall failure, he remained sanguine about its business prospects. "I think that the leaders know that basically chemotherapy has not much of a future. They've given up a long time ago on thinking that this is going to be the wave of the future. It's the wave of the past. They've gambled on other kinds of drugs having to do with genetic engineering and monoclonal antibodies as the future of can-cer treatment. Personally, I think they're dreaming. I think they're squeez-ing every ounce of positive data out of their experiments to make it look far better than it will ever perform clinically. But what matters is what you can sell and get approved. Nothing is touching the chemotherapy juggernaut. Chemotherapy will be used, but once the patents run out, they'll be happy to ditch that and move on to something else. Probably you'll see attacks on chemotherapy starting about the time they're ready to produce a new generation of drugs."[19]

When Cornelius "Dusty" Rhoads launched the chemotherapy pro-gram at Memorial Sloan-Kettering, he consciously founded the enter-prise on patents. "In the near future, patents may well control [medicine's] entire development," Rhoads related to a gathering of patent attorneys in 1940. "The patent lawyers can and do control the support of industrial science."[20] Rhoads professed his intention not only to cure the disease, but also to profit mightily doing it. Patents are the key because they pro-vide seventeen-year exclusive licenses. Additionally, this prohibitively expensive game excludes all but the biggest players.

Radiation is also a major industry. It too is exceptionally profitable, supporting equipment and film manufacturers, hospitals, and a bevy of ancillary technicians and radiologists. When radiation was first introduced in Memorial Hospital in 1924, it constituted the single largest source of income and lifted the institution out of its then impoverished state.[21] By the mid-1970s, there were around 73,000 radiation therapy treatments and implants each year.[22] The average cancer patient today receives four radiation treatments.[23] General Electric sells over $100 million yearly in mammography machines.[24] The mammography industry alone is estimated to generate about $2.5 billion in annual revenues.[25]

Surgery is similarly a vastly lucrative practice, acting as the third financial mooring in the tripod of cancer treatments. The more radical the operation, the more costly. Since surgeons are rewarded monetarily for the magnitude of their handiwork, excess becomes a perverse incentive for financial success.

The amount of unnecessary surgery is high. As early as 1953, Dr. Paul Hawley, director of the American College of Surgeons, stated matter-of-factly in an interview in *U.S. News and World Report*, "You'd be shocked, I think—we are—at the amount of unnecessary surgery that is performed." The reason, according to Hawley? "Money."[26]

"In the United States today," Moss wrote in *The Cancer Industry*, "the direction of cancer management appears to be shaped by those forces financially interested in the outcome of the problem. Distinct circles of power have formed, which, while differing among themselves on many issues, are sufficiently cohesive and interlocking to form a *cancer establishment*. This establishment effectively controls the shape and direction of cancer prevention, diagnosis, and therapy in the United States."[27]

This wide-ranging cancer establishment, as documented by Dr. Epstein and Moss, comprises giant corporations, the American Cancer Society, the National Cancer Institute, the Food and Drug Administration, the American Medical Association, segments of Congress and the federal government, and a web of auxiliary institutions from university research hospitals and laboratories to public charities.

While a small concentrated circle of corporations holds the patents on cancer drugs for private profit, most of the research funding to develop them has come from taxpayer dollars, through the federal government and National Cancer Institute. Institutions such as Memorial Sloan-Kettering have embraced this public-private partnership wholeheartedly. The NCI has been dispensing a budget averaging $1.5 billion a year since the 1971 "War on Cancer" began, with much of the largesse channeled to private corporations as research dollars.

The development of the chemotherapy drug Taxol, which brings Bristol-Myers Squibb nearly $1 billion a year in revenues, was funded with public dollars by the National Cancer Institute for a price tag of $32 million. The NCI then assigned it at no cost to the company, which sells it at twenty times the cost of manufacturing. (It costs about 40 cents per milligram to manufacture and is sold to consumers at around $8.50 per milligram.)[28] As a consequence, many patients cannot afford or are financially destroyed by this government-sponsored drug. Dr. Robert Wittes, after helping develop the drug at the NCI, left the government to assist the pharmaceutical concern in commercializing the product, and subsequently returned to the NCI.[29]

It is by externalizing such research costs (i.e., passing on the bill to taxpayers) that the pharmaceutical business has achieved the highest return on investment of any industry.[30] Simultaneously, drug profits are growing at double-digit rates, with companies reporting increases ranging from 13 to 35 percent a year.[31] For 1997, Bristol-Myers Squibb, the dominant player in cancer chemotherapy drugs, reported earnings of $927 million.[32] Since Taxol's approval in 1992, the drug has generated $3 billion in revenues, about 40 percent of the company's total sales.[33]

Meanwhile, hospitals compete furiously to enroll cancer patients. As Dr. Michael Gruber of the New York University Medical Center commented, "Cancer is to the 1990s what heart disease was to the 1970s. It puts a center on the map, and that begets business."[34]

During the 1990s, the centralization of the drug industry accelerated through several of the biggest mergers in history, many of them global in scope.[35] A handful of companies hold a clear monopoly over the gigantic drug market (as well as the chemical, seed, and biotechnology industries). Merck alone now controls almost 10 percent of the global pharmaceutical drug market.[36] In 1999, even these outsized combinations were dwarfed by mega-mergers. The union of Zeneca and Swiss giant Astra made it the second largest drug company in the world, with sales of $67 billion. It was quickly topped in 2000 by the planned $91 billion merger of Pfizer with Warner-Lambert. Analysts predict more to follow.[37]

Drug companies justify their monopolistic pricing on high research and development costs. Current estimates for testing and approving a new drug through the contortions of the byzantine FDA procedures range from $230 to $500 million in a process often taking ten years.[38] The hidden consequence is that it serves as a barrier of entry against all but the largest corporations.[39] In fact, few "new" drugs are actually developed, as the companies often prefer to redirect existing drugs to new applications or markets.

Ironically, although the pharmaceutical industry first fought fiercely against regulatory procedures requiring proof of safety and efficacy, the laws have turned out to work in its favor. What is less well known is that these provisions were the sole survivors of a much more aggressive congressional press against the perceived monopolistic practices of the drug industry at large. Following multiple mergers among drug companies that created a small clan of behemoths, Senator Estes Kefauver first began an investigation into the monopoly question in 1947. He produced a scathing report entitled "United States versus Economic Concentration and Power." Kefauver and many others viewed this emerging cartel with alarm as a kind of pharmaceutical "club" whose elite members cooperated closely on drug development and licensing, thereby sharing research as well as development and marketing costs. But most importantly, they appeared to be colluding on pricing, a highly illegal activity.[40]

Robert Teitelman, a mainstream financial journalist and editor at *Institutional Investor* magazine, described this showdown between private monopolies and the public interest in his detailed analysis, *Profits of Science: The American Marriage of Business and Technology.* "The issue of monopoly turned on the question of pricing . . . Kefauver focused on what he viewed as a plague of administered pricing—prices set by companies independent of market forces."[41] The senator started probes by the Antitrust and Monopoly Subcommittee in a series of high-profile hearings in 1957 and 1962.

The hearings unveiled damning evidence that the large drug companies set prices well over their costs by virtue of the monopoly power vested in their patents. The committee proved that different companies charged the same price for comparable drugs in apparent price-fixing. "Although competition became cutthroat, the industry's leaders never forgot they were gentlemen when it came to prices," drily observed *Fortune* magazine.[42] "Kefauver concluded," wrote Teitelman, "that the major drug companies did not effectively pass the benefits of research along to consumers, in the form of either lower prices or innovative therapeutics, and that monopoly power and size in pharmaceuticals not only did not nurture innovation but actually retarded it . . . Said Kefauver, 'It is obvious that the selling price for a particular ethical [drug] specialty is not predicated on the cost of materials, but, rather, predicated on what the traffic will bear.'"[43]

Making matters worse for the drug industry, Kefauver provoked a national scandal by exposing the horrors of birth defects caused by the new wonder drug thalidomide. His scoop jolted the nation at the height of an aggressive—and false—national advertising campaign for the drug. Out of this outrage came demands for heightened drug safety laws.

Kefauver went for the jugular. He sought to shrink patentability from seventeen years to three, among many other restrictive provisions. He proposed to compel drug companies to demonstrate both safety and now efficacy. But Kefauver's legislation stalled under crushing political pressure, and only the safety and efficacy clauses became law. As Teitelman concluded, "The drug industry still could feel it had escaped real punishment. By retaining full patent protection, the industry preserved its ability to set prices freely. Ironically, the safety and efficacy provision of the bill only served to raise the barrier of entry against new competitors, and over the long run it fortified the position of the largest companies."[44]

Subsequent investigations by the Federal Trade Commission in the 1960s resulted in criminal charges for price-fixing against a drug cartel composed of Pfizer, Upjohn, Lederle, and Bristol-Myers. But this time, the government found the smoking gun: Internal memos described "pow-wows," a code for price-fixing meetings, and "sinners," anyone breaking rank on pricing.[45]

The patent provisions at the core of the drug cartels remained unchanged, however. Because an herb or formula like Hoxsey cannot be patented, such remedies occupy the status of orphan drugs, with no incentive for companies to develop them. Among other casualties of this quandary are potentially valuable cancer therapies such as vitamin C, hydrazine sulfate (an inexpensive chemical that has shown anticancer properties), and laetrile, the natural extract of apricot pits.

It was actually laetrile that bumped Ralph Moss sideways into his role as gadfly to the cancer establishment. As assistant director of public affairs for Memorial Sloan-Kettering Cancer Center in the early 1970s, he routinely wrote stories and press releases about the wonder drugs coming out of the hospital's research programs. His job also entailed science writing for an in-house newsletter for which he interviewed many of the hospital's star oncologists. His close-up view of conventional treatment became dispiriting, however, as he gradually realized the hospital was far more attentive to drug discovery, career objectives, and patents than to patients.

"Shortly after I was hired there," Moss related, "I interviewed an elderly scientist named Kanematsu Sugiura, who was a very famous pioneer of chemotherapy and also diet therapy. He had been at the center from around the time of World War I, and toward the end of the interview, I asked him what he was working on, and he told me, 'amygdalin,' which is laetrile. I was totally astonished, because I had been given to understand that laetrile was 'quackery,' and believed it. There was nothing in my background that predisposed me to believe that there was anything amiss in the 'War on Cancer.' I asked him why he would be working on that, and he took down from the shelf notes showing that laetrile, in his experiments, slowed the growth of tumors, and more remarkably, it had a dramatic effect in metastases, or spread of cancer, in mice."[46]

Even after the FDA conducted its first seizure of laetrile in 1960 at the successor to Hoxsey's Dallas clinic, by the 1970s over twenty states had legalized its use by cancer patients in direct defiance of the aggressive federal campaign against it.[47] Nevertheless, laetrile was largely frozen out of legitimate testing until Dr. Sugiura's investigation at Memorial Sloan-Kettering.

"Over the course of the next three and a half years," Moss continued, "I watched as my employers just lied about the outcome of Dr. Sugiura's work, and about what had actually been achieved at Memorial with the laetrile experiments. They tried to embroil me in their cover-up of the facts, to the point where I wrote the official press release on laetrile for Memorial Sloan-Kettering. I objected to this in various ways, and, finally, unable to change things from inside any longer, I held a press conference in November of 1977, and said all these things, and was fired the next day, as they put it in the *New York Times*, for 'failing to carry out the most basic job responsibilities,' which is to lie when your boss tells you to lie. From that time on, I've been driven to find out the truth about cancer treatments, conventional as well as nonconventional, and to work through my own anger and own feelings of revulsion at what happened."

When Moss left Memorial Sloan-Kettering, he turned his investigative skills to tracking the rise of this institution that precisely mirrored the new economic order of cancer treatment. The introduction of a postwar, Big Science chemotherapy program demanded a cavernous pocketbook and the formation of an expanded financial confederacy. Moss wrote:

> Such a project was clearly too vast even for the Rockefellers. [Standard Oil Vice President Frank] Howard therefore asked two prominent executives of General Motors to join the project and provide funds for the new center. Together Alfred P. Sloan and Charles Kettering of General Motors contributed several million dollars, and the new research center, the Sloan-Kettering Institute for Cancer Research, was named in their honor in August 1945.
>
> Until that time, Memorial Hospital had been under the control of the Rockefellers, and, to a lesser degree, the Douglases [of radium fame]. With the inclusion of Sloan and Kettering in leadership positions, members of the Rockefellers' traditional rival, the Morgan banking interests, were allowed to share power. Sloan was president of General Motors, long associated with the Morgan interests, and was also a director of Du Pont and of the Morgan Guaranty Trust Company itself. From

> this period forward the world's largest private cancer
> center was ruled by what looks like a consortium of Wall
> Street's top banks and corporations.[48]

Ironically, Moss's analysis of the composition of Memorial Sloan-Kettering Cancer Center's board in 1978 revealed that fully a third were closely tied to large polluting industries including oil, chemicals, and automobiles, some of the very companies that produce many known carcinogens. At the time, General Motors alone was estimated to be responsible for about a third of the nation's air pollution by tonnage. The other principal vested interest of the board was corporate investment: major bankers, venture capitalists, and stockbrokers. Even more significantly, seven of the nine members of the hospital's Institutional Policy Board, which directed its strategic course, had strong ties to companies with immediate interests in the cancer drug or diagnostic markets.[49]

It was also Rockefeller interests that founded the influential American Cancer Society, whose growth was soon supplemented by contributions from Morgan and other financial dynasties. Originally known in 1913 as the American Society for the Control of Cancer, the ASCC instituted a carrot-and-stick public policy of alternately promoting hope and fear. Cultivating cancer consciousness, it drilled dread into the American public with one hand while planting seeds of hope with the other. The society remained mainly oriented to the medical profession until the creation in the 1940s of the Women's Field Army, a pseudomilitary force of theatrically uniformed volunteers who canvassed the nation door to door searching out cancer patients and commanding them to report to their doctors. The Field Army was highly successful at raising the first big bucks for cancer from a frightened public.[50]

In the 1940s the American Cancer Society (ACS) was taken over by a clique of insurgent innovators including Hoffmann–La Roche; drug baron and political lobbyist Elmer Bobst; and Albert and Mary Lasker. Albert Lasker was an advertising man whose most famous campaign was for the American Tobacco Company—"Reach for a Lucky instead of a sweet"—a slogan that, Moss has pointed out, started thousands of women smoking during the 1930s and 1940s. Both Lasker and his wife were also trustees of Memorial Hospital. Mary Lasker engagingly promoted her "noble conspiracy," and "Mary and her little lambs" displayed a golden fundraising touch.[51] At that time, conventional cancer treatment was a dismal failure, bedeviled by the popularity of Hoxsey, Koch, and the numerous competing "quacks" who were attracting large constituencies.

Bobst and the Laskers transmuted Madison Avenue into Medicine Avenue, creating famously effective campaigns that convinced the public to donate large amounts of cash and volunteer time. They devised "Cancer Month," enlisted media mavens from Hollywood, and initiated the Science Writers' Seminar to promote their agendas. The programs quickly built the ACS into the single largest private charity in the country, and its fund-raising clout allowed it to wield powerful influence on the research agendas of the National Cancer Institute. The ACS itself spent a quarter of its bounty on research, all within the close network of allied institutions headed by Memorial Sloan-Kettering.

The ACS created a booklet called "Unproven Methods of Cancer Management" to discredit unconventional cancer therapies. It became a blacklist for "worthless remedies" and "cancer quackery." Whoever had the mishap to appear in its rogues' gallery was assured of losing research funding and becoming prone to prosecution. It would be difficult to overstate the influence the ACS has held over the direction of cancer therapeutics and the concomitant exclusion of unconventional approaches.

Perhaps the greatest irony of the ACS "Unproven Methods of Cancer Management" blacklist is that most of these treatments have not been tested at all. If they are "unproven," they are certainly not *disproven*. Of the approximately seventy-eight methods listed through the 1980s, only 31 percent showed negative clinical findings. There had been no investigation at all for 41 percent. The findings were inconclusive for 16 percent. A total of almost 70 percent provided no definitive documentation for dismissing the therapies. Some 12 percent were actually positive![52]

The "investigation" of Hoxsey cited in the ACS "Unproven Methods" list was the superficial visit paid to the Taylor Clinic (formerly Hoxsey Cancer Clinic) in Dallas in 1958 by the legislative delegation from British Columbia. The group spent three days there while also visiting for almost a week with the AMA, FDA, NCI, ACS, and other vociferous opponents. By any credible standard, this tour does not qualify as a meaningful investigation, yet the ACS imprimatur gave weight to the pronouncement. As recently as 1991, in its *Cancer Journal for Clinicians*, the ACS characterized Hoxsey as "a worthless tonic for cancer." The ACS went on to say, "The Hoxsey medicines have been extensively tested and found to be both useless (the internal tonic) and archaic (the external treatments)."[53]

Several therapies listed in the ACS dishonor roll were later removed. Among them was the Lincoln treatment, as well as Coley's Toxins, about which Patricia Spain Ward wrote for the OTA.[54] Dr. William Coley was a highly prominent New York surgeon who happened upon an immunological approach based on his theory of a viral cause of cancer. Coley's career was virtually ruined as a consequence of his unorthodox researches, though he ultimately managed to remain within the medical fold owing to his exceptionally high stature and remarkable diplomatic skills. His daughter took up the cause after his death and cultivated a large following of wealthy adherents. Eventually the therapy was vindicated to some degree in clinical trials with support from a former vice president of Memorial Sloan-Kettering, as evidenced by its eventual quiet disappearance from the ACS blacklist.

The ACS also publishes a "Reach to Recovery" handbook for its volunteers, who are cancer survivors and who visit other patients with their type of cancer. The program's handbook directs volunteers to "always maintain a positive attitude toward conventional treatment methods," while cautioning not to "promote unconventional therapies."[55]

The ACS has maintained a close collaboration with the National Cancer Institute and the Food and Drug Administration. This ingrown relationship is well illustrated, for example, by the fact that when NCI chief Frank Rauscher left his position there in 1976, he transferred laterally to become vice president for research at the American Cancer Society. (He subsequently became executive director of the Thermal Insulation Manufacturers Association, which promotes the use of carcinogenic fiberglass and lobbies against its regulation.)[56]

The ACS has often come under severe criticism for wide-ranging conflicts of interest. A current member of its board of directors is the vice president of a major herbicide manufacturer.[57] Its financial sponsorship continues to include hefty donations from the same large pharmaceutical companies that produce chemotherapy drugs.[58] Since 1992, when the American Cancer Society Foundation was founded to receive donations over $100,000, its board members have included the president of Lederle Laboratories, the drug division of the giant chemical company American Cyanamid, which produces cancer drugs as well as chemical fertilizers and herbicides. Another board member was the CEO of biotechnology leader Amgen, which makes the chemotherapy drug Neupogen.[59] The ACS itself has shared ownership of the patent on a major chemotherapy drug with a pharmaceutical company, thereby having a clear vested interest.[60]

The ACS has also attracted disturbing attention for the potential abuse of its formidable finances. In 1992, *The Chronicle of Philanthropy* charged the nation's largest public charity with being "more interested in accumulating wealth than in saving lives."[61] The current ACS annual budget is $380 million and its cash reserves total nearly $1 billion.[62] The *Wall Street Journal* found that several local chapters in ten states were spending about a scant 10 percent of funds on community cancer services. For each $1 spent on direct services, the ACS spent around $6.40 on salaries and fringe benefits.[63] Nationally, a mere 16 percent is spent on direct services to cancer patients.[64] Moreover, in 1998 the ACS was found spending close to $1 million on political lobbying, an apparent violation of its legal status as a nonprofit charity.[65]

Protesting such abuses, Dr. Samuel Epstein and the Cancer Prevention Coalition called for an outright boycott of the ACS in 1999. "Instead," wrote the CPC, "give your charitable contributions to public interest and environmental groups involved in cancer prevention."[66]

As demonstrated by the stories of Hoxsey, Dr. Ivy, and countless others, the National Cancer Institute has also acted as a powerful force to prevent the investigation of alternative treatments. Established in 1937 with strong impetus from the success of the Women's Field Army, the NCI was further aided in its extraordinary growth by lobbying from the American Cancer Society after World War II, when its yearly budget began to mushroom from $600,000 in 1946 to the $2.6 billion it garners today. The NCI is angling to raise its annual budget to $5 billion by 2003.[67]

The NCI and ACS have been self-acknowledged partners, directing research agendas, dispensing funding, and excluding unconventional approaches. The basis for President Nixon's National Cancer Act of 1971, which dramatically increased funding to the NCI, was laid by a committee composed of a majority of figures from the ACS and Memorial Sloan-Kettering. The NCI has had a permeable membrane with representatives of the drug industry, particularly in the National Cancer Advisory Board, a key policy-making group that oversees the grant-making process. For example, Dr. Samuel Broder, who served for six years as NCI director, left in 1995 to take an executive position with IVAX, Inc., a major manufacturer of cancer drugs whose CEO was a member of an NCI advisory board.[68] The NCI has applied virtually no funding to treatments other than surgery, radiation, and chemotherapy, or close variants.

Hoxsey's experience with the NCI—seeking a scientific review only to find the agency simultaneously collaborating with the FDA and AMA to prosecute him—has recurred with other unconventional practitioners such as Burton and Dr. Burzynski. The NCI's medical standard seems to fork into a double standard when applied to alternatives. For example, when a single patient in a clinical setting responds to a new chemotherapy drug, that is sometimes considered sufficient cause to launch clinical trials, as happened in the feverish study of Interleukin at the National Cancer Institute.[69] To the contrary, alternative practitioners have been required to supply massive documentation of benefit and safety before even the most preliminary tests can be approved. The standard for safety is equally plastic, especially considering the extreme toxicity of chemotherapy drugs and radiation in contrast with the relative harmlessness of almost all the alternative therapies.

The Food and Drug Administration has been the final circuit in the closed loop of conventional cancer care. As a government enforcement agency, the FDA serves a policing function against presumably harmful or worthless methods of cancer treatment in commerce. The creation of the agency was energetically supported during an era of muckraking when prominent advocates such as the novelist Upton Sinclair highlighted corporate threats to food safety in popular works like *The Jungle*, exposing the horrific practices of the meat industry.

But it was actually a cancer treatment that prompted Congress to enact the first federal law against false claims for drugs. In 1910 the Bureau of Chemistry—predecessor to the FDA—sought prosecution based on the 1906 Food and Drugs Act against the promoter of Dr. Johnson's Mild Combination Treatment for Cancer. The government lost the case because there was no restriction against making therapeutic claims, only against false statements about the identity and composition of ingredients.[70]

In 1912 Congress passed the Sherley Amendment, criminalizing fraudulent and misleading claims of efficacy. However, establishing legal fraud required demonstrating the *intent* to swindle, which is difficult to prove. In 1938 Congress closed the gap by requiring proof of safety, and in 1962 added proof of efficacy as well. Having to prove the efficacy of drugs begat the forbidding labyrinth of baroque requirements now unreasonably obstructing access to the medical marketplace.[71]

The FDA has been frequently exposed as a virtual revolving door with the drug industry. Agency commissioners and officials routinely have come from or departed to the industry they were entrusted to regulate. These apparent conflicts of interest have called into question the agency's leniency in investigating carcinogenic additives in foods as well as many unsafe pharmaceutical drugs.[72]

The FDA has repeatedly been rocked not only by conflicts of interest favoring big business interests but also by credible charges of outright corruption. During the mid-1970s, eleven FDA scientists testified before

Senator Edward Kennedy's Subcommittee on Health and Scientific Research that they were "harassed by agency officials—allegedly pro-industry—whenever they recommended against approval of marketing some new drug."[73]

The investigation stalled for years, partially through the efforts of then Secretary of Health, Education and Welfare Caspar Weinberger, who had earlier spearheaded the seminal California state laws against "cancer quackery." However, the government's own General Accounting Office followed up with a damning audit detailing innumerable conflicts of interest, including ownership of drug company stocks by agency employees.[74] In 1988 several FDA agents were convicted on criminal charges following a covert investigation by Mylan laboratories after the company's generic drugs were rejected for approval by the agency. Private detectives hired by Mylan caught FDA agents red-handed taking bribes in exchange for expediting drug approval.[75]

But above all, the FDA's power has resided in its role as gatekeeper. Its ability to deny Investigational New Drug status has obstructed unconventional treatments from testing. Without access to testing, they cannot be researched, much less validated and made available, and thereby become subject to criminal prosecution. As in the cases of Hoxsey applying to the NCI, or Dr. Burzynski to the FDA for Investigational New Drug status, rejection of their applications was immediately followed by FDA prosecution. Raiding a clinic while it is applying in good faith for a test sends a clear message. Whether or not convictions occur, the costs and distraction are enormous, and reputations can be irrevocably damaged.

In this light, condemning alternative practitioners for their lack of research or documentation is an exercise in cognitive dissonance. While approving about forty highly toxic cancer drugs, *the FDA has yet to approve a single nontoxic cancer agent or one not patented by a major pharmaceutical company.*[76]

Apart from the obvious financial forces, there is also an ideological bias at work. Virtually all the alternative therapies are biological in nature, and until very recently the drug industry has dismissed such approaches. Financial journalist Robert Teitelman offers an intriguing analysis. "In the midst of the triumphant march of physics and electronics in the 1950s and 1960s, it was easy to overlook the difficult marriage of biology and medicine. While the effects of advances in quantum physics on radar, television, and semiconductors were vividly clear, few biological advances produced much, if anything, in the way of new medicines.

Although many considered the 1940s and 1950s the 'golden age of drug discovery,' mostly due to the development of antibiotics, vitamins, anti-histamines, and the Salk polio vaccine, biology could take little of the credit. And when the pace of new drugs slowed again in the 1960s, the 'failure' of biological research bore some of the blame."[77]

As Teitelman argues, biologists had such scant knowledge of identifiable "mechanisms" that their discoveries yielded little if any practical application:

> In the drug industry, chemical compounds which, given the advanced state of an organic chemistry enhanced by the insights of quantum mechanics, could be tailored with increasing skill, were developed and tested first in animals and then in humans. If they proved effective, they were packaged and sold. Why they worked was normally beyond the industry's scope. The tools were relatively advanced, but the users of the tools were still mostly blind.
>
> Drug discovery was an industrial process as much as steelmaking or automobile making. Drug companies did not primarily study disease, they formulated thousands of chemical compounds annually. Pharmacologists did not labor to understand how a compound and a disease interacted—how could they, given the sketchiness of biological knowledge?—they sought to test as many compounds as they could to see what worked; the more money spent, the more compounds screened, the greater the probability of discovering the next penicillin. Advances in chemistry helped. The drug industry was producing more new drugs not because it better understood underlying biological reality but because it had learned to manipulate small molecules chemically and to organize screening more efficiently. Given the incomplete state of biological knowledge, mass screening was an alternative that was both cheaper and safer.

Drug development was the epitomy of a vast bureaucratic process that mirrored the companies' own structures for organizing industrial protocols. Of course many of the true breakthroughs came not from industry labs but from isolated academics or lone inventors. "Drug discovery was *not* rational," Teitelman suggests. "It resembled, as one observer said, 'molecular roulette.'"[78] But favoring the giant companies were the requirements of the grinding drug discovery process for financial clout and a large bureaucracy, attributes not available to universities or individuals. Only in the 1980s, with the accrual of knowledge in molecular biology, did the biotechnology revolution hatch tangible results with practical applications.

Biotechnology is now the buzz of a brave new world of medicine, although it hasn't delivered yet. Perhaps one reason is that biomedical research continues to operate with the same industrial, mechanistic mentality despite fundamental conflict with the principles of biology. For instance, recent research on specific inherited "breast cancer genes," anticipated by many as a route to early detection and prevention, has instead uncovered a vast complexity of interactions all over the biological map that clearly are not going to provide predictability, much less a neat, single-action mechanism at work.[79]

In 1999 a teenager died shortly after receiving an injection of a gene-altered virus, raising a very serious red flag.[80] Nor do early genetic-engineering experiments in other fields bode well. Efforts to produce "super-pigs" with lower fat content bore animals that were "excessively hairy, lethargic, riddled with arthritis, apparently impotent and slightly cross-eyed,"and that could barely stand up.[81] Dolly, the famed clone in sheep's clothing, is aging prematurely and rapidly and no one knows why.[82]

Genetic medicine's strategy follows the logic of reductionism, pursuing single-action mechanisms in contradiction to biology's web of conditional interconnectedness. As the giant profit-driven drug companies have systematically bought up biotech companies, the old industrial outlook continues to inform research.[83] While genetic medicine could conceivably one day yield safe, valuable therapies, they are unlikely to emerge out of the old methods and ways of doing things. Given the unforeseen harms caused by treatments such as radiation and chemotherapy, tinkering with mechanistic genetic therapies could prove to be even more dangerous to human health. Biologist Mae-Wan Ho has termed the situation the "marriage of bad science and big business."[84]

Despite such radical emerging technologies, Congress recently diminished the regulatory powers of the FDA after drug companies lobbied to relax the standards of safety and efficacy while shortening the lengthy, expensive timelines required to gain drug approval. Using dangerous and fearsome diseases such as cancer and AIDS as justifications, the pharmaceutical manufacturers want to save money and lessen their liability despite lowering the bar for drug-safety testing and effectiveness. A new law took effect in 1999 that implements these changes.[85]

Overall, the National Cancer Act's "War on Cancer" has served mainly as a generous government economic development initiative for drug companies and medical-supply corporations. As former NCI director Samuel Broder characterized the situation, "The NCI has become what amounts to a government pharmaceutical company."[86]

Virtually none of this vast public funding has furthered the investigation of alternative approaches, although copious federal monies have stoked the litigious siege against "quackery." How might matters have turned out differently if the hundreds of millions of dollars spent prosecuting alternative cancer therapies were instead applied to evaluating them?

Patent medicine was supplanted by patented medicine during the twentieth century against the backdrop of vast financial gain. But this trade war fought over money is an old story in medicine, a flashback to the earlier competition between allopaths and empirics. Or as Yogi Berra once said, It's déjà vu all over again.

19

Two Centuries of Trade Wars: The High Priests of Medicine

O nly during the twentieth century did allopathic medicine's joint venture with big business privatize health care, transforming the medical commons into the rich preserve of corporations. But the underlying pattern of obstruction by doctors against outsiders has a long genealogy that sheds considerable light on its present condition. "Doctors have always been anxious to convince the public that medicine, in any of its aspects, is far too complex and perilous a matter to be meddled with by laymen," wrote Barbara Griggs.[1]

One of the blackest episodes in medical and human history occurred from about 1300 to 1700 in Europe when hundreds of thousands of women were murdered as witches, often by burning at the stake. One of the central consequences was the wholesale loss of the folk medicine traditions carried by women as village herbalists and midwives. When the church condemned their therapeutic craft as black magic, it subsumed medicine as its nearly exclusive domain, often along with the property these women owned. The notion of the high priests of medicine was not metaphorical.[2]

By the 1500s members of the exclusive club of physicians spent an arduous fourteen years obtaining a degree at elite institutions such as England's Oxford and Cambridge, and resented the widespread competition from "uneducated" folk healers. The doctors organized to obtain nothing less than a royal decree from the king ensuring the strict regulation of medical practice by banning other practitioners around London. With the new royal act in place, the physicians pulled rank in the hierarchy of practitioners. They sued the surgeons, the surgeons sued the barbers, and all of them savaged the lay practitioners for practicing medicine without a license.[3]

However, as fate would decree, King Henry VIII was an amateur devotee of herbal medicine, and his Parliament countered with a radical "Act" legitimizing the practice of lay herbalism in 1542. "It shall be lawful for every person being the King's subject, having knowledge and experience of the nature of Herbs, Roots and Waters . . . to practice, use and minister . . . according to their cunning, experience and knowledge in any of the diseases . . . without suit, vexation, trouble, penalty, or loss of their goods."[4]

The King's Act did not stop there. It roundly chastised the doctors, who, "minding onely their own lucre, and nothing the profit or ease of the diseased or Patient, have sued, troubled, and vexed divers honest persons, as well as men and women, whom God hath endued with the knowledge of nature, kind and operation of certain Herbs, Roots and Waters, and the using and ministring of them, to such as has been pained with customable diseases."[5]

The royal act became popularly known as the Quacks' Charter, fully legalizing a new stratum of herbal healers. But the battle pitting doctors against "Empiricks and unlicensed Practisers" was far from over.

By the 1830s in the United States, heroic medicine was losing favor with the public. Allopaths apprehensively watched their legal monopoly melt away as states successively authorized the budding pluralism of alternative medical practices. For the first time, empiric practitioners gained legal footing equal to their allopathic counterparts, allowing them to sue to collect their fees. Allopathic doctors, now stripped suddenly of the legal armor of their monopoly, found themselves vulnerable to intense economic competition.[6]

Homeopathy had begun its steep ascent, introducing a complex, sophisticated, and harmless pharmacopoeia. Homeopaths had undertaken a rigorous and elaborate system of "provings," administering doses of a plethora of natural products to observe the medical symptoms they caused, then preparing infinitesimal doses of these same substances to treat those afflictions. The therapy became popular not only with the public, but also among the social elite, including the clergy, intellectuals, the business community, and the press. It also found a vast constituency among women, often including the very wives of the allopaths.[7] The situation became doubly irritating to the doctors when homeopathy began to attract numerous members from their own fold, including prominent physicians. By 1900 as many as a sixth of homeopaths came from allopathic medical schools.

Also thriving was the vast array of herbal healers growing out of the movement of "Indian doctors" and "root doctors" who had adapted the extensive Native American botanical pharmacopoeia. Prominent among these were the Thompsonians, founded by Samuel Thompson, a New Hampshire farmer who systematized a healing regimen using botanical remedies and steam baths. He patented and franchised the program very successfully across the nation, rapidly making over 100,000 sales by 1839 and boasting three million adherents, about a sixth of the populace. Thompsonians founded their own drugstores and infirmaries to disseminate this popular medicine of the masses.[8]

Throughout this era when the populist ideals of Jacksonian democracy saturated the land, antiauthoritarian and anticorporate sentiments were widely expressed in the proliferation of lay medicine and resistance to the professional elitism of doctors. As Paul Starr wrote, "It was the aim of the Thompsonians, whose declared sympathies were with the laboring classes, to overthrow this tyranny of priests, lawyers and doctors. The genius of the Thompsonian system was to express a protest against the dominant order in its therapeutic as well as its political ideas."[9] When Harry Hoxsey later railed against the "High Priests of Medicine," he was firmly rooted in a vital American populist tradition.

By 1850 Thompsonianism gave way to the rise of the Eclectics, whose first medical schools had now taken hold. By the 1880s the Eclectics had over 10,000 practitioners, about on a par with homeopathy. Despite their smaller numbers compared to the 100,000 allopaths, the empiric ranks were undeniably draining away a great deal of business.[10]

It was in response to this compelling economic threat that the American Medical Association arose in 1847. The profession envisioned a national organization as the solution to its crisis. Under the leadership of New York's Dr. Nathan Smith Davis for the next fifty years, the stated purpose of the AMA was to "improve medical education," and the AMA branded as a quack any practitioner not having a "scientific," that is, allopathic, medical training.[11] The AMA banned the publication of homeopathic case histories from its medical journals. It forbade medical doctors to conduct consultations with homeopaths, and barred them from medical societies altogether.[12] The subtext was to delegitimize the empirics and stave off any prospect of vigorous competition. As one nervous allopath wrote, "Quackery occasions a large pecuniary loss to us. The United States must be regarded as the very elysium of quackery. They assume an equality, and by fraud and deception, too frequently triumph and grow rich, where wise and better men scarcely escape starvation."[13]

The AMA rationale was that improving medical education would renew public confidence and distinguish "scientific medicine" from quackery. The public, however, was singularly disinterested in this transparent subterfuge against free market forces. As Starr wryly noted, "Quacks, as Everett Hughes once defined them, are practitioners who continue to please their customers but not their colleagues."[14]

For the balance of the century, allopathy's public favor would decline and languish while the empirics prospered. Doctors were acutely aware of their poor image from using dangerous poisons in contrast with the empirics' generally innocuous materia medica. What temporarily restored public confidence in the doctors was not a reconstruction of medical education, but a shift in therapeutics. Deeply influenced by homeopathy, the allopaths began to relinquish bloodletting, diminish their heroic doses, and rely increasingly on empiric remedies.[15] As one allopathic practitioner wrote, "For more than half a century, there has been a decided movement in the profession in opposition to an indiscriminate heroic treatment. He who gives the least medicine, and that of the least offensive kind, is coming to be regarded as the best physician. Men of high reputation in the profession have lost confidence in therapeutics and therapeutic agents, and rely mostly on nature and hygiene."[16] This position remained a controversial one within allopathy, however, and would not prevail.

Fearing a loss of control, the allopaths' response was to unify as a sovereign profession in a national organization, the AMA, to control medical licensure. Owing to the proliferation of empiric sects and the egalitarian nature of post-Jacksonian democracy, most state medical licensure laws had been dismantled by the mid-nineteenth century. Because a mere diploma admitted a practitioner into the medical marketplace, the AMA focused its efforts on creating a secondary system of state and ultimately national licensing boards to regain control and also stanch the excessive numbers of doctors flooding the marketplace and depressing income.

The AMA reconstituted itself as a confederation of state and county medical societies. Requiring membership at the county level in order to gain access to the others forced physicians to pay dues at each tier. Local membership also became a prerequisite for obtaining hospital privileges. Within a few brief decades, 60 percent of doctors belonged to the AMA, and "organized medicine" was writ large by 1920.[17]

Though really aimed to undermine the empirics, the AMA's clarion call for improved medical education was appropriate. Allopathic education was itself greatly in need of upgrading. There was a disturbingly high failure rate of allopathic graduates applying for jobs in the armed services. In one case, only about a third of applicants made the cut.[18]

But the educational "standards" also represented a strict loyalty oath to the allopathic set of practices, engendering "a multitude of star chambers all over the land," as a New York doctor wrote in 1883 about the AMA's national Code of Ethics.[19] Added a New York professor of municipal law, "Will the law allow patients to be punished from employing those whom the law pronounces qualified? It is a conspiracy against the public health."[20]

When the AMA expelled the New York Medical Society in 1883 for abolishing the clause barring consultations with homeopaths, the *New York Times* objected strenuously. "The AMA says that if a patient's life cannot be saved except by such a consultation, then the patient must die, and no doctor who will allow a homeopathist to help him can be recognized by such an association."[21]

When the New York Medical Society then lobbied the legislature in 1890 for a single medical board to approve doctors as well as homeopaths, a body that would be dominated by a majority of allopaths, the *New York Times* again protested. "We may imagine what would be the result if the 'single board' were applied to examinations in theology. The homeopaths and the eclectics claim the same right to license their own graduates that the different churches possess, and there does not seem to be any good reason why it should not be conceded to them."[22] The homeopathic recommendation for separate boards triumphed and was replicated in other states.

The AMA, a private, unincorporated entity, was testing the boundaries of legality as well as medical ethics. Though still a weak professional trade association, it had fixed on the template that would guide it to a medical coup d'état. Its "garrison-state mentality" against nonallopathic practitioners, as Coulter termed it, would inform a ruthless winner-take-all strategy for the next one hundred years.[23]

As the nineteenth century drew to a close, a powerful constellation of financial forces aligned to propel allopathic medicine to unsurpassed hegemony. Following the Civil War, the drug industry was born. It began by providing the Union Army with calomel, but soon adapted itself to the expansive pharmacopoeias of the empirics. The pharmaceutical industry sprang from the ensuing patent medicine boom, which was largely founded on botanicals and homeopathic remedies. By the 1880s, newly formed companies with names like Squibb, Parke-Davis, Merck, Abbot, and Eli Lilly were producing prodigious quantities of standardized preparations including bloodroot, barberry, mayapple, and salicylic acid, an aspirin precursor. Allopathic companies joined the lucrative bandwagon in force. Purely homeopathic remedies were of little interest since they were so inexpensive that practitioners gave them away free.[24]

"The 'patent medicines,'" wrote Harris Coulter, "were compounds whose ingredients were nearly always kept secret, but whose names were copyrighted or protected by trademark and which were advertised as specific remedies for one or several disease conditions. The medical profession distinguished these substances, whose ingredients were secret and which were advertised directly to the public as remedies for specific conditions, from the products of the 'ethical' firms which were—in principle—advertised only to the profession and whose ingredients were disclosed. The 1847 [AMA] Code of Ethics stated categorically, 'Equally derogatory to professional character is for a physician to dispense a *secret nostrum*.'"[25]

Because its Code of Ethics barred secret remedies and direct advertising to the public, the AMA now risked openly contradicting its central articles of faith. Manufacturers sought several routes around the conundrum. They produced "proprietaries" whose ingredients were disclosed but that were nevertheless legally protectable. The huge popular success of this new marketing stratagem created an unstoppable commercial force. Some companies further evaded the secrecy issue by revealing their ingredients privately only to the editors of medical journals. Doctors knew less and less about what they were prescribing, relying on the good graces of silent tribunals in journal offices or on drug manufacturers' own promotions. The drugstore became the emblem of the era.[26]

These "proprietaries" laid the foundation for the new patent medicines from Germany, synthetic drugs protected by actual modern patents. The term *patent medicine* quickly assumed an entirely novel meaning for a pharmaceutical industry now poised to dominate the medical landscape.[27]

Before long, drug companies themselves acquired and published medical journals, pouring their proprietaries through the funnel of official medical publications to disperse through doctors. They also lavished advertising dollars on independent medical journals, becoming their fiscal anchor. By the turn of the century, only one out of 250 medical journals relied solely on subscription revenues from its professional constituency.[28]

The nascent drug industry joined forces with the American Medical Association, and it was into this turbulent setting that Dr. George Henry Simmons came to the AMA. As the AMA *Journal* stated in 1902, "What the medical profession needs is a leader, to take it out of the valley of poverty and humiliation, a Mitchell, as the miners have, or a Morgan, as the trusts have."[29] The *Journal* was already turning a profit by 1900 from copious advertising from drug companies.

The AMA neatly inserted itself between medical corporations and the marketplace. "This strategic gatekeeping role permitted the AMA, in effect, to levy an advertising toll on the producers," Starr wrote.[30] Drug company ads boosted the revenues of the AMA *Journal* 500 percent in ten years, rising from $33,760 in 1899 to $150,000 by 1909, and to $9 million by the 1950s, when it accounted for half the AMA's revenues.[31] The money fueled the allopathic trade association's old vendetta against the empirics, whose pluralism left them scattered in organizational disarray against the one-pointed assault by organized medicine.[32]

Yet while the AMA was starting to become prosperous in 1900, doctors themselves remained impoverished. According to Coulter, "Conditions of practice were steadily worsening, with the average allopath earning only about $750 annually. The life expectancy of the physicians was said to be the shortest of any professional man. About forty physicians were committing suicide every year, the principal causes being poverty and financial insecurity." Medical practice was reduced "to a frenzied scramble for subsistence."[33]

Dr. Simmons identified two key sources of the profession's woes: the oversupply of doctors and competition from "quackery." To resolve the difficulties, he turned his attention to opening the arms of the AMA to the "sectarians" with an offer of membership if they would but renounce allegiance to any one school. His tactic worked. As Dr. J. N. McCormack, a close Simmons associate at the AMA, wrote in 1903 about the sectarians, "Many of them are recognized as physicians of ability and as powers for good in the community, and if they are willing to meet the conditions of our invitation, made fair and honorable for them and us, and come into an organization in which they are hopelessly outnumbered, there seems every reason for accepting them."[34]

To gain professional acknowledgment, empirics and homeopaths joined the AMA in large numbers, diffusing their impact and fogging the distinction that made them singular in the public eye.[35] Swallowed whole by the AMA, the empirics lost their political leverage and identity. Dr. McCormack was later quoted as remarking, "We must admit that we have never fought the homeopath on matters of principle; we fought him because he came into our community and got the business."[36]

Now the AMA resurrected its long-standing call for the reformation of medical education. By controlling medical education, it seized the opportunity to stanch the oversupply of doctors and raise their income. But of equal importance, the organization could now deconstruct the licensing apparatus of its competitors. Forming the Council on Medical Education, Dr. Simmons began to design medical standards pointedly structured to favor allopathy.

In 1907 the council visited medical schools around the nation including Eclectic and homeopathic institutions, since it now admitted them to its ranks.[37] There was an uproar when the empiric schools caught wind of the low ratings that threatened to entirely discredit them. Dr. Simmons did not publish the results, which also damned a goodly number of allopathic schools, but he finessed the strife by passing the controversy laterally to the Carnegie Foundation for the Advancement of Teaching, a seemingly objective body. Established with funding from Andrew Carnegie, the architect of the steel monopoly, the foundation sent its representative Abraham Flexner, along with an AMA official, to resurvey the embattled terrain. The result was Flexner's pivotal 1910 *Bulletin Number Four*, a report on medical education in the United States and Canada. Its outcome was the demise of empiric medicine.[38]

The determinations of the Flexner report, which were even harsher than the AMA's recommendation to eliminate half of medical schools, guided state medical examining boards in their standards. Graduates from medical schools found wanting were excluded from practice, leading to the extinction of these institutions. The AMA Council on Medical Education soon emerged essentially as a "national accrediting agency," as Paul Starr noted, and its "decisions came to have force of law. This was an extraordinary achievement for the organized profession."[39]

While there was certainly substandard medical education on both sides of the fence, in practical terms the report served as a political hatchet to chop away the competition that the AMA had been seeking to eliminate for sixty years. Although there were other important factors that contributed to the justifiable demise of many medical schools, the AMA's use of the Flexner report principally served its own self-interests. "Physicians finally had medical practice pretty much to themselves," Starr wrote. "With the political organization they achieved after 1900, doctors were able to convert that rising authority into legal privileges, economic power, high incomes, and enhanced social status."[40]

A bad rating also meant the inability to gain funding from Andrew Carnegie and John. D. Rockefeller Sr., the prime philanthropists of medical education. Abraham Flexner's brother Simon was president of the Rockefeller Institute for Medical Research, the single largest funder of medical education. The Flexner report became the "manifesto of a program that by 1936 guided $91 million from Rockefeller's General Education Board (plus millions more from other foundations) to a select group of medical schools."[41]

Medicine had never before been lucrative, yet suddenly it was pregnant with sufficient promise to attract the "robber barons" of the late nineteenth century. They applied the industrial logic of mass production to the emerging medical treatments. The AMA lashed itself to the wheel of these overwhelming financial forces to transform medicine into an industry. The fortunes of Carnegie, Morgan, Astor, and Rockefeller financed surgery, radiation, and synthetic drugs, the lucrative keystones of the nascent medical economy.[42] The Rockefeller Institute for Medical Research, which the philanthropist used to mitigate his notoriety, became the principal sponsor of medical research and helped make it an industrial, mass-market phenomenon.

Surgery commanded high fees for doctors, who advocated radical and frequent operations. It spawned the vast and gainful hospital system, profitable new technologies, and a sprawling infrastructure composed of anesthesiologists, staff, and nurses. The number of hospitals grew from just 200 in 1873 to over 6,000 by 1920.[43]

As radium fever swept medicine, the price of radium rose over 1,000 percent almost overnight. James Douglas, head of the Phelps-Dodge Mining Company, as we saw earlier, donated a $100,000 wing to New York's Memorial Hospital with the explicit agreement that radium would now be used in every case in the institution newly configured to service nothing but cancer. Radiation therapy soon spread to other elite institutions. The doses were heroic, and another lucrative technology entered the hospital system.[44] Douglas himself barely missed his financial objective of cornering the national radium market, foiled only by the Du Pont family's adroit manipulations and huge countervailing resources.

The drug industry became the most profitable business in the world. Rockefeller emulated the monopolistic corporate model of Germany's I. G. Farben, with which he had close business ties. The giant conglomerate, which controlled almost all German chemical and drug businesses, served as the prototype of corporate organization adopted by its emerging U.S. counterparts. Creating a joint venture with the German combine in 1927 centered on important patents, Rockefeller's Standard Oil of New Jersey (Esso) activated the U.S. pharmaceutical industry on a large scale.

At the time, Germany led the world in medical science and research. Oddly, it was Hitler's Nazis who conceived the most aggressive and advanced war on cancer of the era. During the 1930s, Nazi Germany initiated widespread though socially selective public health campaigns against industrial carcinogens, radioactivity, and smoking, while promoting organic foods, vegetarian diets, and herbal and natural medicine. German cancer research was by far the most developed in the world, and drew international recognition.[45]

I. G. Farben had been doing extensive experimentation with cancer, witnessed personally by the influential vice president of Esso, Frank Howard. Joining the board of Memorial Hospital in the 1930s, Howard was closely involved in the formation of the Research Committee, which by 1941 began to develop chemotherapy from nitrogen mustard gas. He led the full-scale chemotherapy enterprise there after the war's end.[46]

The involvement of John D. Rockefeller in the demise of empiric medicine was sharply ironic. Rockefeller's father, William "Wild Bill" Rockefeller, had gotten his start in the Pennsylvania oil fields bottling mineral oil and selling it as a cancer cure. He traversed the countryside with leaflets reading, "Dr. William A. Rockefeller, the Celebrated Cancer Specialist, Here for One Day Only. All Cases of Cancer Cured unless too far gone and then they can be greatly benefited." His product Nujol (as in "New Oil") was eventually incorporated into his son's drug companies as a mineral oil laxative, although it actually appeared to cause constipation.[47]

John D. Rockefeller himself, however, was a stalwart devotee of homeopathy, shunning medical doctors and refusing to consult anyone but a homeopath well into his robust nineties. Thus it seemed an impenetrable paradox that Rockefeller's fortune would prove instrumental in nearly destroying homeopathy and empiric medicine. The Flexner report unequivocally recommended the closure of all the homeopathic medical schools at a moment when Rockefeller was personally irate over the extensive dissension and disarray within the diverse homeopathic community. His advisers apparently convinced him that "scientific medicine" would eliminate sectarianism by incorporating the best of all worlds without bias.[48]

In any case, Rockefeller's General Education Board channeled huge amounts of cash into allopathic schools, and the twenty-two homeopathic colleges dwindled to seven by 1918, while the nine Eclectic schools were reduced to one.[49] Of 162 allopathic medical schools at the turn of the century, fewer than half remained by the 1920s, all firmly under AMA control.[50] The number of graduates dropped precipitously, as the law of supply and demand now fattened physicians' pocketbooks through the nation's diminished doctor-patient ratio. Dr. Simmons proved to be the visionary leader *JAMA* had called for, his adept plan now a reality.

In a brief twenty years, the AMA came to dominate medical practice through brute financial force, political manipulation, and professional authority enhanced by rising public favor with "scientific" medicine. The AMA emerged as the supreme arbiter of medical practice, making binding pronouncements regulating even the most picayune details.[51] American medicine surged forward as a profit-driven enterprise of matchless scope.

By the time Dr. Morris Fishbein assumed the mantle of Dr. Simmons, who had himself started out as a homeopath, the AMA was at the helm of a strapping new industry flying the allopathic flag. The code word for competition was *quackery*.

Harry Hoxsey, a backwoods shaman born in the Golden Age of the Doctor, really never stood a chance against Dr. Fishbein's industrial-strength crusade. It is remarkable that Hoxsey fought as long and successfully as he did. The overall failure of allopathic cancer treatment certainly contributed. Another principal reason was that the public still continued to embrace empiric therapeutics. It was estimated that an astonishing 85 percent of people continued to use "drugless healers" into the early 1940s, according to surveys conducted by the Chicago Medical Society and others.[52]

By the 1980s the commercial juggernaut of industrial medicine had successfully built an institutional fortress excluding all but its own. Nevertheless, allopathic medicine still bore the same endemic flaws that have repeatedly undermined it for centuries. In cancer especially, its heroic therapeutics were largely failing, and despite an effective public relations campaign, patients often considered the treatment worse than the disease. Allopathic unwillingness to look at alternative methods was increasingly hard to justify, and once more, patients were migrating in large numbers to the next generation of unorthodox cancer therapies.

In the end, people involved in orthodox science and medicine are no more or less human than those in other professions, all of which are fraught with ego, greed, jealousy, and power struggles. But it is no accident that in this century the word *orthodox* shifted from a purely theological term to a clinical one. For, despite the obvious trade war between doctors and alternative practitioners, the therapeutic battleground is also an ideological one, a fervent contest of belief systems.

For example, as one opponent of alternative therapies stated, "Purveyors of questionable therapies seem to hold the view that it is the job of science to disprove crazy ideas. Dwindling research funds should not be utilized to disprove the fads, frauds, and fancies of alternative medicine. However, the medical profession needs to be adequately prepared to educate the public on those issues lest 'disappointment in us will surely drive many into the hands of the magicians.'"[53]

But who are these "magicians"? Are they researchers such as I. Semmelweiss, who was hounded mercilessly to his death for observing that doctors were killing their patients by not washing their hands before childbirth and surgery? Or Louis Pasteur, who met violent opposition for proposing the germ theory of disease? Or Galileo, whose opponents viewed his strange telescope as a heresy and refused even to look through it to verify what he saw? Those who say that such closed-minded oppression couldn't take place today need only examine the long trail of medical follies culminating in the AMA's conviction of conspiracy against the chiropractors.

And so the question remains: What if Hoxsey, who certainly fit the stereotype of a quack, actually had something? Or Gerson, or Burton, or Burzynski, or any of the several dozen other alternative cancer therapies whose anecdotal evidence indicates that they might show enough benefit to be worth investigating? What happens if orthodoxy again refuses to look through the telescope?

Among other consequences, real quackery will persist. Only rigorous evaluation that is open-minded and evenhanded can finally determine true merit. "How is our Congress to legislate intelligently when its technological advisers themselves wear blinders and practice deceit and suppression?" Patricia Spain Ward asked plaintively. "We've lost a lot of time. Just think of how many people have died. We could have been so much further ahead by now."[54]

The real impetus driving the OTA investigation was public pressure, the sheer force of numbers of people using alternative cancer therapies, with or without the approval of organized medicine. A landmark national survey published in the *New England Journal of Medicine* revealed over a third of the American public using alternative medicine by 1990 when the OTA report finally came out. In an economic system that exalts the market, consumers were voting with their pocketbooks, spending an estimated $14 billion a year on alternative practitioners, primarily out-of-pocket.[55]

The final OTA report to Congress, while still heavily criticized by the alternative community, did affirm that indeed unconventional cancer therapies merited further investigation. The report set in motion a radical political shift that materialized sooner than anyone expected with the creation of the Office of Alternative Medicine in 1991 within the federal National Institutes of Health. Congress directed the OAM to begin at last the objective review of alternative cancer treatments and other unconventional therapies. It would be a muddy road for thick wheels, but at least there was forward motion.

The medical civil war was far from over, but for the first time there was an unequivocal federal directive to explore alternative therapies. "I've really looked at it always," cancer patient and activist Bob DeBragga once told our camera, "*always* from the patient's point of view. And if there's something in orthodoxy, like a little bit of radiation, or the proper surgery at exactly the right time, with good nutritional support, this is what I want. What I want is whatever is best for the patient. And I don't care whether it's called orthodox, unorthodox, fringe—I don't care. There's just too many people dying. Too many people dying."[56]

Bob DeBragga died one month after the September release of the OTA report. Given six weeks to live, he outran his prognosis by twelve years using alternative therapies. He lived to see the promise of a collaborative medical future.

A Truce in the Medical Civil War: The Office of Alternative Medicine Looks at Hoxsey

By the time the Office of Technology Assessment finally published *Unconventional Cancer Treatments* in 1990, after four years and a half-million dollars, the report had the dubious distinction of being the most protracted and expensive in its history. It recommended specific action points for the National Cancer Institute including obtaining and disseminating sound information on alternative treatments, facilitating "best case" reviews of patients successfully treated by these practices, including those in a national remissions database, and allocating meaningful funding to start actual testing.

Gar Hildenbrand, former executive director of the Gerson Institute and an OTA advisory panel member, had remained intimately involved with the political maneuvering as a watchdog for the alternative community. In an interview with me, the compact, forty-eight-year-old advocate, who abandoned a budding career as a playwright to engage in medical politics after his own lupus was successfully treated by the Gerson therapy, recalled the prickly atmosphere. "When Roger Herdman [of the OTA] went before the NCI's National Cancer Advisory Board, he said to them, 'The American people have spoken and Congress has heard the people, and now you must listen. The news that this report bears is that you must now pay thoughtful attention to the alternatives.' One of the board members leaned back in his chair and said, 'Doctor, we hear you telling us we've got some kind of disease, but we don't feel sick.' That set the tone for the next several years of jockeying."[1]

Within a year it became obvious that the NCI was not acting on the congressional mandate. As a semiautonomous agency, it did not report to the National Institutes of Health but only to the rarefied National Cancer Advisory Board and an insular president's panel. Its relative political immunity bolstered its arrogance, but it was increasingly vulnerable to unaccustomed pressure for its failure in its primary mission of eradicating cancer. The institution's defiance of the congressional directive left but one pathway for redress: Follow the money. Congress authorizes the NCI budget, and can pull rank to get what it wants.

Two populist politicians from Iowa, six-term U.S. Representative Berkley Bedell and Senator Tom Harkin, decided it was time to take preemptive action. Bedell had a strong personal motive for cutting through the tangle. A direct, outspoken former entrepreneur who had founded a highly successful fishing tackle company, he contracted Lyme disease while fishing. The illness compelled him to retire and landed him in the hospital several times. Despite medical treatment, his condition worsened. He opted to explore an alternative therapy.[2]

Bedell, whose deceptively homespun, country-boy persona masks a razor-sharp investigator's edge, tracked down a Minnesota farmer who had empirically devised a remedy for Lyme disease. Injecting a milk cow's udders with some of Bedell's own blood, the farmer extracted whey from the animal's colostrum, the first milk from nursing, and fed it to him. The former congressman got well, though the farmer was charged with practicing medicine without a license. (The farmer was released after a hung jury.)

Subsequently, Bedell was diagnosed with prostate cancer. The disease recurred after conventional treatment, and again he sought relief with an alternative therapy. He used a nontoxic immune-stimulating drug called 714X, originated by Gaston Naessens, a Canadian biologist who had performed elaborate research over many years using an advanced microscope and a decidedly unconventional approach that landed him in the Canadian courts. Again Bedell got well.

Bedell brought his recovery using a "quack" therapy to the attention of his colleagues, among them Senator Tom Harkin, who had been in Congress with him for twelve years. Harkin was strategically well situated as chairman of the Appropriations Subcommittee, which authorized funding for the National Institutes of Health. Bedell and Harkin joined forces to sponsor legislation that amounted to an end run past the NCI. In 1991, they created the Office of Alternative Medicine (first called the Office for the Study of Unconventional Medical Practices), under the auspices of the gargantuan National Institutes of Health. The legislation passed. Although its funding of $2.2 million was minuscule within the

$10 billion NIH funding, it did represent the seed of a new order—a homeopathic dose of sorts.

In contrast with the NCI, the NIH was more open to new ideas, exhibiting a freshly felicitous attitude to the foundling of alternative medicine. The landmark event produced a sharp turn in media perception. The *New York Times* expectantly noted the "mainstreaming of alternative medicine."[3]

The NIH recognized that evaluating unconventional therapies might necessitate unorthodox research strategies as well. Among the proposals was an idea originally put forth by Lawrence Burton that "field teams" actually come to his clinic and observe patients and the treatment in a real-world clinical setting. OAM Director Dr. Joe Jacobs, who held a markedly conventional orientation, was less than enthusiastic about this unorthodox prospect. Under pressure, Jacobs finally agreed and sent teams to visit several alternative clinics, especially oriented to cancer because of the congressional priority. It quickly became clear, however, that the leadership of OAM itself was recalcitrant and biased. When $750,000 for a trial of Dr. Burzynski's antineoplastons simply evaporated without a trace, Bedell and Harkin plugged the breach. Threatening to suspend OAM funding entirely, they called for the resignation of director Jacobs, who by now was at odds with most of the respected members of the alternative medicine community.

Gar Hildenbrand recalled a meeting he witnessed between Senator Harkin and a high NIH official. "The official has been called into the senator's office. Senator Harkin has his popcorn machine in his lobby, and the official picks up a bag of popcorn and sits there munching popcorn like he's at a movie theater. Then Senator Harkin comes in doing his best Gary Cooper, and he just fills the office with light because he's very warm. He says 'I had allergies. I was in D.C. and I was working, and my allergies were horrible. I've been taking Seldane for years, one in the morning and one in the evening, and it wasn't working any more. So my doctor put me on six Benedryl in the morning with the Seldane and six Benedryl in the evening with the Seldane, and it was still not cutting the allergies, and I was miserable. I couldn't think. My sinuses were draining.

"'Then I had to go to Iowa and spring was happening all over again. When I came back to Washington, Berkley brought in this little ninety-year-old guy with an even older friend who proceeded to tell me that if I would take bee pollen—I forget how much I took but it's on a piece of paper on my desk over there—if I take this bee pollen and a glass of water, my allergies would get better. If I took it, and ten minutes later nothing happened, then I should have another glass of water and another hit of bee pollen. I can't remember how many times I did it, but it's on a piece of paper on my desk. I did it a number of times, and then I got called away for a vote, and while I was placing the vote, I realized that my allergies had let up. I took more of it—I think I took some that night and I know I took some more the next morning—I can't remember how much, though it's on a piece of paper over there on my desk. And you know what? They've never come back. I don't take any Seldane. I don't take any Benedryl. I just take bee pollen and my allergies are gone and I want you to study it,' he tells the official.

"Harkin then says, 'I got a problem because people are always coming up to me and saying, "Hey, Tom, how's it going over there with your Office of Alternative Medicine at NIH?" I think you people are laughing at me.'

"Berkley won two times," Hildenbrand concluded. "He's batting a thousand and that's why the office happened. Tom was sensitive and Berkley had personal experience. You know what we call those: N=1. When it happens to you, the number—the sample size—that is significant is one. All the confusion goes away when your body gets well."

The NIH hired professional mediators and held a meeting to reconcile the two hostile camps. As participant Ralph Moss described the drama, "So many bad things had happened. It was almost like sitting down in Bosnia or something. There were people in that room whose lives had been ruined by the actions of the establishment, whose careers had been ruined, whose work had been stolen, who had been put in jail, who had been called every name in the book. There were those at the meeting who were saying that we should 'just forget' everything that had happened, just get past it. It's very hard to do. I could do it—except I need some guarantees that we're not going to see a repeat of the same. So I'll wait, probably another twenty years, and see what happens."[4]

After a short transitional phase, the OAM came under the leadership of Lieutenant Colonel Wayne Jonas, M.D., in February 1995. An expert on research methodology, the boyish-looking Dr. Jonas came from a position in the Army as chief of the postgraduate Fellowship Research Training program at the military's respected Walter Reed Institute of Research in Washington, D.C. He held a long-standing interest in alternative medicine including homeopathy, acupuncture, and nutrition. His arrival was welcomed by the alternative community, and for the first time, an atmosphere of trust started to develop.

Bedell was insistent, however, about radically changing the research culture. Gar Hildenbrand described to me how Bedell, who joined the OAM advisory board, counseled the NIH to resolve the dilemma. "Berkley

says that the idea of writing the Office of Alternative Medicine into existence came to him when he was reflecting on the way that he had built
Berkley and Company, his fishing tackle business. He said his R&D guys
were in the laboratory all the time and the company was floundering. He
told them they needed to go out, and they didn't go out, so he tied going
out to their wages, which made it very, very interesting to them to go out.

   "As soon as they went out, they began to find that other competitors of
theirs were doing really good stuff, so they reverse-engineered it and gained
dominance again. The NIH was told by Senator Harkin, 'You go out the
door and you look at what your competition is doing and you come back
and you report on it.' They didn't even know how to do that. This is all
that has been recommended to NIH, but they had no idea how to mobilize
research, which is why they went to the Army. The Army is all about mobilization. The NIH has been this ivory tower and staunch bureaucracy
that has operated on cronyism for all these years, and had no idea. What
Wayne Jonas developed was a way of reaching out with remote sensors to
the university research centers and the wonderful people who have gathered around who are very committed to moving the assessment of alternatives forward. These are going to feed the outside into the NIH so that it
cannot be insulated any more. That's its problem—it's been so insulated.
When is the last time you heard of a breakthrough from NIH?"

   According to Harkin's directive, Dr. Wayne Jonas linked the OAM
with ten (now thirteen) independent partner centers around the country,
including Columbia University, Harvard, Stanford, and the University
of Maryland. Also awarded a very substantial grant was Bastyr University, the preeminent naturopathic college, where a major AIDS study got
under way.

   It was politically clear, however, that meaningful progress required
the participation of the National Cancer Institute. With NCI funding,
the School of Public Health at the University of Texas in Houston was
chosen to manage the OAM cancer section, partially because of its close
relationship with M. D. Anderson, the nation's most influential cancer
center along with Memorial Sloan-Kettering.

   Appointed director of the Center for Alternative and Complementary Medicine Research in Cancer was Mary Ann Richardson, Ph.D. A
straight-talking Texas native, Richardson was formerly in the oil business. Around the same time the industry crashed in the mid-1980s, she
did too, in a serious accident. "I was injured and got in touch with my
own healing process," Richardson told me when I visited her in Houston.[5] Having been interested in alternative medicine for fifteen years, she

returned to school to do graduate work in public health. Just as she was completing her Ph.D. dissertation, news of the OAM's request for the first round of small, pilot cancer proposals reached her. After the longest wait for a response to any request for proposals in NIH history, Richardson's proposal was selected to locate the OAM cancer section at the University of Texas School of Public Health in Houston.

"The request for proposals let people come out of the woodwork," Richardson recalled. "There's an underground of people interested anyway, but then there was money offered by the NIH." The center spent the first year reading reports and literature, sorting through options and strategies. The group identified leading alternative cancer therapies as priorities for study in 1996. One of them was Hoxsey.

How did Richardson choose Hoxsey? "Hoxsey is famous," she explained, brushing back a mane of brown hair from her windswept face. "I actually went down and visited one summer when I was doing research. It was amazing because here's Mildred smoking, and about ten feet away there's a guy getting a treatment. Mildred was very gracious. She gave me Hoxsey's book and the video, and we talked. She's a Texan, so here was another Texas girl. She was telling me about how, especially with breast cancer, you just separate the tumor from the breast [using the salves]. She asked a patient to 'Show Dr. Richardson your breast.' It was clearly separating the tumor. She told me, 'In about a week we'll be able to scoop the whole thing.' Mildred is a very strong woman and definitely believes in what she's doing. She was totally devoted to the people as a nurse. She truly believes."

Impressed with what she witnessed, Richardson proposed the OAM Hoxsey research study. I had spoken once previously with her in late 1996 about possible Hoxsey research, suggesting that she be in touch with Catherine Salveson. After we finished the film in 1987, Catherine made a commitment to see Hoxsey tested one day and gained Mildred Nelson's consent to advance the process.

"When I first went to Bio Medical in 1983," Catherine told me, "I was essentially a public health nurse coming from the point of view of working in a multicultural rural state where people used a lot of alternative treatments. I personally had a lifestyle that included alternative treatments. I had been to China a couple of times, where herbal medicine is an art, and worked with Native American tribes in the Southwest. I was really coming from a point of view of folk medicine, cultural medicine, and people's right to natural treatments that were basically harmless."[6]

Catherine subsequently earned a master's degree and Ph.D. in nursing, with a specialty in researching alternative therapies, and then joined the faculty of Oregon Health Sciences University, a large nursing college and leading research institution. By 1997 she was ready to pursue the Hoxsey research. "I now see that what we're looking at is not about folk medicine. It's about mainstream medicine, and it's really about a balancing and a return to where we were at the turn of the last century when there was room for more than one point of view in health care. Also, research and information and markets have opened up for a lot of alternative treatments."

The politics of AIDS have also fundamentally altered the focus and importance of medical research. "Especially at the beginning of the epidemic," Catherine elaborated, "the use of alternative treatments by people with HIV disease was the norm because there wasn't anything coming out of the pharmaceutical arena, and people were dying. They could not tell these young people that they couldn't use an alternative treatment because they were going to die and doctors didn't have anything else to offer them. In large measure, the HIV epidemic fueled the patients' rights movement."

The other crucial shift affecting alternative treatments also came out of the HIV epidemic when the activist group ACT-UP stormed the NIH in the mid-1980s. "It was the first time that any patient group for any disease had ever set foot into the NIH except by invitation," Catherine pointed out. "These bench researchers who lived in these ivory towers suddenly were afraid to leave their fancy buildings because there were thousands of angry young people in the streets at the campus in Bethesda screaming at them to stop padding their résumés with research credentials: we need drugs that will help cure AIDS.

"That had a huge impact on the NIH to start the Office of Alternative Medicine. That was also the turning point with the development of an underground network among wealthy, prominent, educated people with HIV—gay men—to scour the planet for anything that could help them and bring it into this country, not in a surreptitious way. They set the tone that patients had the right to help save their own lives and be allowed to take whatever risks they choose."

During this period, there was bitter contention about the regulatory role of the public health system altogether. The doctrine of *in loco parentis* ("in place of the parent") guided the FDA and other public health regulatory bodies to enforce mandatory medical treatments whether patients wanted them or not. Among the most controversial cases were those involving children or people with religious objections to procedures such as blood transfusions. One infamous case revolved around young Chad Green, a child with leukemia whose parents declined chemotherapy in favor of several alternatives including Hoxsey and Gerson. A court ordered the boy removed from his parents' custody and legally compelled him to have chemotherapy. The family went underground and took him back to Mexico.[7]

Public opinion firmly opposed such medical Big Brother tactics. The storming of the NIH and concurrent public resistance to the doctrine of *in loco parentis* radically changed the way that new drugs are evaluated by the FDA, resulting in "compassionate care" and "fast track" guidelines. Where it used to take up to fifteen years for a drug to complete testing requirements and gain approval, now the AIDS drug AZT and a number of others got through much more quickly. A fresh precedent was established to permit doctors to give patients experimental drugs even when they did not know whether they were effective. They could dispense them in the hope they would be beneficial, and watched the patients very closely for any adverse effects on "fast track" access. "That's what alternative treatments are," Catherine suggests. "We cannot verify the effects when the research is not complete. The research becomes paramount."

When Mary Ann Richardson approached Mildred Nelson about performing research, Mildred referred her to Catherine, who joined the OAM project as a co-investigator. In the spring of 1998, an OAM team consisting of Richardson, an epidemiologist, and a biostatistician met Catherine at the Tijuana clinic to begin a "historical cohort study." They selected the roster of cancer patients from the first quarter of 1992—a five-year marker—and began the tedious task of ascertaining what has happened to these people since.

The review of these approximately 150 cancer cases is a very preliminary step and cannot reveal anything definitive. It could provide potential leads by finding positive outcomes, and it does dip a toe in the research waters whose ripples may lead to more in-depth testing. After almost seventy-five years, the federal government is at last formally investigating Hoxsey and other alternative cancer therapies.

Hoxsey is, after all, the preeminent herbal treatment for cancer, and its social history and widespread use make it a prime candidate for research. About 1,200 people a year including 600 cancer patients now come to the Bio Medical Center, qualifying it as probably the largest of the alternative cancer clinics. The numbers alone justify scientific investigation. But what exactly does such an evaluation involve? The step seems to symbolize a new era in medical research, but what are the real chances of scientific objectivity and social fairness?

For such a test to have credibility, the research design must be capable of withstanding scientific rigor. But is testing an unconventional therapy such as Hoxsey different from standard protocols?

One numbing conundrum is that conventional medicine sincerely considers it "unethical" not to first administer standard cancer therapies to all research patients, treatments that can severely damage a patient's immune system. Since Hoxsey relies on stimulating the body's immune response, this scenario means starting with a negative bias. Mildred Nelson often turns away patients who have had prior chemotherapy because their immune response is so severely impaired that the Hoxsey treatment can no longer help them.

There is also a fundamental conflict of medical paradigms at issue. A revealing parallel is the difficulty of testing traditional Chinese medicine by conventional standards. Classical Chinese medicine posits the existence of *chi*, a vital life energy somewhat analogous to the *vis medicatrix naturae*. The basis of acupuncture, for example, is to invigorate the person's *chi* by using small needles to stimulate a grid of meridians at highly specific points relating to bodily systems. Western medicine does not accept the existence of *chi*. Tests have validated medical effects on these energy meridians, which do not correspond to any recognized nerve, circulatory, or other physiological pathway, but no one has yet been able to isolate or quantify *chi* itself in a scientific sense.[8] Similarly, because immunology is a new and poorly understood realm, even defining which effects of the Hoxsey tonic to measure is a question, although there are some accepted markers.

Another major problem stems from the fact that classical protocols for medical testing are designed mainly for evaluating synthetic drugs. Generally these tests seek to isolate a single "active ingredient" theoretically responsible for an effect based on a specific molecular mechanism. Something like the Hoxsey tonic has multiple ingredients acting in synergy through potentially very complex mechanisms. As Gar Hildenbrand illustrates, "We're not going to know a molecular mechanism. The human genome hasn't been sufficiently mapped yet. If we take the entire mega-computer network that is working worldwide grinding away at mapping the human genome, after we've finished mapping and try to beef it up a little bit to do nutrition and the interactions of nutrition with the genome, you're going to need fifteen or twenty times that computer system. There are ten thousand phytochemicals in a carrot. What's doing what? In each of the Hoxsey herbs, there are another ten thousand phytochemicals.

"Carbon-based life-forms are very, very intricate, so the molecular mechanisms are very, very deceptive and not at all what they seem to be. Also, we are rapidly reaching the point where we have to confess that we are moving from the realm of chemistry into a marriage of chemistry and particle physics to explain how things stay alive. Show me one person who can design a relatively competent randomized clinical trial and cope with molecular mechanisms that have to do with physics. In fact, show me a person who can design a randomized clinical trial correctly. Did you know that there is no technology transfer for randomized clinical trial methodologies per se? In the near future, there will be courses taught to medical students on how to construct randomized clinical trials, but there aren't any today. It's extremely haphazard."

There are several appropriate approaches that could be applied to testing Hoxsey, according to Mary Ann Richardson. The first is taking a chemical "fingerprint" of the Hoxsey tonic to verify certain marker compounds showing constituents or properties with known anticancer or immune-stimulating activity. These "biological response modifiers" as a class are viewed as having myriad effects and, as such, require a far more thoughtful and flexible research methodology. Since Hoxsey has already been used by people for seventy-five years, it seems unnecessary to test it first on animals, as is normally done. Similarly, the questions of dosage and toxicity are already established because of its long practical history.

A clinical trial with human subjects might then test for prolonged survival, disease-free survival, or improved quality of life. The content of the tonic must be characterized to allow it to be standardized for consistency from batch to batch. Because of intense variability in plant products, it is important to ensure that what is tested at the outset would be the same product used years later.

Another vital research agenda is quality of life. Many patients are as concerned about the quality of their life as the quantity. Since most alternatives such as Hoxsey are nontoxic and do not contribute to further physical suffering, these treatments merit investigation as palliative agents as well.

A serious complication for testing the Hoxsey tonic is that patients going to Hoxsey use a gestalt of treatments, not just the tonic. They follow a complementary diet, receive nutritional support, and often use other immune therapies. In addition, they have the unique experience of the Bio Medical waiting room, an environment brimming with hope, positive expectation, and prayer. It would be impossible to duplicate such a setting in a clinical trial and absurd to try.

The obvious question is: Why not conduct a study at the clinic? That overall model is precisely what the OAM started considering. When the OAM held several meetings to probe protocol design, what emerged is the POMES process: Practice-Based Outcomes Monitoring and Evaluation

System. The concept goes back to former Congressman Bedell's directive to get out of the office and venture forth into the world as it is. Since patients are already receiving treatments in real-life settings from the most skilled and experienced clinicians, it makes particular sense to conduct reviews on-site.

The founders and practitioners of alternative therapies are naturally the most knowledgeable about their own protocols. It is common for hands-on clinicians to achieve results that may elude other researchers much less familiar with the subtleties of the therapy. The experiments must ultimately be replicable by others, but the initial tests are far more likely to show positive outcomes if the actual practitioners are closely involved in designing and implementing them.

Generally members of the alternative medical community like Mildred Nelson have acted as clinicians, treating patients without paying much heed to the complexities of gathering the data essential for stringent research. As such, with some important exceptions, the alternative cancer community is mostly not well prepared for meeting the rigors of research agendas. The lack of expertise in clinical testing by most unorthodox practitioners presents a serious hindrance to the ultimate acceptance of alternative therapies. (Only about seventy formal clinical trials have been held on alternative practices, most of them relating to traditional Chinese medicine.[9])

Recognizing the problem, Gar Hildenbrand set about becoming an epidemiologist, a tedious and painstaking profession that fastidiously documents case histories to identify correct diagnoses, courses of treatment, and other factors that may influence the progress of disease or recovery. He compares epidemiology to prospecting. His work has since focused on documenting the Gerson therapy and designing credible testing methodologies. He has worked with the OAM and now Berkley Bedell's National Foundation for Alternative Medicine reviewing patient records from treatments including the late Dr. Lawrence Burton's IAT and Dr. Burzynski's antineoplastons.

One study Hildenbrand designed and published looked at melanoma patients using the Gerson therapy. The five-year Gerson survival rates were considerably higher than those reported with conventional treatment, particularly in advanced cases, where 70 percent lived five years using Gerson as opposed to 41 percent using conventional treatments.[10]

But is scientific proof really the issue? Is there a double standard, as critics charge, a higher bar for proving alternative therapies? Even presuming the best of all worlds of scientific rigor and honesty, bulletproof tests of alternative therapies still may not overcome the social bias of orthodoxy. Gar Hildenbrand illustrates with the story of what transpired when Dr. Wayne Jonas presented positive results from three clinical trials of homeopathy to a largely conventional audience. "Lieutenant Colonel Wayne Jonas, director of the Army's postgraduate research training fellowships program at Walter Reed, was the number one man in research training—this guy knows a thing or two about research. He chose the clinical trials in homeopathy because they were immaculate. This was real observation, and these clinical effects were real. There was no way they could have happened by chance.

"As Jonas concluded this portion [of his presentation], he saw the hands begin to go up in the house. One by one the good old boys stand up and say things like, 'Doctor Jonas, if we're to accept what you tell us about these clinical trial results, we have to throw away all of our classical chemistry and all of classical physics. Maybe there was a problem with the study design?' To which Wayne replied, 'In fact, this design is tighter than the one used for your last clinical trial.' You could just feel the hubbub growing. When the event was over, the good old boys were still storming and angry. I thought, 'Isn't this amazing?! Not only did homeopathic medicine provide clinical responses in the people in those clinical trials, but just hearing the word *homeopathy* got a rise in the net blood pressure of the good old boys network. That's a medical effect I'd like somebody to test: causing hypertension in the NCI just by presenting findings on homeopathy.

"That's a good example of what the problem is," Hildenbrand concludes. "It's not about science, and that's why I became an epidemiologist, because the only way we can wage this argument is on the facts. The facts, the data, the testing—these things don't lie. They're not always conclusive right away. When you do retrospective findings, you don't prove cause and effect, but you demonstrate a very strong association. The history of medicine is a trail of associations that have led to stronger findings and harder research. There are two groups of people in the sciences who will be useful in trying to change the way that this beast behaves: epidemiologists who know their cancer staging and how to catalog charts, and medical sociologists and anthropologists who are asking all the important questions about the social influences that lead to the screwups in the evaluations."

Neutralizing social bias is basic to performing fair tests, and the POMES process solves this dilemma in several ways. Tests will be monitored by an oversight board composed of a balance of representatives from both conventional and alternative medicine. In addition, experts in international conflict resolution and arbitration including a board of appeals are embedded at every level to mediate disputes. Evaluators will work with practitioners on-site and engage them meaningfully in the tests themselves. The trials will be as much about overall medical protocols and cancer management practices as about substances and molecular mechanisms. They will also focus on *outcomes:* Did anyone actually get well?

"The alternative treatments didn't have a chance in the kind of trials set up by the NCI," Ralph Moss told me, highlighting the case of Essiac, the Canadian herbal cancer formula of burdock, sheep sorrel, slippery elm bark, and Turkey rhubarb. "First of all, they never tested it. Second, when they did a little trial at Sloan-Kettering, they got some sheep sorrel, froze it for a couple of months, defrosted it, and then injected it into mice. They didn't see any results and they announced that they had tested Essiac tea and found it ineffective. Or with Burzynski, they changed the protocol in midstream in the middle of a clinical trial where they were telling patients in advance—I've heard this from patients—that this was a worthless treatment that they were going to be given because it was part of their requirement to do this clinical trial. That was the atmosphere under which the Burzynski trial was undertaken. The NCI, FDA, and Memorial Sloan-Kettering on their own changed the protocol in such a way that it was guaranteed for failure. The oversight committee of POMES would put an end to that. It would provide a body that's higher than either the NCI or OAM or the alternative researcher in that situation. It would have to approve the protocols. It would have to guarantee that there would be fair play."

As a precursor to full-scale testing, the OAM has also proposed "best-case reviews," much like what Lawrence Burton originally sought. When a therapy can demonstrate verifiable clusters of cures, it can serve as a qualifier for further evaluation. In fact, all that best-case review is intended to show is verified cancer and verified survival with acceptable quality of life. Ultimately, survival is the decisive measurement.

Called *outcomes research*, this approach skirts the thicket of deceptive statistical measures such as "tumor response rate" where the tumor shrinkage has no correlation with extended survival, to reach a simple conclusion: Did the patient have cancer and get better? That is, after all, the main issue. What is the outcome?

While alternative therapies are routinely discounted because they are scientifically unproved, amazingly, 85 percent of prescribed standard medical treatments lack scientific validation altogether, according to the *New York Times*.[11] Richard Smith, editor of the *British Medical Journal*, suggests that "this is partly because only one percent of the articles in medical journals are scientifically sound, and partly because many treatments have never been assessed at all."[12] Surgery and radiation, for example, were grandfathered in as standard treatments without double-blind, placebo-controlled, randomized clinical trials, for the most part.

A recent editorial in the *Archives of Internal Medicine* comparing conventional with unconventional medicine cites a startling 1986 assessment by the American College of Chest Physicians of cardiovascular disease therapies. The study found that only a quarter were actually proved effective by scientific evidence, whereas a 55 percent majority had insufficient data to support their use. Even after lowering the bar two years later, the college still gave 56 percent a failing grade.[13]

Clinical trials are often poorly supervised as well. As the *New York Times* reported in May 1998, "Federal investigators said today that patients who participated in clinical trials of new drugs were often exposed to unsafe and unethical practices because no one policed the research to protect their interests." The federal report noted that medical review boards were unable to oversee the overwhelming volume of tests properly.[14]

Scientific abuses abound. It is not uncommon for researchers to depart from the protocols approved by the review board, a breach that automatically should invalidate a study. Eli Lilly was found using homeless, often alcoholic men to test the safety of experimental drugs, a direct violation of the FDA's rules for voluntary, noncoercive drug evaluation subjects.[15] Doctors and drug companies have often recruited participants for research with misleading advertisements in buses and subways and on university campuses by offering free treatment or money.

Flawed testing may also do egregious harm. People over sixty-five, who comprise over half the number of U.S. cancer cases, do not tolerate toxic chemotherapy drugs as well as younger patients, and because few seniors are included in clinical trials, little is known about chemotherapy's actual effect on the elderly.[16]

The underlying function of these tests is economic: to approve patentable drugs and devices. Such commercial pressure can result in shoddy protocols and double standards, as demonstrated by the testing of chemotherapy drugs against one another rather than against a control group not receiving the actual drugs. The "proof" from such clinical trials simply does not meet formal scientific standards.

Fraud and abuse are widespread in the medical research industry, according to a two-part *New York Times* investigative series in early 1999. "In the early 1990s, the economics of drug development changed. Managed care put the squeeze on drug prices, leaving companies one option: increase the number of drugs they were selling. As a result, the companies began a rush to drug development." Because clinical trials are the sine qua non to bring new drugs to market, these companies "opened the financial floodgates" by putting a bounty on the heads of test subjects and giving physicians juicy financial incentives to bring them in the door. Even doctors without research credentials or experience can net from $500,000 to $1 million by headhunting for subjects. The consequence during the 1990s, according to the *Times* investigation, has been that 70 percent of doctors conducting experiments have been involved in three or fewer studies, "a number unlikely to give them mastery over the process." A quarter of all doctors who did human experiments in 1997 conducted only one experiment. "The push to finish trials quickly and move the drugs onto the market has overshadowed every other goal," the *Times* concluded.[17]

As a result of these sorts of scandals and other abuses, federal health investigators have begun two inquiries to determine whether the swiftly changing system of clinical trials adequately protects the interests of patients and test subjects, particularly in research funded by industry. The focus will be on recruitment procedures and oversight by clinical investigators.[18]

For cancer especially, there is often intense pressure from both doctors and patients to use therapies before they have been sufficiently tested. One particularly poignant instance has been the broad use against advanced breast cancer of high-dose chemotherapy followed by bone-marrow transplantation. This harrowing procedure is unspeakably painful and can be life-threatening. After doctors began offering the treatment only as a last resort in the late 1980s, the federal government mandated insurance companies to pay for it despite a lack of studies with control groups. Then four major studies appeared in 1999 concluding that the procedure does not prolong survival overall, but a commercial pipeline was already in place.[19] As the *New York Times* reported, "So now oncologists and companies will press ahead, continuing to sell a painful, expensive procedure that the best available science says is no improvement over standard care, which is less traumatic."[20]

Even those pharmaceutical drugs that undergo ostensibly credible academic research are increasingly suspect because universities are so closely tied to corporate "gifts" that come not with strings but with ropes. According to a 1998 article in the *New York Times*, "In an anonymous survey, more than half of the university scientists who received gifts from drug or biotechnology companies admitted that the donors expected to exert influence over their work, including review of academic papers before publication and patent rights for commercial discoveries."[21] The study, jointly conducted by researchers from Harvard and the University of Minnesota and published in the AMA *Journal*, said that many of the scientists had received valuable corporate gifts that were very important to their work, a factor that could easily influence their impartiality.[22]

In 1997 U.S. companies shelled out a whopping $1.7 billion on university-based science and engineering research, a fivefold jump from 1977. For academic scientists and institutions, the money represents critical revenues and sometimes a stake in patented discoveries. Yet often authors of published studies fail to report their financial ties. A review of 210 journals that have a formal disclosure requirement showed that 142 did not publish a single disclosure in all of 1997. A survey of the problem published in the *New England Journal of Medicine* found that while only 3 percent of the authors of one prominent study declared relevant financial ties to their subject, 96 percent should have.[23]

Another analysis showed that when chemical companies paid for studies, about three quarters of the results were favorable to their products, whereas only one quarter were favorable when independent researchers conducted comparable tests. A recent *JAMA* article and editorial openly admitted that reports of research on drugs tend to exaggerate the benefits and can harm patients. Similarly, among published studies of new drug treatments, 98 percent of those with drug-industry funding were positive, compared against 79 percent without industry support.[24]

Such a case occurred when the Monsanto corporation gave large research grants to the University of Florida. The ensuing positive research data led to FDA approval for the company's controversial bovine growth hormone (to increase a cow's milk production). However, the studies failed to acknowledge farmers' disturbing reports of adverse reactions, which the company later admitted. Two investigative reporters followed the trail, documenting how Monsanto spent millions in grants to the University of Florida, whose studies led to the drug's approval. They then detailed a revolving door between Monsanto executives and the FDA. The reporters went on to interview two Canadian regulators who charged Monsanto with offering them a $1 to $2 million bribe for approving the drug without further testing. Fox Television news killed the story after the station received aggressive threat letters from Monsanto attorneys. When the reporters were then fired, they pointed out that Monsanto was a client of a major advertising company owned by Fox chief Rupert Murdoch, whose stations advertise Monsanto products nationally.[25]

Whatever the obstacles may be, alternative cancer treatments are here to stay, and leading mainstream medical institutions are beginning to acknowledge them through research. When I visited Mary Ann Richardson in Houston, I drove from the airport to meet her at the School of Public Health at the University of Texas. The university is adjacent to M. D.

Anderson medical center, which covers an entire city neighborhood and services about 13,000 cancer patients a year. (In its 1950s heyday, the Dallas Hoxsey Clinic was treating 12,000 patients.)

At Richardson's request, epidemiologist Nancy Russell took me upstairs to see the Learning Center on the cancer ward. The center was created in 1997 as a resource for cancer patients seeking information about alternative therapies. The windowless room was stacked high with bookshelves offering literature ranging from nutrition to attitudinal healing. Prominent on the shelves were works by Dr. Bernie Siegel and Dr. Andrew Weil. Several computers were available to dial into cancer databases and the Web. Patients and their families pored over books and surfed the Net. The center now gets a whopping 1,000 people a month seeking information on alternatives.[26] Nestled in the heart of a leading cancer institution, the Learning Center represents an implicit admission that alternative cancer treatment is part of the new medical architecture.

Now that funding is available, alternative medicine is increasingly defining a leading edge of research. Both M. D. Anderson and Memorial Sloan-Kettering Cancer Center have been testing green tea, or more accurately several of its "active" ingredients, for anticancer properties.[27] Because various studies have shown that green tea reduces the risk of colorectal, lung, esophageal, and pancreatic cancers, the Lipton tea company is also testing the substance at the University of Arizona.[28]

In association with the NCI, M. D. Anderson is set to evaluate shark cartilage, which is reputed to have anticancer activity and is widely used by a cancer underground in the United States and abroad.[29] (Sadly, this market surge is further endangering several shark species.) Through an OAM grant, the University of Toronto is testing mistletoe, a folk remedy for cancer espoused by the Austrian spiritual philosopher Rudolf Steiner, originator of Waldorf education and biodynamic farming. Mistletoe has already shown antitumor effects in both people and animals in studies in Germany.[30] And after being fully acquitted on thirty-four counts of mail and insurance fraud in 1997, Dr. Burzynski launched seventy clinical trials of antineoplastons with human subjects with brain cancer, tests whose early results are very promising.[31]

"There are some doctors who are never going to accept this," Mary Ann Richardson told me, "and then there are some who are very open and willing to evaluate alternative treatments. Their patients are using them. They know we need to provide information to the patient. There is cross-pollination and an interest to find out what works and integrate it, and find out what doesn't work and get rid of it. I think we have a real opportunity right now. We need to do it right and show that we're serious."

Adding to the commotion is the entry of major corporations into the alternative marketplace. Procter & Gamble is now sponsoring the research of Dr. Nicholas Gonzalez in New York City under the auspices of Columbia University's College of Physicians and Surgeons and a $1.4 million grant from the NCI. Dr. Gonzalez took up the work of Donald Kelley, the dentist who reputedly cured himself of terminal cancer using pancreatic enzymes and other nutritional means. Dr. Gonzalez has undertaken stringent research with the therapy, which purports to cure otherwise incurable pancreatic cancer. A preliminary study found that the subjects lived an average of triple the usual survival rate for inoperable pancreatic cancer.[32] Of eleven patients, two are alive and well with no detectable disease, one for 3.5 years and the other for 4.5 years. The engagement of Procter & Gamble, a Fortune 500 company, vaulted the formerly reviled treatment to instant plausibility.[33] When large corporations begin to take a stake in alternative cancer therapies, it signifies the maturation of a market and consecrates a political realignment.

How will this change play out? Hildenbrand envisions an optimistic medical future. "I see it happening incrementally over time in such a way that it's unstoppable. The focus of research shifts, and it will be driven by outcomes. It will be one of the most enthusiastic periods of scientific growth that NIH has ever experienced, when all bets are off and the job will be to find the truth. Not to find a circumscribed, relative lower-case 't' truth, but to find the big 'T' truth. That's what science needs. I remember [Nobel Prize–winning scientist] Albert Szent-Györgyi said, 'When you go hunting, you never know where the bird's going to fly up, so you've got to be prepared to turn in any direction.' Scientific research is like that. You stumble over things. You don't discover them because you intend to. You stumble over them and you have to be prepared to shift.

"Many of these treatments will pan out. The silver bullet hasn't been suppressed, but it hasn't been invented by the suppressor either. The trick will be—like the chimpanzee in the cage given segments of an extendable stick—to reach through the bars and get the piece of fruit. The trick is to learn how to put those segments together so we can reach beyond our cage. I could be wrong. Someone could come along with 'the cure' tomorrow, but, so far, I haven't seen it."

The signals of the shift to embrace alternative therapies are unmistakable. In 1997 the American Cancer Society discontinued publication of its "Unproven Methods" blacklist of alternative cancer therapies. In early 1998 the National Cancer Institute dropped its comparable Cancer Information Service statements defamatory to unconventional cancer treatments. These developments belie intense public and political pressure.

Both institutions are refashioning their public information outlets in collaboration with members of the alternative medical community, including former adversaries such as Ralph Moss, who was appointed to an influential NCI panel that provides information for the Physicians Data Query service.[34] Moss, who has authored a consumer's guidebook to nontoxic cancer treatments and maintains a Web site, expects such information may now be integrated into these official databases, which reach hundreds of thousands of doctors and cancer patients.[35]

In late 1998 the Office of Alternative Medicine was elevated to the status of a National "Center" for Complementary and Alternative Medicine (NCCAM) within the NIH. Its budget almost tripled to $68 million, with over $10 million allocated for actual alternative cancer research.[36] The National Cancer Institute quickly funded a Division of Complementary and Alternative Medicine with advisers including Ralph Moss. The White House added its own Commission on Complementary and Alternative Policy to study and make policy recommendations to Congress.[37]

"It's interesting to contemplate the dilemma that the National Cancer Institute is in," Moss conjectures. "If they do decide to do the tests, then there's always that possibility—and I think it's a damn good possibility—that some of these treatments are going to turn out to be quite valuable. If they decide not to do the tests, there's going to be tremendous fury in Congress and the public, because what then are they about? If they're not about scientific testing, what good are they? Why are we wasting our money?

"I'm tremendously excited. The creation of OAM was one thing, but OAM has shown it cannot on its own solve these issues. It couldn't move forward without the NCI for political reasons. NCI demanded participation and then, when they got the participation, they froze in their tracks. They couldn't deal with it. Now they have to be nudged forward. What we're saying is: Prove them or disprove them. We've had seventy-five years of Hoxsey. Does it work? Doesn't it work? Nobody knows. How do you know? Short of good studies, how does one decide issues like that? We don't want people doing something if it's not going to work for them, not in terms of just conventional treatment, but alternative treatments as well.

"The best-case scenario is that some tests will be carried out with the imprimatur of NCI, NCCAM, and probably other collaborative centers like the University of Texas and Columbia. Some of those will show that there's no effectiveness, and some of them will probably show that there is effectiveness in some treatments. The ones that are shown to be effective that are funded by and based on NCI-reported research are then going to be published in major medical journals. The first one that validates a nontoxic treatment is the beginning of the end of this Middle Ages that we're in. Because once one goes through the door, then a lot of others are going through the door, and that's what they're afraid of. They're afraid that, if a Hoxsey were proven to be effective, the public will run to it because nobody wants the chemo drugs. If chemo is the only choice, then they'll reluctantly take it, but the minute it's known there is something nontoxic out there, everybody's going to want it.

"It's the first time we've ever really been in a situation where we can feel somewhat confident that the trials will be fair trials," Moss concludes. "We don't get a 100 percent guarantee, but I think a vigilant board would be able to detect fraud on either side, especially on the part of the establishment if it tried to squelch some positive findings. The proponents will either live with it or they won't. If they don't like the results, then they can still object, but I think the public will accept the results, whatever they are, if they're really from an impartial body. I don't see how we can lose."

Despite Moss's optimism, this "thorniest briarpatch in American medicine" is still a tangle even Br'er Rabbit might not want to be thrown into. Profound social issues continue to impede the research and acceptance of alternative cancer therapies. What is it really going to take to change the system?

21

Look Out, America! Here Come Alternative Cancer Therapies

When we released the *Hoxsey* film over a decade ago, the mention of alternative cancer therapies elicited arched eyebrows. The prospect that an herbal treatment might alleviate or cure cancer drew polite retreat or outright hostility.

Since that time, a grassroots health-care revolution has been ripening and today the blush is on the fruit. Alternative medicine, formerly a fringe niche, is going mainstream. The use of alternatives by vast numbers of people in the United States is visibly influencing markets and politics. The popular use of herbal remedies in particular is increasingly palatable to conventional medical practice. At last, the arch polarization in medicine seems to be diminishing, even the long-taboo realm of unconventional cancer treatments.

Yet altering deeply ingrained national policy is like turning a battleship in rough seas: It doesn't happen quickly or without getting drenched. Redirecting the medical course will be an extended voyage fraught with submerged snags. Nevertheless, there are several "policy cures" that would reduce both incidence and deaths at this critical turning point when cancer is poised to become the leading killer and the dominant specialty of American medicine.[1]

The public interest mandates treatments that are affordable or even cheap. Yet many alternative therapies such as Hoxsey, which are inexpensive or cannot be patented, essentially occupy the status of orphan drugs, medicines no one develops because they lack sufficient profits to attract corporate engagement. The total of $3,500 paid by Hoxsey patients barely covers the expense of a day in a conventional cancer ward, not even including drugs or radiation.

If such treatments prove effective, it is the government's role to sponsor their development in the public interest. Securing adequate funding from the National Cancer Institute to test alternatives is a paramount reform. Various analysts have proposed a congressional mandate to devote a third of the NCI budget annually to studying alternative cancer therapies. Given the prospective promise already exhibited by some of these treatments, the likelihood of major advances would appear higher than with current conventional therapies. If the resistance to the NCI toward alternatives proves intractable, the inauguration of a separate body within the NIH may be necessary for the task.

Major reforms are also required in the regulatory arena. Certain historical FDA tactics must be eliminated. While treatments are seeking investigation, they should not be subject to raids, seizures, import alerts, and policing actions. Nor should doctors face the revocation of their licenses by licensing boards for associating with "unproven" treatments under evaluation.

There need to be strong penalties against obstructing and sabotaging tests of alternative treatments. If scientific researchers were made liable for manipulating data, knowingly making false statements, and undermining experiments, they could face heavy fines and potential loss of their licenses or positions. Such scientific abuses could also prompt automatic "investigational use" status of the therapy, triggering a disincentive against hanky-panky.

Science writer Robert Houston has identified these and other key areas of reform in his insightful monograph *Repression and Reform in the Evaluation of Alternative Cancer Therapies:*

- Compel the government to pay court costs above a certain deductible to discourage politically motivated prosecutions.

- Relax proof of efficacy standards in proportion to the safety of the treatment and degree of failure treating the affliction by conventional methods.

- Apply "fast-track" and "compassionate care" standards.

- Compel insurance coverage where reasonable proof of efficacy exists.

But perhaps *curing* cancer is not even the fundamental issue. "Treatment is damage control," provocatively states Samuel Epstein, M.D., the author of 280 scientific articles and ten books, including the groundbreaking 1978 book *The Politics of Cancer,* which documented the link between industrial pollutants in the environment and rising cancer rates.

He estimates that *70 to 90 percent of cancers are caused by environmental and occupational exposure to carcinogens.*[2]

In precise, rapid-fire British diction, Dr. Epstein makes an irrefutable case for concentrating foremost on *cancer prevention*. "Losing the winnable war of prevention against cancer is a paradigm of failed healing. It reflects institutionalized failure to prevent cancer in spite of overwhelming documented evidence on its avoidable causes."[3]

Cancer prevention is by far the most cost-effective and humane approach to the disease. It is the proverbial elephant in the hospital room, yet the National Cancer Institute has explicitly excised prevention from its core focus on basic research, diagnosis, and treatment. NCI Director Dr. Richard Klausner objected to the suggestion of emphasizing cancer prevention as "a very unhelpful and false argument."[4] The NCI has consistenly prevented prevention.

Dr. Epstein has studied the area of cancer prevention for well over four decades, presently as a professor of occupational and environmental medicine at the School of Public Health at the University of Illinois Medical Center. "For the NCI," Dr. Epstein wrote, "cancer prevention means trying to change lifestyles without in any way seeking to reduce unknowing exposures to industrial carcinogens in air, water, food, the home, and the workplace."[5]

For his highly public and aggressive activism in this arena, Dr. Epstein landed on the 1980s White House "hit" list that targeted thirty prominent scientists to remove them from government advisory committees and boards. Such a hit list from the Environmental Protection Agency (EPA) said simply: "Get him out, horrible."[6] Conversely, in 1998 his work on cancer prevention was honored with his selection for the prestigious Right Livelihood Award, called the "alternative Nobel Prize."[7]

The NCI has allotted a seemingly impressive $255 million a year for prevention out of its $2.6 billion budget (soon to be $3.2 billion).[8] However, Dr. Epstein points out that the huge bulk has been directed at a "blame-the-victim" policy focused on reducing dietary fats and cigarette smoking.[9] While these factors do contribute to cancer incidence, they are overstated. Critics including Dr. Epstein say that the NCI's assessment that 35 percent of cancer is attributable to a high-fat diet is based on very shaky data. In fact, a fourteen-year Harvard study of nearly 89,000 women published in *JAMA* in 1999 found no evidence that a high-fat diet promotes breast cancer, or that a low-fat diet prevents it.[10] Of the 180,000 annual cases of breast cancer, which strikes one in eight women (the leading cause of death among women aged eighteen to fifty-four), up to 70 percent cannot be explained by these traditionally accepted risk factors.

Moreover, in almost all studies of smoking and lung cancer, the crucial variable of occupational exposure to carcinogens has been neglected. Why, for instance, has its incidence among nonsmokers more than doubled in recent decades?[11] Although smoking is a major health hazard and contributor to lung cancer, the narrow focus on tobacco is also an opportune smoke screen for masking other, more problematic causes of cancer: agricultural and industrial pollution. Many analysts consider these the principal factors in the mushrooming of U.S. cancer rates in this century, from one in twenty-seven people in 1900 to one of every two men and three women.

When Harry Hoxsey first began treating cancer in Illinois in the early twentieth century, the fearful disease was beginning its steady ascent against the emergent industrial backdrop of coal mines and smokestacks. That legacy has since ballooned. As a recent report in *Cancer Prevention News* stated, "There is overwhelming evidence that the dramatic increase in cancer rates is linked to increased chemical production over the last century. Annual production rates for synthetic, carcinogenic, and other industrial chemicals increased from one billion pounds in 1940 to more than 500 billion pounds annually during the 1980s. The evidence that chemicals cause cancer comes from animal and human tests."[12] Over 75,000 such chemicals are now in use, and the chemical industry introduces between 1,000 and 2,000 new ones each year. A scant 3 percent have been tested for safety, and over forty such industrial chemicals are recognized human carcinogens.[13]

The report found strong grounds for linking the spike in breast cancer rates with increased levels of pesticides and other industrial pollutants such as DDT, chlordane, and PCBs. Over fifty carcinogenic pesticides are used on major crops, and residues of just twenty-eight of these have been directly associated with over 20,000 cancer deaths every year in the United States.[14] Recent tests of twenty-seven kinds of domestically grown foods in the United States cited seven fruits and vegetables—apples, grapes, green beans, peaches, pears, spinach, and winter squash—as having toxicity at hundreds of times the other foods analyzed.[15] By age five, most children eat foods containing half a lifetime's limit of known carcinogens.[16] It is a formidable irony that the National Cancer Institute advises the public to eat five servings a day of fresh fruits and vegetables as a cancer-preventive diet, while failing to note the presence of carcinogenic agrochemicals contaminating them.

A recent study in England of more than 20,000 children showed an increased incidence of leukemia and other childhood cancers among those living near industrial sites. Cancer is now the most common form of fatal childhood disease where once it was a rarity.[17]

A compelling public health case study of cancer prevention comes from Israel. After research showed that three organochlorine pesticides found in milk and dairy products caused multiple forms of cancer in rats and mice, a public revolt convinced the Israeli government to ban the three poisons. In the following eight years, breast cancer mortality rates, which had been rising every year for twenty-five years, fell almost 8 percent for all age groups and more than a third for women aged twenty-five to thirty-four.[18] In response, the American Cancer Society issued a joint statement with the Chlorine Institute against the Israeli ban on these chemicals. As recently as 1998, the ACS failed to cite environmental factors in its influential "Cancer Risk Report: Prevention and Control."[19]

By 1948 the chief of the NCI's own Environmental Cancer Section, Dr. Wilhelm Hueper, had already documented strong connections between cancer and environmental and occupational exposure. The NCI's response was to command this expert on the carcinogenic effects of toxic dyes and radiation to cease his research on occupational cancer—on order from the surgeon general, no less.[20] Dr. Hueper, known as "the father of American occupational carcinogenesis," was the inspiration for the cancer chapter in Rachel Carson's *Silent Spring*, which first widely exposed the dangers of cancer-causing chemicals in the U.S. environment.[21] He did retain his post as founding director of the Environmental Cancer Section at the NCI until his retirment in 1964. On the day he left, the section was eliminated and the authoritative library he had collected was dispersed.

The NCI today attributes just 4 percent of cancer mortality to occupational exposure, and allocates only $50 million a year to study avoidable carcinogens in the environment and workplace. It has focused on the mechanisms of cancer rather than its causes, and deflected the issue of prevention by calling it the province of federal regulatory agencies.[22]

One solution is a mandatory NCI cancer prevention budget of meaningful proportions, coupled with objective studies of the relationships to cancer of environmental pollution and industrial toxins. Dr. Epstein has further spearheaded citizen "right-to-know" initiatives providing detailed analyses of carcinogenic substances permeating the environment and food supply, such as those documented in his book *Safe Shopper's Bible*, covering numerous brand-name products containing known carcinogens.[23] Representative Henry Waxman of California has proposed notifying consumers through their water bills about the carcinogens present in their tap water, as well as their concentrations.[24] Several municipalities including the City of San Francisco and Albany County in New York have adopted "sunset" laws to phase out the use of toxic chemicals in public buildings and grounds, parks, schools, and roadsides.[25]

Recent research has revealed that many standard pharmaceutical drugs cause cancer. Since 1994 new data on carcinogenicity testing published in the *Physician's Desk Reference* for only 241 fairly recent drugs have shown nearly half causing cancer in mice or rats. "It would appear," wrote Dr. Epstein, "that prescription drugs may pose the single most important class of unrecognized and avoidable cancer risks for the entire U.S. population." Over 2.4 billion prescriptions were written in the United States in 1997.[26]

Radical improvements in curtailing heart disease underscore the value of preventive medicine. "Death rates from cardiovascular diseases have plummeted by 60 percent since 1950," the *New York Times* reported in 1999.[27] While there were important advances in treatment for heart attack and stroke, the principal factors were preventive measures such as quitting smoking, better control of blood pressure, and decreases in cholesterol levels. "It was a familiar story to those who study public health," said the *Times*. "The great advances of the 19th century were also controlled by a collection of societal changes, like maintaining clean water supplies and quarantining the sick, resulting in declines in diseases like tuberculosis, cholera, and diphtheria before there were drugs to treat the illnesses or vaccines to prevent them." Meanwhile, the article paints the depressing contrast to the rise in cancer mortality rates between 1979 and 1997 from 179.6 to 201.6 deaths per 100,000.

"Cancer, in other words," wrote medical historian Robert Proctor, "is not a constant of the human condition but a product of the substances to which we are exposed at home or at work and the lifestyles we lead."[28] It is a disease of civilization, and as such can be greatly controlled with prevention. Much of its "cure" is political rather than medical.

The NCI's second and equally controversial approach to "cancer prevention" has been the use of "chemopreventive drugs." With great fanfare, the NCI in 1998 curtailed a clinical trial of the drug Tamoxifen because it considered the early results so positive: a 45 percent reduction in breast cancer among women taking the drug.[29] However, a second study in England published in the *Lancet* found no difference in breast cancer incidence in women treated with Tamoxifen versus a placebo.[30] Critics point out that the drug itself, a structural analog of DES (diethylstilbestrol), is a "rip-roaring carcinogen" that apparently caused uterine cancer in a significant percentage of the women, who were not informed prior to the trial of its potential harmful effects. These "side-effects" include coronary embolism, deep brain thrombosis, uterine cancer, and cataracts.[31] Further research has shown that Tamoxifen can actually stimulate the growth of cancer cells after two to five years of use.[32]

As Dr. Epstein has observed, there was a reduction in the incidence of invasive breast cancer of about 1.7 percent over the abbreviated study period, but the incidence of complications went up 2.2 percent. He characterizes the situation as "disease substitution rather than disease prevention." He further warns that the very short, aborted study period leaves many unanswered questions about longer-term negative effects.[33] Nevertheless, Tamoxifen was officially approved for breast cancer prevention in late 1998, and the manufacturer, British conglomerate Zeneca, announced its plan for an aggressive mass-marketing campaign directed at women.[34]

In a perverse spin on corporate vertical integration, Zeneca founded and helps fund National Breast Cancer Awareness Month. Formerly Imperial Chemical Industries, Zeneca reaps half its profits, about $500 million annually, marketing Taxomifen, now the world's best-selling cancer drug, and sells it through the eleven cancer treatment centers it owns. The company earns the other half of its profits from herbicides, fungicides, pesticides, plastics, and industrial chemicals, including $300 million a year from the sale of the carcinogenic herbicide acetochlor. Its Perry, Ohio, chemical plant is the third largest source of potential cancer-causing pollution in the United States, emitting 53,000 pounds of known carcinogens into the air in 1996.[35] However, Breast Cancer Awareness Month is focused solely on early detection through methods such as mammograms, conspicuously failing to mention environmental causes.[36]

Like Zeneca, many of the same giant chemical-pharmaceutical conglomerates that produce chemotherapy drugs also manufacture carcinogenic agricultural and industrial chemicals. As described earlier, their top executives populate the boards of Memorial Sloan-Kettering Cancer Center and other major cancer treatment hospitals, while moving back and forth from the private sector to the NCI and FDA in a revolving door between government and industry. The late industrialist Armand Hammer, whose companies are major producers of carcinogenic chemicals and include Hooker Chemical, which caused the infamous Love Canal disaster, himself chaired the elite President's Cancer Panel under Ronald Reagan.[37] Meanwhile, General Electric and Du Pont, the two top leaders in toxic Superfund sites in the United States, sell over $100 million annually of mammography machines and film for cancer "prevention."[38]

"Science has a face, a house and a price," wrote Robert Proctor. "It is important to ask who is doing science, in what institutional context, and at what cost. Understanding such things can give us insight into why scientific tools are sharp for certain kinds of problems and dull for others. It might also help us see why the war against cancer is going so badly."[39]

Proctor points to what *Time* magazine called "Hertz rent-a-scientists" whose real job is to produce uncertainty. It is the "triumph of what PR men call Gibson's Law: 'For every Ph.D. there's an equal and opposite Ph.D.'"[40] Armies of paid scientists produce doubt on behalf of the industries that will suffer if forceful public health measures are enacted toward cancer prevention.

Authentic preventive measures could detract from the profitability of these polluting industries and expose them to liability potentially on the scale of the tobacco industry. In fact, the United States is the world's biggest exporter of carcinogens, from tobacco to pesticides and pharmaceuticals.[41] Has this institutionalized conflict of interest biased the focus of public research away from fundamental prevention?

Environmental conditions also raise several serious problems for Hoxsey as a botanical product. The shadow side of the herbal boom today is that companies facing surging demand are turning to sources in China and Eastern Europe, where there is severe environmental pollution. Additionally, herbs imported into the United States are commonly fumigated with toxic chemicals according to FDA regulations. The presence of environmental or agricultural toxins in medicinal herbs compromises their safety and efficacy. Combined with inferior plant products flooding the market, the result could produce a backlash against these medicinal herbs.

Heavy demand for herbs is already placing strains on the environment. Many botanicals are wildcrafted (picked in their natural habitats), leading to the depopulation of numerous wild plants. Conservative estimates now suggest that one in eight plants is threatened with extinction worldwide, in the United States one in every three.[42] Among these is Hoxsey's prized bloodroot, one of at least nineteen popular herbs mainly occurring in the wild that are at serious risk today.[43]

While dedicated groups such as United Plant Savers are making an effort to bring attention to this crisis, a large-scale shift to cultivation is essential to prevent this spiraling loss of biodiversity. Yet even today's largest U.S. medicinal herb farms are relatively small. If the Hoxsey tonic were medically validated tomorrow and made accessible to the U.S. public, the commercial availability of the herbs would be hopelessly insufficient to meet the demand. Increasing the supply of organic herbs grown without toxic agricultural chemicals is critical.

The supply of qualified practitioners is also a concern. Very few doctors are trained in herbal medicine. Fortunately, there is currently a surge in the numbers of both naturopathic and osteopathic physicians who have traditionally employed herbal medicines extensively. Both professions are projected to occupy a substantial niche among doctors in the next ten years.

There are already three naturopathic medical colleges (and a fourth in development) that can barely meet the demand of applicants. Five states in the last five years have passed new licensing laws relegitimizing the practice of naturopathy after its earlier demise at the hand of Dr. Fishbein's AMA.[44] In the past thirty years, osteopathic schools have swelled from five to nineteen, netting 45,000 practicing osteopaths by the year 2000.[45] This trend may help fill the need for qualified doctors knowledgeable about herbal and alternative practices. Both Jim Duke and Mark Blumenthal point out that their audiences for herbal education are increasingly pharmacists, physicians, and medical students and their professors.[46]

Health and environment are ultimately inseparable. Cancer is a public health issue much like tuberculosis at the beginning of the twentieth century, a situation that was corrected less by medical advances than by public health measures. Because cancer is now seen as a cumulative lifestyle disease, "treating" it must begin with societal prevention as well as supporting people to improve their personal lifestyle choices.

Another serious policy concern is the trustworthiness of official cancer statistics, which seem to emanate more from spin doctors than medical ones. In 1998 the NCI presented optimistic data showing a 3 percent drop in cancer incidence since 1991, heralded as the first decline since the 1930s.[47] Critics charge, however, that the supposed improvements are statistically questionable. In fact, many forms of cancer are disturbingly on the rise, including cancer of the uterus, breast, prostate, and brain, as well as melanoma. Liver cancer has grown by 71 percent since the 1970s. Testicular cancers among men from age twenty-eight to thirty-five have skyrocketed by 300 percent since 1950, and breast and prostate cancer by 60 percent. Childhood cancers have risen 40 percent in the past twenty years.[48] As Dr. Epstein has pointed out, the overall cancer incidence has jumped by 60 percent between 1950 and 1998.[49] In this light, the NCI's statistics appear colorized.

Although the U.S. cancer death rate increased over 10 percent between 1950 and 1991, the NCI also announced encouraging cancer data in 1998, citing a 3 percent reduction in deaths since 1990. The NCI claimed the alleged drop occurred from improved treatment, but credible analysts including Dr. John Bailar and Dr. Epstein charge that, once statistical manipulations are stripped away, the number is only about 1 percent. Much of even this seeming improvement is likely attributable to earlier diagnosis and the large numbers of white men quitting smoking.[50] Dr. Bailar says flatly that cancer is "hardly more curable now than thirty years ago." He points out that cancer deaths are still 6 percent higher today than in 1970, just before the $30 billion "War on Cancer" began.[51]

A recent study reported in the AMA *Journal* called official cancer death rates even more sharply into question. After matching autopsies against cancer diagnoses as the cause of death, the study found a whopping 44 percent discrepancy, corroborating similar studies done in earlier decades. In other words, doctors failed to diagnose or detect cancer in very large numbers of deaths. Autopsy rates today are only about 5 percent in many community hospitals, compared against 50 percent in the 1960s.[52] What this means is that cancer death rates are being underreported, perhaps by large margins. "Thus, a recent decline in autopsy rates could be adversely affecting the quality of health care," reported the *New York Times*.

Many public health officials are calling for greater accountability in the National Cancer Institute's own claims. In 1994 a group of sixty-five public health scientists led by Dr. Epstein and two past directors of federal agencies spoke out at a press conference at the National Press Club in Washington. "The NCI should be enjoined from making or endorsing claims for cancer cures unless these are clearly validated on reduced mortality rates and unless they conform to standard regulations on claims of therapeutic efficacy."[53] These experts are demanding the NCI be held accountable if it is found doctoring statistics.

But behind these chilling numbers are the fragile lives of real people facing cancer. The most divisive medical policy issue entangling Hoxsey and alternative therapies is a concern raised first by cancer patients: their medical civil rights. Facing a life-threatening illness for which conventional medicine often has little or nothing to offer, patients are angry at the severe restrictions blocking their access to other options.

Legislation before Congress called the Access to Medical Treatments Act (S-1035) would guarantee medical civil rights by authorizing doctor and patient to decide jointly and without constraint what is best for the patient, based on informed consent. Drafted by Berkley Bedell, it has support from forty congressional sponsors. The bill's passage would cut through the knot of regulatory and research obstacles to give patients access to potentially helpful (and generally harmless) therapies.

In the film, we put this controversial question of freedom of medical choice to FDA spokesman William Grigg. "There really is no lack of freedom of choice in telling people that they can't lie, they can't advertise falsely, that it's against the law to sell you the Brooklyn Bridge. It may limit your freedom to buy the Brooklyn Bridge and pay a lot of money, but it doesn't limit your freedom in any real way."

"The only people that object to it is the competitor," Hoxsey's lawyer Jimmy Martin countered philosophically. "You know, the medical association is a competitor. If somebody who's sick wants to take some medicine, why not let him take it? It was established that it couldn't hurt. All the doctors ever contended was that it wouldn't cure anything, and it didn't hurt. The doctors said, 'We don't know what to do, we can't cure cancer; it's incurable.' But still they didn't want Hoxsey to be telling these patients, and giving them some medicine.

"Sometimes," Martin mused, "I would think, 'Well, maybe there's something to it [Hoxsey].' And then I'd think, 'These doctors, they ought to know more about it than me.' But I've always wondered, if I had developed cancer and some doctor told me that I'd better get my affairs straightened out—that I couldn't live long—I believe I'd have done like them. I'd have been grabbing at straws and I'd go see Hoxsey—see if he couldn't do something for me."

The reality is that growing numbers of cancer patients, possibly as many as two thirds, are choosing alternative therapies regardless of the obstacles.[54] These issues can sound rather depersonalized until they are connected to the human faces of cancer patients fighting for their lives. Here is a sampling of how Hoxsey patients feel about their medical civil rights.[55]

Mrs. Margaret Griffin, the seventy-nine-year-old Pennsylvania survivor of lymphosarcoma who went underground to obtain Hoxsey in Dallas after being given up to die over thirty years ago, had this to say. "I think we should have freedom of information and freedom of choice. It should be made available to the public, and then let them choose what route they're going to take. We're all adults in charge of our own destiny, and we should be allowed to go whatever route we think would be best for us. Of course I'm angry. I can't even put it into words. I keep writing letters trying to contact people. They should burn in hell for what they're doing to the people of the world. I think really we need anarchy in the streets. Then maybe we'll get something done."

Stephen Crutcher, who avoided surgery to remove most of his jaw, palate, teeth, and gums and went instead to the Bio Medical Center in Tijuana, spoke more gently. "I don't think Hoxsey is a miracle cure and it's probably not going to work for everybody. But I think everybody should at least have the opportunity to be aware of it and know that it's there and given the opportunity to try it. Or talk to people and have the information available so that they can look at different ways instead of just surgery and radiation and chemotherapy. If it worked for one person, then it warrants looking into, because it could probably work for others. I think it's something that should be available here. You shouldn't have to go out of the country. We're supposed to have the best medical systems in the world. This is kind of ironic."

Gwen Scott, the New Zealand breast cancer survivor given up on by her doctors, is unshakable about her medical civil liberties. "I actually do have that right. Whether it's the law, whether it's illegal or not, is unimportant. I go by more universal law than man's law. I do have a right as a patient, and if other people don't think I have, well, it's their problem, not mine."

Scott confronted her doctors about their own attitudes toward her medical freedom. "I said [to my oncologist], 'But you told me that you supported me.' He said yes. And I said, 'But you don't approve.' And he said, no, he didn't approve. I said, 'That's okay. I can live with that.' I can have his support. It doesn't matter whether he approves or not. It really is none of his business. So we get on fine.

"My general practitioner didn't seem to have a great respect for anybody that didn't think the same way as he did. He did say to me that I had no right to experiment with my body. When anybody says something like that to me, it's a bit like red to a bull. I just thought that, God, they've been experimenting with it enough and it was my turn now. It was my body, after all. I told him that, and refused to leave his office until he wished me a Merry Christmas and shook my hand. Now I have another GP here."

A year after we interviewed Florence Gibson, the African-American breast cancer Hoxsey patient whose optimism and inner resolution gave her all the hallmarks of a survivor, we were stunned and saddened to learn that she succumbed to the disease. We asked her husband, Frank, if he would be willing to share on camera his feelings about her death. He agreed. We traveled to his home with trepidation, having no idea how he would react to the tragic loss of his childhood sweetheart while using Hoxsey.

Surrounded by heart-shaped photographs of their marriage, Frank Gibson seemed composed and spoke with the same gentleness we had felt in happier times in Mexico. "It was kind of like a little outing for she and I, because we were together. We'd go down to San Diego, and we'd go to the movies. We went to the movies more in the last year of her life than we did the previous thirty years. Every time we went to San Diego, we'd go downtown and go to a movie just like we did many years ago.

"Initially, the quality of life was actually enhanced because we were just the two of us together, and it was kind of neat in that respect. I've only known one or two people that underwent traditional treatment. From what they said—the discomfort, nausea and stuff that they had—there's no comparison. As far as the discomfort we had, the only discomfort we had, as far as this treatment goes, was going five hundred miles to get it.

"In November of 1984, the year that I lost her, the doctor wrote down 'terminal.' Until then I never even thought of it as terminal anything. She made it plain to me that she did not want to try anything else, that she was content to stay with the treatment she was receiving. She maintained that attitude up to the very end, that we had done the right thing."

Finally the rush of remembrance released Frank's heartbreak. Struggling to hold back tears, he swallowed hard to push his words out. "I couldn't say this doesn't work, and obviously I couldn't say this does work. This is what we chose, and we felt good about it. It's unfortunate it didn't work the way we wanted it to, but as she said, 'I could have been dead already if I'd gone the other route.' Those were her words. I think we're all right now, just content that she did what she wanted to and thought was best. I think that's the consolation that I have, that I helped her to accomplish the ends to do what she wanted to do."

"I hate to see people go for alternative therapies," the skeptical but tolerant Dr. Bernie Siegel told us, "when they have a very good chance of being cured at that moment in a conventional way. I know that they're increasing their risk, and they may die pursuing something that doesn't work. But, I have to say, it is their life, not mine. I can state honestly what I think, and I say to a lot of people, 'I wouldn't do what you're doing.' They don't run out the door with that. They say, 'Okay, but this is my choice and this is what I want to do.' But if they have a strong conviction, then I will say, 'Okay, follow your conviction.' And I know that if it doesn't work, they'll be back saying, 'Let me try the other.' "[56]

The abiding truth for cancer patients is that they want unrestricted access to all treatments. According to Ralph Moss, only about 5 percent entirely abandon conventional cancer care even when pursuing an alternative.[57] What patients want is the best of all worlds, an expanded menu of options supported by access to credible information. The stereotype that orthodoxy has long put forth of poor, credulous cancer patients ripe for exploitation by clever promoters is false. In a study by sociologist Barrie Cassileth, the profile of patients using alternative cancer therapies describes well-educated, middle-income, often female clients who have done a considerable amount of research to make their choice.[58]

A collaborative medical model is emerging today that cobbles together an eclectic mixture of varying treatments for appropriate conditions, respecting the patient's orientation, quality of life, and desires. Conventional cancer centers now often incorporate dietary and nutritional programs, attitudinal healing and counseling, and even herbal medicines. There are many caring doctors who would be more responsive to their patients' wishes if they did not fear for their professional standing, and if sound information were available to help support those choices.

Gar Hildenbrand, who deals on a daily basis with desperate, frightened cancer patients caught in the medical crossfire, suggests a tempered activism. "I would say in the short run that patients should do what they want to do instead of what they're told to do. We have to have the locus of control back in the individual, and that's going to take some deprogramming. We're fortunately no longer subjected to *Dr. Kildare, Ben Casey*, and *Marcus Welby* on TV, but that did a lot of damage. This was a time when Hollywood would have the physician slap the patient, and the patient would say, 'Thank you, doctor, I needed that.'

"What has given birth to the alternative medicine movement on Capitol Hill is the defiance of the American people. People are just saying, 'I'm not going to do that,' and they go elsewhere. What we have in place is a desperately clinging monopoly, but what in reality is going to happen is the empowerment of competition and the restoration of pluralism in medicine, and it's people-driven. Use the representative republic and the democratic structure of the country. Handwritten notes to representatives and senators are never thrown away."[59]

The Hildebrands now work with former congressman Berkley Bedell, who formed the National Foundation for Alternative Medicine, a private nonprofit group to conduct independent testing of alternative therapies worldwide. "What science wants and what people want in terms of trials are completely different," the activist ex-legislator states. For example, Bedell objects to the stipulation that patients must first undergo conventional cancer treatments as part of a protocol. Meanwhile, he strongly continues to lobby for passage of the Access to Medical Treatments Act.[60]

The underlying demographic truth Bedell is addressing is that masses of patients are flocking to alternative medical treatments, and organized medicine is compelled to respond. As the AMA *Journal* reported in 1998, almost two thirds of the nation's 125 regular U.S. medical schools now teach elective courses on alternative therapies, a number that bounced to seventy-five from forty-six just two years earlier.[61] The AMA *Journal* decided to publish an entire issue on alternative medicine in 1998 after discovering that the subject was the seventh-ranked item of interest to its readers (although its own editors had rated it sixty-eighth out of seventy-three categories).[62] To most people's surprise, the special issue presented four positive studies out of six on alternative practices, including two relating to herbs showing efficacy.[63]

Dr. Fishbein could hardly have imagined this "plant and vegetable debris" washing up on the pages of his cherished *Journal*. Clearly alternative medicine is here to stay, but how will the system incorporate it?

"Pay Your Money and Take Your Choice": The Corporatization of Alternative Medicine

In just a hundred years Dr. Fishbein's medical-industrial complex has developed into a kind of medical-corporate state, a highly concentrated set of interlocking interests geared to the bottom line. The same motivation of profit that has generally hindered the acceptance of alternative therapies is now paradoxically propelling their adoption. This economic matrix will fundamentally determine how unconventional cancer treatments such as Hoxsey will or won't be absorbed into mainstream medical practice.

"Alternative medicine is clearly the largest growth industry in health care today," wrote Jane Brody in the *New York Times* in 1998.[1] When Dr. David Eisenberg of Harvard updated his 1990 survey, he found an estimated 42 percent of the American public using alternative therapies in 1997. The number of visits to alternative practitioners jumped by nearly 50 percent and exceeded total visits to primary-care physicians. Spending was conservatively estimated at $21.2 billion, with at least $12.2 billion paid out-of-pocket by eager customers. Total out-of-pocket expenditures for alternative therapies was comparable with 1997 expenditures for all physician services.[2]

Cresting the wave is herbal medicine. When *Time* magazine published a 1998 cover story on "The Herbal Medicine Boom," the report was tellingly positioned as a business story. An estimated sixty million Americans are now using medicinal herbs in a market exceeding $4 billion, characterized by an annual 35 to 40 percent growth rate.[3] The aggregate stock value of publicly held herb companies went up 44 percent in 1997, the highest of any category except top-performing high-technology stocks.

Herbal growth rates are rising fastest in mass-market outlets such as Target, Kmart, and goliath Wal-Mart, which now produces its own herbal line. Taking a stake are many large drug companies including Bayer, Warner-Lambert, and American Home Products.[4] Seizing the global edge are several multinational drug giants such as Novartis, BASF, and Bayer, which are already experienced at selling medicinal herbs in Europe and Latin America.[5]

Accelerating the renaissance of herbal medicine is the steady validation of certain herbs for serious medical conditions. Ginkgo, reputedly the oldest tree in the world, has been found effective against Alzheimer's disease in studies in Germany. Even a more reserved study published in 1997 in the AMA *Journal* showed its effectiveness in limiting symptoms associated with Alzheimer's. The National Center for Complementary and Alternative Medicine is now preparing to launch a $15 million study of its effects on dementia.[6]

St. John's wort has made headlines for its efficacy against depression. A meta-analysis of twenty-three German studies found the herb more effective than synthetic antidepressant drugs such as Prozac and Zoloft for cases of mild depression.[7] German physicians now prescribe St. John's wort at least seven to one over these synthetic drugs. U.S. sales netted about $400 million in 1997, though still a distant second to Eli Lilly's Prozac sales of $2.5 billion in 1996.[8] The NIH has now started research on this plant.[9]

Black cohosh, studied in clinical trials in Germany for over forty years, has shown effectiveness for menopausal and premenstrual symptoms.[10] The herb was an old standard of the Eclectics, who used it for female reproductive complaints.[11] It was also the principal ingredient in the famous Lydia Pinkham vegetable compound, the classic women's patent medicine earlier in the twentieth century. (The compound's 20 percent alcohol content may have also provided attitudinal healing of sorts.)

Germany leads the developed countries in its acceptance of herbal medicine. The German equivalent of the FDA has systematically compiled over 380 monographs on individual herbs, detailing both their safety and efficacy. Its Commission E collated all the herbal folklore as well as scientific studies into a reliable database. The monographs were published in the *German Federal Register*, intended as package inserts to permit physicians, pharmacists, and customers to have access to credible information. An estimated 70 percent of German doctors prescribe herbs, and their prescriptions now account for over half the country's $3 billion annual herb sales.[12] Fully 1,400 preparations of the 8,250 in a recent edition of the German pharmacopeia, the *Rote Liste*, are of herbal origins.[13]

"Germany is not some backwater," comments Mark Blumenthal, whose American Botanical Council published the groundbreaking Commission E monographs in the United States. "This is an industrialized nation that for sixteen years spent time and expertise reviewing the safety and appropriate use of herbs as drugs and medicines. It is the most rational system in the entire world for how to evaluate herbs as medicines for their safety and efficacy. It's a model we can use in the U.S."[14] Dr. Varro Tyler, Distinguished Professor of Pharmacognosy Emeritus at Purdue University, has called the system "rational herbalism."

Yet the very success of alternative medicine yields a new array of pressures and problems entering the medical marketplace at a moment of radical restructuring. The inevitable logic of the powerful political and economic forces set in motion a century ago is coming home to roost in unprecedented corporatization at the same time that medicine is undergoing profound therapeutic changes.

The AMA continues to play a complicated and shifting role in this transformation. Where once Dr. Fishbein successfully represented the AMA as a benevolent guardian of the public health, the perception is widespread today that it is first and foremost a trade association, a doctors' union whose top order of business is its members' financial and professional well-being.

Although today's AMA is in many ways an organization in crisis, its power should not be underestimated. It remains one of the largest and most powerful national political forces, the proverbial "eight-hundred-pound gorilla on Capitol Hill."[15] Its annual $180 million budget makes it the second biggest of the 4,000 lobbies in Washington.[16] The AMA's core mission of preserving the power, privilege, and financial prosperity of doctors has established it as an organization "notorious for confrontation, ultimatums, and hardball politics".[17] Its political action committee, AMPAC, has given over $100 million over the last twenty years to 83 percent of federal congressional representatives and senators. The AMA actually owns the very building in the nation's capital that the government leases for its federal political action committee monitoring program.[18]

In 1997 the *Journal* attracted $21.4 million in advertising revenues, the great majority from drug companies, as has been the case for a century.[19] Drug ads still comprise a whopping 20 percent of the AMA's total operating revenues, a situation that consumer advocate Dr. Sidney Wolfe has called "massive prostitution."[20] While the *Journal* promises a "fire wall" between advertisers and editorial content, the great majority of drug company–sponsored scientific studies it publishes is positive, omitting the large numbers that are negative or inconclusive. The *Journal*, after all, solicits advertisers to pay top dollar for its pages, whose 750,000 circulation still commands the greatest market share of doctors (including fifteen international editions in 150 countries). The lure of advertising profits continues to compete with the impartiality of "scientific medicine."[21]

The AMA medical publicity machine Dr. Fishbein founded is running in perpetual overdrive today. The "*JAMA* Report," a video news release, goes out weekly on satellite to every TV network and local station in the United States, reaching between 25 and 110 million viewers. Most major newspapers routinely scan *JAMA* for breaking stories, as do wire services and radio. The AMA also floods about 2,500 press outlets worldwide with weekly e-mails and faxes.[22]

The credibility of the AMA's vaunted Code of Ethics, which ostensibly puts the profession of healing above business, is in tatters today. In 1998 the AMA once again was mired in negative publicity as the Seal of Acceptance experienced its latest devaluation. After the AMA granted the Sunbeam corporation an exclusive product endorsement for the manufacturer's medical devices without even testing them, the medical association was set to receive millions of dollars in licensing fees, which it planned to use to offset declining membership dues. Outrage from the medical community and other competing companies crashed the nakedly commercial transaction. The mass media roasted the AMA's signature cupidity.[23]

Member dues, the leading source of AMA income, show a precipitous drop to between 25 and 38 percent of doctors. This plummeting proportion is comparable to where the organization stood shortly after the turn of the last century, when Dr. Simmons launched the massive drive that made nonmembership professional suicide.[24]

Ironically, the AMA's century-long political-economic prowess on behalf of its members has borne the seeds of its own decline. The fact that doctors have flourished as the country's richest profession has contributed greatly to the impoverishment of the nation's health-care system, whose costs are hurtling past the $1 trillion mark toward fiscal insolvency.[25] The AMA overachieved in its quest for a doctor-centered, fee-for-service system. As a result, the white coat is being displaced by the suits of corporate medicine, and Dr. Fishbein's AMA is history.

The AMA's failure to deliver affordable, effective health care to a large plurality of Americans opened the gate wide for privatization. As Paul Starr presciently wrote in the Pulitzer-winning book *The Social Transformation of*

American Medicine in 1982, "The failure to rationalize medical services under public control meant that sooner or later they would be rationalized under private control. Instead of public regulation, there will be private regulation, and instead of public planning there will be corporate planning. Instead of public financing for prepaid plans that might be managed by the subscribers' chosen representatives, there will be corporate financing for private plans controlled by conglomerates whose interests will be determined by the rate of return on investments. That is the future toward which American medicine now seems to be heading."[26]

But it was not only national health insurance and competition from the empirics that Dr. Fishbein opposed so vehemently. The AMA also fought domination by corporations, and was remarkably effective at preventing corporate competition from offering health-care services for well over half the century. Laws enacted around 1900 forbade corporations to engage in the commercial practice of medicine. The justifications were that, unlike a doctor, a corporation could not be licensed to practice medicine, and that the commercialization of medicine conflicted with "sound public policy."[27]

Dr. Fishbein characterized the prospect of corporate medicine as "racketeering."[28] In truth, the AMA had a horror of corporations relegating doctors to the status of employees, diminishing them to just another labor input on a corporate balance sheet. The AMA was singularly adept at positioning itself as a protector of the public health by invoking the sanctity of the doctor-patient relationship while neatly inserting itself as gatekeeper to the medical marketplace.

Because of its unique professional sovereignty, the AMA remarkably managed to limit emerging corporate medical industries to outlying sectors such as the drug business and medical-supply companies. By the 1970s, however, as Starr wrote, "Enormous increases in cost seemed ever more certain; corresponding improvements in health ever more doubtful."[29] The consequences were heightened critical scrutiny and government intervention.

As annual national health care costs skyrocketed from $13 billion to $71 billion between 1950 and 1970, the critical condition of medical economics presented an irresistible target for commercial medicine.[30] Large corporate ventures seized the opportunity, promising efficient business management to control costs. The result was the adoption of Health Maintenance Organizations (HMOs).

"The organization culture of medicine," wrote Starr, "used to be dominated by the ideals of professionalism and voluntarism, which softened the underlying acquisitive activity. The restraint exercised by those ideals now grows weaker. The 'health center' of one era is the 'profit center' of the next."[31] Although the AMA initially opposed HMOs, it finally saw the prescriptive writing on the wall and had to accept corporate medicine. HMO plans today enroll over 60 percent of the population.[32]

In many ways, Dr. Fishbein's worst fears about the corporatization of medicine are being realized. In a 1995 article in *The Nation* titled "The Madness of the Market," Robert Sherrill wrote, "Forget the kindly doctor of *The Saturday Evening Post* covers. He's dead. The guy who carries the little black bag these days is the corporate executive, and the bag is full of production charts, not a stethoscope and pills."[33]

Managed care has proved to be a deeply flawed system both financially and socially. U.S. health care costs have reached the highest per capita of any developed nation in the world. At the same time, health-care quality has generally declined. While corporate profits have risen, the United States ranks seventeenth in male life expectancy and sixteenth in female life expectancy.[34] Over 16.1 percent of Americans—43.4 million people—do not have health insurance.[35] Managed care has become "managed cost."

In October 1998 more than four hundred doctors in Dallas terminated their contracts with Aetna Inc.'s HMO in the biggest rebellion to date against a health insurance company. The doctors were irate over their lack of prompt access to company records on patients' treatments, medications, and trips to the hospital. They were also frustrated by the company's very slow payment to doctors, as well as by mandatory contract terms that often dictate treatments but ascribe liability to the physician. Moreover, the doctors were revolting against being constrained from informing patients about other options not covered by the company.

Aetna struck back by stopping the doctors' access to all its Dallas patients.[36] In 1999, in retaliation against HMOs at large, the AMA called for the formation of a formal doctors' union.[37] Large managed-care companies are now backing down, allowing doctors greater discretion, but the situation is likely to remain a tense tug-of-war.[38]

Health care under managed care is not very safe, either. According to the *Journal*, over 100,000 Americans are killed each year by the pharmaceutical drugs they take in hospitals, making the appropriate use of pharmaceuticals just in hospitals the fourth leading cause of death in the United States (behind heart disease, cancer, and stroke). These deaths are generally not attributable to actual errors by doctors or patients, but rather to drugs' "side effects." There were an additional 2.2 million non-fatal adverse drug reactions, about 7 percent of hospital patients.

Some studies suggest that almost 40 percent of surgical operations in the United States are unnecessary. One medical researcher calculated the human costs: "More deaths are caused by surgery each year in the United States than the annual number of deaths during the wars in Korea and Vietnam."[39] In fact, wherever doctors' strikes have occurred, the death rate has dropped.[40]

Each year, hospitals essentially kill the equivalent number of people as three jumbo jets crashing every two days through missed diagnoses, medication use, and other preventable mistakes.[41] Medical mistakes produce about a quarter of the mortalities from heart attack, stroke, and pneumonia.[42] At a cost of $4.5 billion a year, some two million Americans annually get infections in hospitals, a rate that rose by 36 percent in 1995.[43] In 1999 the National Academy of Sciences asked Congress to create an agency just to monitor medical errors after finding that between 44,000 and 98,000 people die each year because of mistakes in hospitals alone, more than the death toll from highway accidents.[44]

Doctors and nurses alike are held to assembly-line production quotas, and nurses especially are being overworked because their low pay makes them more cost-effective than doctors for a managed-care bottom line. Federal investigators recently revealed that a study of hospital inspectors found them failing to detect substandard care or to identify incompetent doctors because the inspectors "strive to foster a collegial atmosphere."[45] Writing recently in the *New York Times*, Dr. Sandeep Jauhar characterized hospital-acquired complications as having reached "epidemic proportions."[46]

Despite the FDA's adoption of "fast-track" approval of new pharmaceuticals, the agency has produced scant additional funding to monitor drugs afterward. Adverse reactions often do not show up until drugs are widely used, yet the FDA allots only $140,000 annually for the Medwatch system, which is charged with monitoring reactions to all drugs sold in the United States. Until late 1997 Medwatch was not even computerized.[47] In 1999 federal investigators found flaws grave enough to recommend mandatory reporting by hospitals of all adverse drug reactions in which patients are injured.

Simultaneously, the drug industry has been booming. Over the past four years, the pharmaceutical sales force for the top forty companies has shot up from 35,000 to over 56,000. The industry spent $5.3 billion in the United States alone in 1998 sending "detail men" into doctors' offices and hospitals, and another $1 billion on marketing events for doctors. That translates into nearly one drug salesperson and almost $100,000 for every eleven practicing physicians in the United States, according to the *New York Times*. National spending for prescription drugs has more than doubled in the past decade to $78.9 billion, while drug costs have risen on average 17 percent a year in the last few years.[48] Drug companies are now permitted to market directly to consumers, a kind of doctor by-pass loosing a flood of promotions.

Economists project that the amount spent on drugs in the United States will nearly triple from $62.2 billion to $171.1 billion from 1996 to 2007.[49] Total global drug sales reached $251.3 billion in 1998, up 7 percent.[50] The *European Financial Times* estimates the number at $300 billion, and notes "operating margins of up to 35 percent for the most successful companies."[51] Overall drug company profits average over 16 percent, triple that of the average Fortune 500 company.[52]

Meanwhile the United States boasts the highest medication prices in the industrial world, an average wholesale price 32 percent higher than Canada's, the next most costly country.[53] As for the exorbitant costs of drug development, which the drug industry cites as the cause for such swollen prices, a feeble seventeen major new drugs were developed between 1987 and 1991, and twelve of those were paid for by government research subsidies.[54]

Moreover, in 1995 the National Institutes of Health under Director Harold Varmus (now executive director of Memorial Sloan-Kettering) struck from its contracts the "reasonable pricing" clauses, a protection against profiteering by pharmaceutical companies on drugs developed with public funding.[55] His rationale was that this limitation was discouraging private industry from drug development. The drug industry bemoaned the fact it spent a hefty $9 billion on drug development in 1995. To put matters in perspective, it spent $10.8 billion on sales and marketing, about 20 percent of its total budget and twice that of other consumer-products industries.[56] In addition, the pharmaceutical industry spent $74.8 million on political lobbying in the United States in 1997, the largest of any single lobby group.[57]

Just when drug company mergers and acquisitions have narrowed the band of players to about a dozen giant companies, a parallel trend is shrinking the number of managed-care corporations.[58] A mere six conglomerates now control nearly all medical insurance. (Medicine is not an isolated example of corporatization. Fifty of the world's hundred largest economies are corporations. The five hundred largest corporations control 25 percent of the entire world's output.)[59]

This consolidation has not led to the political promise of lower prices or increased competition. A recent federal report by the Health Care Financing Administration estimates that *health-care spending will double* from $1.035 trillion in 1996 (13.6 percent of the GNP) to a staggering $2.133 trillion in 2007 (16.6 percent of the GNP).[60] The United States pours almost twice as much of its GNP into health care as most Western

European countries, yet it doesn't produce a healthier population. Citizens in the Netherlands and Scandinavia live longer, and the majority of Europeans have better infant mortality rates.[61]

With poignant irony, Dr. Paul Ellwood, the social architect who first advocated HMOs, dramatically reversed his position in 1999. Speaking at Harvard, Dr. Ellwood criticized the "unacceptable" quality of American health care, and called for government intervention after all. Part of his turnaround occurred after receiving poor care following a life-threatening riding accident. "It doesn't make any difference how powerful you are or how much you know," he said. "Patients just get atrocious care and can do very little about it."[62]

This newly configured medical-corporate state renders the fate of alternative medicine doubly enigmatic. Alternative practices are generally much cheaper and should substantially reduce costs in a beleaguered system. A study done by Dr. Larry Kincheloe at an HMO in Oklahoma City found that his group could save between $500,000 and $750,000 a year by shifting to herbal medicines for conditions in which their efficacy is well documented.[63] The potential cost savings from alternative therapies are likely to emerge as a principal vector in their growing acceptance, yet they also threaten an entrenched and highly profitable set of vested interests.

Given burgeoning market demand for alternative treatments, large insurance companies including Kaiser Permanente and Oxford have added them to their mosaic, and most others are looking seriously at doing so. Surveys by the companies themselves have shown that one third of their clients are already using alternatives.[64] Because credible proof of efficacy remains the sine qua non for insurance coverage, the contest around the testing of alternative cancer and medical therapies has very high stakes for medical economics.

As these giant companies join the fray, the real crucible is the economic matrix onto which alternative treatments will be grafted. Just when the therapeutic civil war in medicine may be subsiding, corporate monopoly is ascendant in the trade war. At the *fin de siècle* of another Gilded Age, heroic doses of greed are quickening the vertical commodification of health care as it gropes to assimilate alternative medicine as a booming new profit center.

How alternative medicine will navigate this profit-driven corporate concentration is a puzzle. Treatments such as Hoxsey are often inexpensive, and could be offered cheaply. They do not glitter with the kinds of astronomical venture capital profits that enchant the drug and biotechnology markets. Patented high-end "herbaceuticals" are already emerging as a countertrend to cheaper, unpatentable whole plants.[65] Many patients also seek alternative medicine as much for caring as for curing, and there's not a big profit margin to be had in caring.

Billionaire financier and investor George Soros views health care as a vivid example of where the market simply does not work.[66] Making money off human suffering, Soros suggests, may be an inappropriate arena for pursuing Wall Street returns. In early 1999 in a speech at Columbia University's College of Physicians and Surgeons, the philanthropist pledged $15 million for a new program to de-emphasize profit in medical care. "Health-care companies are not in business to heal people or save lives," the capitalist commented. "They produce health care to make profits."[67]

Gar Hildenbrand concurs. "What we really need is a major allocation of taxpayer money from the NIH to be mandated for public-interest research that would not generally be funded by the pharmaceutical companies and drug developers. Otherwise, we're literally using taxpayer money to duplicate or expand their work and give gift horses back to industry. I don't think medicine really belongs in the marketplace because you lose science to the business agenda."[68]

Today's medical system is shooting the rapids into a new millennium, and futurists see several currents that they expect will sharply alter the course of U.S. health care over the next twenty years. Clement Bezold's Institute for Alternative Futures think tank prepared a revealing 1998 report on Complementary and Alternative Medicine.[69] (*Complementary* therapies are used as adjuncts to conventional treatments. *Alternative* therapies serve as actual substitutes.)

Bezold predicts radical changes on the medical horizon:

- Health care will be increasingly driven by outcomes. Practitioners will become "outcomes generators," and their performance will be tightly tied to producing positive results. Consumers will judge treatments by their outcomes. Outcomes measures will reinforce better functional results, long-term efficacy, minimal side effects, and cost effectiveness.

- Because patients generally want less invasive therapies, overtreatment by aggressive practices such as chemotherapy drugs that do not produce good outcomes is vulnerable to curtailment, even just on economic grounds.

- Mounting environmental concerns will continue to drive research showing how toxins defeat the immune system, and the definition of outcomes will broaden to include prevention. The future orientation of a group such as the American Cancer

Society may shift toward promoting wide-ranging cancer prevention strategies, while providing public information on the panoply of scientifically justifiable complementary and alternative treatment approaches.

- Public health spending will be under pressure to reflect these priorities, while the large market for alternative therapies will amplify corporate engagement.

- There will be a trend toward "customization," individualizing therapies to the singular needs and desires of each patient. The advent of treatments uniquely tailored to genetic matches will accelerate this tendency. Because customization is consistent with the nature of most alternative therapies, alternatives will ride the trend.

- Medicine will become more patient-centered, expanding to include the patient's values, belief systems, and subjective responses.

- Restrictive medical regulations will decline. Clinical trials will wane in the face of increased emphasis on outcomes from less expensive and less cumbersome models such as the best-case series and advanced computer modeling.

- The cost savings of alternative treatments will be a major factor in their ongoing acceptance.

- Freedom of medical choice will emerge as a compelling political issue in tune with market economics, customization, and patient demand.

- Immunotherapies will continue to move to center stage among therapeutic approaches.

Dr. William Fair, the Memorial Sloan-Kettering urologist who has successfully managed his own cancer using alternative therapies, envisions the reinvention of cancer therapeutics. He proposes not so much curing as *controlling* cancer, much as diabetes is held in check.[70] It's a course very different from the single-minded assault to kill every last cancer cell in the body that has characterized allopathic treatment for the past hundred years.

Dr. Fair's model hearkens back to a fundamental conflict of medical opinion from a century ago between Louis Pasteur and his scientific rival Béschamps. Where Pasteur identified pathogenic germs as the cause of disease, Béschamps contended that "the terrain is everything."[71] In his view, it is principally an imbalanced metabolism that allows dangerous pathogens to gain dominance or stimulates otherwise harmless germs to mutate and turn malignant. A healthy terrain, he proposed, defeats pathogens or holds them harmlessly in check in a dynamic balance.

In other words, as Dr. Fair implies and Hoxsey and the empirics have said, the medium may be the message in biology as well. People can live with cancer, by using strategy over brute force, by fitting together the extendable segments of advancing knowledge, by enhancing the terrain. Or, as a doctor friend once remarked as only a doctor could, perhaps our purpose as human beings on Earth is to build immunities.

It is only very recently that medicine has entered the dawning age of biology. In this light, it is unsurprising that the drug industry has failed to find a magic bullet for cancer. Answers will more likely lie in the vastly complex ecology of the biological realm, where the cancer industry has not been looking. Rather than magic bullets, the most promising directions are toward strengthening immunity and revitalizing the terrain. Nontoxic customized approaches may ultimately prevail for what many now believe is not a single disease but a complex of many kinds intimately bound up with environment, diet, lifestyle, and personal belief systems.

If there is one thing to count on, it's that any scientific theory will eventually be proved wrong. Most great discoveries have come from empirical observers. Much of the contribution of the rationalist or allopathic school has been to systematize those insights and codify them into systems accessible to other practitioners.

What seems sure is that medicine in the age of biology enters the domain of *vis medicatrix naturae*. Perhaps something like the Hoxsey tonic and Dr. Burzynski's antineoplastons and the Gerson diet are the true medical biotechnologies.

Alternative medicine runs deep and wide in the American psyche. There is growing recognition that medicine's destiny is a collaborative one, a return to the pluralism that existed just a century ago. What patients want is free access to unbiased information and heterogeneous choices. They also seek a healing partnership with their doctors and a plethora of other practitioners.

While physicians have fought fiercely for their professional sovereignty during the twentieth century, the greater social issue today is the sovereignty of the patient. In a market economy, goes the old saw, the customer is always right. When we filmed the AMA's Oliver Field, an architect of the aggressive repression against Hoxsey and myriad "quack" therapies, we were surprised at his response to the question of freedom of medical choice. "This is a free country," he told us. "You pays your money and you takes your choice. If it's wrong, you're the one who's going to suffer."[72]

It was odd to hear the former head of the AMA's Bureau of Investigation, which the AMA converted into a research archive in 1990, echo the words of his past nemesis, William Hawley Atwell. "So I wish to say," the judge ruled in 1949 in Hoxsey's victory over Dr. Morris Fishbein, "pay your money and take your choice. Those who need a doctor, if you think one side is the best, go and get him. If you think the other side is best, you certainly have the right to go and get him. This is a free country; that is what we stand for in America."[73]

The Other
Heroic Medicine

I visited the Bio Medical Center twice in early 1998 for this book, but I had returned there several times in the intervening years. Once, around 1990, an associate with lymphoma asked me to accompany him to the clinic. With a history of cancer in my own family, I decided to get a checkup myself.

I felt very vulnerable in a wispy blue smock sitting with anxious new patients in the waiting room. We had our blood work, X-rays, and other tests, got dressed, and waited some more. I was grateful to learn that I was healthy and did not have signs of cancer. I went on the tonic for the next six months anyway, since Mildred believes that it also acts as a preventive. I was faithful to the regimen, which was not that difficult. I liked the root-beer taste of the tonic and felt good about doing it. The symptoms of my associate's lymphoma disappeared in three months, and he is still alive after nine years though he still struggles with the disease.

In 1996 I brought some other colleagues to visit Mildred. One was Oren Lyons, a chief of the Iroquois Indian nation and a global spokesperson for indigenous peoples' rights. Also joining us was John Mohawk, another Iroquois who is the former editor of *Akwesasne Notes*, a highly respected Indian news publication. Both Oren and John are professors of American studies at the State University of New York at Buffalo, and they live in the dual worlds of traditional indigenous culture and postmodern mainstream society. They came because they were deeply concerned about a close friend dying of a brain tumor. They were also intrigued with Hoxsey as an herbal treatment whose origins owe much to traditional Native American plant lore.[1]

We chatted into the evening in Mildred's trailer. Mildred believed her mother was part Cherokee, growing up in the Oklahoma Territory in Indian country. Oren and John talked about how the young people today don't go down to the riverbed any more where the herbs grow, how volumes of their rich Native heritage of botanical knowledge are vanishing.

Oren described the indigenous view of herbs, which are considered sacred plants whose permission must first be asked before they can be used. He observed that native peoples have generally not grown medicinal herbs, but wildcrafted them in the natural settings where they concentrate their special power. Both John and Oren expressed interest in cultivating the Hoxsey herbs on Indian lands, where today there is a small but vigorous rebirth of traditional herbalism, and where cancer is epidemic. Oren spoke slowly in the same idling pauses punctuating Mildred's languid storytelling. From a traditional perspective, he said, it is the spirit that heals, though the herbs and the medicines help.

Mildred was captivated by the conversation, enthralled talking about plants, animals, traditional culture, and, always, cancer. She was having increasing difficulty obtaining high-quality herbs, which for many years were supplied mainly by Mormon, Amish, and Mennonite growers who farmed without chemicals. But their children were losing touch with the land, too, and the botanical future looked unstable.

When I arrived back at the San Diego airport in January 1998 for work on this book, I drove to the familiar International Motel. In the morning, I waited for the cancer van, which Raul was still driving after almost twenty years. Fifteen years since I had first come, the scene had not changed much, the streaming pathos of cancer patients seeking desperate measures after being given up to die. Raul kept up a cheerful patter, saluting numerous pedestrians on the Tijuana streets as his cousins, trying gently to lighten the load.

Tijuana is now a Mexican metropolis, swollen with growth and beset with modern problems. Contractions in the Mexican economy have pushed peasants out of the countryside, and many come north seeking survival and opportunity. Shantytowns ring the city, water is scarce and polluted, and the populace lives in fear of rampant drug running. Only months before, the outspoken editor of a Tijuana newspaper had been wounded in an assassination attempt to silence his crusade against narco-terrorists. A year earlier, Mexico's leading presidential candidate had been gunned down at a rally here in broad daylight, probably by agents of the drug cartel he openly opposed.

Climbing the steep hill toward the clinic, the van passed veils of barbed wire and tall spikes shielding the houses in what has become a swanky neighborhood in an uneasy community sharply divided between haves and have-nots. The bright orange, green, and white stripes of a jumbo Mexican flag hung listlessly over the city below, sagging in the gray diesel air. In the near distance shimmered San Diego, glistening on the azure Pacific, a world apart of gated communities, scenic red trolleys, Sea World, and a giant Navy base.

Entering the clinic, I saw many familiar faces, but there was a palpable void—Mildred was not there. She was in the trailer next door, indisposed. For the past three years, Mildred has had serial health problems—bronchitis, pneumonia, a broken rib, the pains of aging. I passed some time in the waiting room, looking out across the ordinarily brown hills of Tijuana now saturated to a verdant green by the punishing rains of El Niño. A cluster of patients sat around a TV monitor watching our *Hoxsey* film, playing on a continuous loop all morning. I watched the patients watching the film. Heads shook at the high drama of Harry Hoxsey battling Morris Fishbein. Eyes moistened at the victories of other cancer patients, at Mildred's fierce compassion. Hope filled the air.

I went next door to visit Mildred. She was resting in bed, looking very frail, slipping below a hundred pounds. It was unnerving and painful to see her so debilitated; I was accustomed to the zestful woman who walked through walls. Like Harry Hoxsey, she has lived three lives in one. The strain was finally showing. For all her loving strictness with her patients, she herself makes a lousy patient. It was all anyone could do to get her to eat.

We chatted awhile, and Mildred was as lucid and combustible as ever, making big plans for the clinic. She had been shuttling back and forth to the respite of her Oregon cattle ranch, her other great passion and the only place she could get proper rest away from the stress of the clinic. She was looking forward to calving season on the land.

"I grew up the oldest of seven children," Mildred recalled. "My father was a rancher west of Forth Worth, Texas. I started to school on horseback, and all the years growing up, I might not have the horse I wanted, but I was never without a horse. In the years that went by, mother got sick and I had the responsibility of the children, but I still didn't like anything to do with the house. I wanted to be out and be around the horses and the cattle. I became quite accustomed to that type of life.

"By the time I was ten years old, we were in the Depression. By the time I got out of high school, with seven kids there wasn't a lot of money, but a neighbor that had lived nearby had been in a discussion with a friend of the family, and they had decided, because Mom had been sick, that I would make a very good nurse. I was asked to go to Fort Worth to drive. I'd go down driving, and when we'd get about halfway there, she said, 'Oh, do you know why we're coming down?' And I said, 'No, I'm not coming for anything—I'm just driving you.' And she said, 'Oh no, we're going to see if we can get nurse's training.'

"I go marching in with her," Mildred laughed, "knowing I couldn't possibly get into nurse training, but nevertheless put my application in. The day before I was supposed to be there, I get the notice, and hadn't even told my parents that I had done this. When I showed the letter to Dad, he said, 'Why don't you spend the money for something you want to do? You will never go with this discipline to be a nurse.' And I said, 'No, I'll do it.' He said, 'You won't last six weeks. You have not had that type of discipline or that type of a life. You might as well spend your money for something you want. You won't last six weeks.' And I said, 'Yes, I will.' After I got the first six weeks in, then it was a snap. That's how I started in the field of nursing."[2]

I bummed a ceremonial cigarette and we talked on. I am always curious about how Mildred sees the state of cancer, witnessing as much of it as she does. Cancer used to be an old person's affliction, she said, but now it's striking younger people all the time—teenagers, little children. For the first time, she sees breast cancer in very young girls, and lots more melanoma in general. The disease seems more virulent. People are diagnosed and they're dead in six months—that seldom used to happen. Perhaps, she speculated, people's immune systems are so weakened by toxic pollution, stress, and bad diet that they just go faster. Cancer is rising in Mexico, too, and the country is not prepared for it. More Mexicans are coming to the clinic these days. It's bad.

Mildred confirmed her commitment to Catherine to follow through on the Hoxsey research, though, ever tough and canny, she expressed the same guardedness that has allowed her to survive doing Hoxsey all this time. It was a different world, I suggested, when she left the country in 1963. Medicine seems to be changing, more open to alternatives, more inclusive. Cautiously she agreed, while maintaining her insomniac vigilance against the treatment's exploitation or misuse.

Mildred's concerns about commercial exploitation are valid in today's medical marketplace. There are already several Hoxsey-clone formulas being sold that are not the Hoxsey formula, one of which is improperly prepared in alcohol. Catherine Salveson helped Mildred obtain a trademark on the Hoxsey name, and suppliers of these other tonics are being notified to cease using "Hoxsey" in their promotions.[3]

In the late 1950s, after losing the final court battles, Harry Hoxsey threatened to release the tonic as a patent medicine without any claims for cancer. This scenario has been enacted more recently by Essiac, the Canadian herbal cancer remedy. After the death of founder nurse René Caisse, the formulas went into an official trust with exclusive rights to the formulas, preparation, and name. The product is now marketed widely in health-food stores without any health claims.[4] Although there is another competing product, it is easily distinguishable from the authorized article.

Through Catherine's academic position at Oregon Health Sciences University, the nursing school authorized her to initiate medical research on Hoxsey. It seems eminently appropriate that the treatment that has been shouldered by a nurse should come back through a nursing organization. "The nurses are more open-minded," Mildred commented. "Of course, they are the ones who are beside the patient, all hours of the day and night going through this thing, and with the families. I think really they have a much broader scope of the heartbreak and everything that goes with it than even the doctors."[5]

As a fellow nurse, Catherine has studied Mildred Nelson closely. "Mildred is not practicing as nurses are licensed to practice. Nurses practice under statutes and state law. Their practice is very carefully monitored by boards of nursing and by codes of practice from the profession. Mildred does not follow anyone's rules except her own. She doesn't practice under anybody's authority. In that regard, she does not practice nursing, but she was trained as a nurse and she started as a nurse, and nursing is about caring. Nursing is about commitment to the patient no matter what the outcome. In that regard, she's a nurse's nurse if there ever was

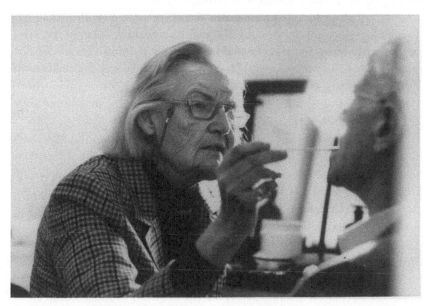

Mildred Nelson treats an external cancer, 1985,
Bio Medical Center, Tijuana.

one. She calls herself a nurse. To my mind, even though she doesn't have a legal, professional license, she's as much of a nurse as anyone who's ever been trained as a nurse and who cares for people.

"In the thirty-five years she has been in Mexico, she has personally monitored and been involved in the care of thousands of people. She has participated in the care of all of these people, and has insight and understanding about cancer, and she does a lot by her instincts. She has also watched people die and get well, and, as a compassionate healer paying attention, she is committed to trying anything. She would try a litany of treatments of anything that she could get her hands on that she thought would help people. When she finds out it's not helpful, she stops it. The bedrock underneath all her commitment is the tonic. Everybody gets the tonic. Beyond the tonic, she is always looking for how to craft a treatment for each individual. If that means being woken up in the middle of the night to talk to somebody about their nausea, she's there. I've never met anyone as a healer who has her level of personal knowledge and just plain commitment. She has been on twenty-four-hour call forever, and you can't ask for much more.

"I love Mildred Nelson. Even if there were no Hoxsey or if Hoxsey were gone, I have come to know and love this woman as a member of my family. She has inspired me. She has given me courage. She has helped me learn how to stand up for myself as I watched her and what she's gone through. She has taught me about compassion."

As I sat with Mildred, a line of patients awaiting the external medicines was starting to loop down to the trailer, where she would treat them from her chair in the living room, a bowl of Pine-Sol by her side. I agreed to come back that evening, and returned to the waiting room to visit with more patients.

On the prominent black onyx fireplace in the center of the waiting room was a new metal plaque. It read, PATIENTS' TRIBUTE TO MILDRED NELSON AND THE HOXSEY TREATMENT. Mildred's patients universally adore her. I have never heard an unkind word about her from a patient, other than objections to her smoking.

Gwen Scott from New Zealand spoke highly of Mildred. "I stayed another day so I could meet and personally talk with Mrs. Nelson, and we had about an hour together. To meet Mrs. Nelson herself was very, very humbling and an amazing experience, just in knowing that you're very, very privileged to be there and taking that treatment. I didn't know what to expect, and I just found her so down-to-earth and so natural. I think her wisdom and her common sense and her frankness and the absolute truth of whatever she had to say—to me she was like someone who could be respected like Mother Teresa or some of these great people. And then there's the legacy of Hoxsey and the generosity of Mrs. Nelson in the charitable way of the payments and the fact that she never sends out accounts or anything like that."[6]

The sentiment is reciprocal: Mildred lives for her patients. "Probably the most important thing," Mildred said, "is the fact that I do care about them, and their getting well is very important to me and to their families. Oftentimes we gang up on them and get them started on the right track. The poor little people that come in when there's no family, no one that cares, nobody to help, no one to encourage—the attitude means a lot. They are going against everybody else's wishes and they're sort of on their own. Nobody is really believing that what they're going to do is going to help them. It was usually the ones that were more ill than the others that you became more concerned about. As you'd watch them get well, then you felt so close to them. Like maybe they kinda belonged to you?"

Hoxsey has never claimed to be a cure-all, and Mildred also sees a lot of death. "As our patients come in, they are already classified terminal. You do everything you can for them. You have to be honest with them. You have to take care of them the very best that you can. Some of them you feel sure will not make it because they are too far advanced for anything to happen. There's quite an emotional thing that's involved. No one likes to give somebody bad news or death news. We try to do it as discreetly as we can with as much confidence to the patient as they can have. The children that come in, whether they are actually considered terminal or just ill, are the ones that really eat your heart out. Those days, most of the day is spent crying instead of a happy-go-lucky day.

"There are the ones you lose. If it's after you've been around them for quite a period of time and you lose 'em, it's very similar to losing a member of the family. You become very attached. I constantly say, 'I'm not gonna attach myself to a patient again,' but you do. Every one of 'em. As time goes on and you're around them more and more, they become quite dear to you. We're much like a family, and you feel that you have lost something very precious when you give one of 'em up. You're never ready to give 'em up. I don't care if they've lived thirty years after you treat 'em, you're not even ready to give 'em up then.

"The average people through the medical profession say [about Hoxsey], 'Oh, they're robbing them, they're stealing from them,' but they don't sit here and listen to conversations that go on between the doctors and the patients. One little ray of hope, and, as ill as some of them are, as small as our hopes are that they will recover, some of them make it. Others die. There is nothing in medicine 100 percent for all people. After the doctors have finished with all of their treatment, have given them up, they come down here. We see them through the very end with it, and the doctors say, 'Oh, they're going to kill you.'"

For many patients, experiencing Mildred's clinic is transformational. Gwen Scott described her first visit there. "To be there when people are told that their cancer has gone and see the emotions of others and feel it: You just need heaps of hankies. There was an American lady who was very loud and very noisy. She was henpecking the husband and the son quite a bit, and it was not a lady that I normally would talk to, but I found her sitting quietly on the bed. From having made such a noise to being such a quiet person, she really needed me to go and talk to her at that time when she was quiet. She was waiting for her first three-month result, and it dawned on me then that all the noise and bickering were her way of coping with her concerns.

"She was sitting there quietly waiting for the results from her first scan. Because she was so large, when she did walk into the lounge at the clinic later on, it created an incident. The whole room sat up. There was nobody talking. It was really quiet, and there was this huge lady standing in the middle of the room with tears in her eyes, saying, 'They've got it. They've got my cancer. My cancer is reduced in size.'

"Just to be there and see that woman and see that family and see their emotions, that was that first trip for me. There was one girl who said, 'If it meant my getting cancer all over again just to be here, I would choose to have cancer all over again.'"

Catherine Salveson sees Mildred Nelson's Bio Medical Center as an expression of a larger pattern in the transformation of American medicine. "Part of the rise of alternative medicine has to do with the fact that women are the ones who decide the health care of the family. It's the mama and it's the wife who pick the doctor, who pick the health-care plan, who make the decisions about what you're going to get when you have a bad cold, whether you get echinacea or whether you get Advil. Part of what's happening with alternative medicine is that women in general are being empowered regarding their role in health care.

"In most medical schools now, there's gender parity, about 45 percent women. Women are more open-minded about alternatives than men are. They just think differently. The acceptance of alternatives into medicine is also happening because there's been a feminization of medicine.

"When Hoxsey was doing battle, there were no women's faces on the wall at the AMA. It matters. The people who make the decision about what you give somebody when they're sick—if they know I give this pill to my family, to somebody I love, and they're going to be sick as a dog, or,

I give them this other one and it takes them longer to get well but they feel okay—I'm not going to give them those pills.

"Women are more noncompliant than men," Catherine concludes with a sly twinkle. "They don't always do what the doctor tells them. Ask any gerontologist. They'd much rather take care of an old man than an old woman. An old man will do what he's told. An old lady often won't. She'll do what she damn well pleases and what her neighbor does and what she heard about in church. And what's cheap. Mildred is a woman. I think part of why Hoxsey has endured is the myth of Mildred. Everybody had to walk past her desk. She would look up and look them in the eye, even if she never said anything to them. Those piercing eyes were like tossing somebody a life rope. She was like that silver thread, that placental cord saying, 'No! You don't have to get dead.' The fact that she was a woman and a mother mattered."

When I returned that evening to see Mildred, she was propped up in bed watching a University of Texas football game with the sound turned off. A fierce little dog named Trouble sat protectively by her side, growling whenever I leaned in too close.

The dawning of 1996 marked the fiftieth anniversary of Mildred's "working with Hoxsey," and 1998 clocked her thirty-fifth year in Mexico, a North American woman in a Mexican man's world operating a "quack" cancer clinic. Since going to Tijuana, she has treated upwards of 30,000 patients. How does she look back on her life work? "Working with the clinic, getting it to where it is today, has been a rewarding experience that I wouldn't want to give up or trade for anything else. It's been lots of hard work. There are heartaches with it every day, but there's also daily rewards. Most people forget to count their blessings, and then you see how many there have been through the years. When you look back at the number of people that are here today that would not have been, there isn't an awful lot that could make you wish that you had not done what you have done for a lifetime."

I once asked Mildred what she looked forward to. "Getting as many people well as I can. We were not put here to be petty or be selfish. What we do for somebody else is the important thing in getting through this life."

As a nurse, Mildred also holds a perspective on her relationship with her patients distinct from that of most doctors. "Much of the time, the patient and the doctor do not have a good relationship. Doctors are afraid to have a relationship with the patient. Most of them are aware that, going down the route that they do, they'll lose the patient. They don't want the pain of losing a friend or somebody that they're really close to. As a result, the patient is very aware that he is avoiding them in many ways.

When the patient would like to talk to him, discuss different things with him—their beliefs, their fears, their anxieties—the doctor says, 'Good morning, how are you?' and he's gone. He tells the nurse to give them something, and the patients are very uncomfortable with it.

"I think doctors should know a little more about their patients: their thoughts, their wishes—what the patient wants, what they're entitled to. In most places today, they're given a number and they're treated as though they were a number. This isn't all of them, but the majority. Especially in your areas where there's a lot of research going on, the patient becomes the statistic and they know it. They feel it. They don't like it. They are individuals. They are interested in living. Instead of the doctors saying, 'Well, you've got thirty days to live, is there anything we can do for you?,' they could have a little compassion and a little thought for the patient, and make life much easier in the end.

"If doctors had this type of relationship with the patient, and found out what pleasure it is to accomplish something that everybody else said that you can't do, then yes, they'd all enjoy it. The patient would be happier, and the doctor's happier. Today, they're patients. Tomorrow they're not patients; they're people who are friends and relatives. I think that there are more people in the medical profession who are becoming aware of the fact that they are really missing something in their care for patients. Whether it's cancer surgery or whatever, they seem to be afraid to have a real doctor-patient relationship for fear they're going to get hurt. When it comes to hurting, we hurt every day."

I returned to the Bio Medical Center a few months later. It was calving season and Mildred was at the ranch, recuperating and overseeing the mass spring birthing. Her sister Liz Jonas was now presiding. Liz stepped in to manage the clinic in 1997 during Mildred's increasingly extended sick leaves. Another open-hearted Texan, Liz did not expect to be operating her sister's cancer clinic. She is not a medical person, but does have a strong business background as a business administrator and CPA for the Tandy Corporation, owner of Radio Shack. She has also managed the family affairs for many years.

"I was meant to be here," Liz told me philosophically.[7] It has been challenging, since she commutes back to Texas often, trying to keep work and family together. She believes that ultimately the clinic will return to the United States.

In the waiting room, the anxiety over Mildred's absence was palpable. A hushed muttering passed through the room in periodic waves, wondering whether she would return. Just how sick was she? What would happen to the clinic and to their medical lifeline?

Many years before, while making the film, we asked Mildred about the future of Hoxsey. At the time, she'd already had two strokes, and the fate of the treatment was a real concern. "The future of the Hoxsey treatment? Of all those people out there, there has got to be somebody that will want to do it, to give part of themselves to take care of people who are sick. That person will come along while I'm physically able to train 'em and teach 'em. When the day comes, I will teach 'em. So that isn't a worry to us. If that doesn't happen, then I'm sorry it is lost, and it wasn't intended to go on."

Mildred did train several people, but they didn't stay. One set up a competing clinic; another gave up and went back to the States. A New Zealand physican who studied with her extensively was ultimately blocked from practice abroad. There is no successor, and much of the profound reservoir of empirical experience Mildred has gained over fifty years will go with her. The clinic will probably survive, at least for a while. Liz Jonas is a very competent businesswoman dedicated to her sister's legacy. There is a strong core of highly competent doctors and staff who have worked with the program a long time. But Mildred Nelson, like Harry Hoxsey, is one of a kind.

"I don't know what the future of Hoxsey is," Catherine Salveson sighs. "Mildred Nelson has encouraged me to go ahead and do the research. The future of Hoxsey is very much tied to this research because, if anything were to happen to Mildred, the forces that are currently in play are very unpredictable. If the research is in place, then it doesn't matter as much what happens with the rest of the clinic and the infrastructure that she has built in Mexico. There will be a second infrastructure, the research infrastructure, that will contain the treatment.

"There's no question in my mind that this tonic helps people," Catherine adds. "I also know that the kind of person who goes against their doctor and who goes to a 'Third World' country to a 'quack' clinic to take a weird tonic is an unusual person. Many people come from a support system, whether it's a spiritual support system of being a Mormon, Jehovah's Witness, Amish, or a Seventh-day Adventist, or simply a person who is determined to live or has a relative who's determined to keep them alive.

"I also know that these herbs have value in helping people who are fighting cancer. I believe that people who had cancer are alive in part because they took this tonic. That's why I'm so committed to doing this research and helping bring this treatment back to the United States so it can be available to people more easily."

If the therapy were validated, a vigorous alternative medicine community now exists to carry it on. Intense interest exists among the burgeoning numbers of naturopathic physicians, who are already using Hoxsey-like formulas and studying the medicines.

If Hoxsey is lost, it certainly won't be the first time a promising alternative cancer therapy has succumbed to medical politics. Most of the hundred or so such therapies over the course of the twentieth century vanished with their founders. The shadow side of "scientific medicine" has been its recurring pattern of condemnation without investigation.

Clearly, conventional cancer treatments have an important place in medicine and save many lives. But a hundred years from now, medicine will likely come to regard some of these methods the way it now remembers the use of mercury and bloodletting. Scientific theories are provisional, based on steep learning curves and embedded in the temper of the times. Dr. Abigail Zuger recently wrote a medical meditation of sorts in the *New York Times* contemplating the hundredth anniversary of the 1899 *Merck Manual*, the "venerable" medical textbook which at that time recommended many highly toxic drugs that today are museum-quality horrors. "We have harnessed our own set of poisons for medical treatment; in a hundred years a discussion of cancer chemotherapy may read as chillingly as endorsements of strychnine for tuberculosis and arsenic for diabetes do today."[8]

Yet although allopathic medicine has largely failed against chronic killers such as cancer and heart disease, it excels at surgery, emergency care, the treatment of trauma, and certain bacterial infections. Many of its diagnostic tools are without compare. When operating empirically, allopathic medicine can be superlative. To deny its many vital contributions is equally counterproductive. Medicine now has the extraordinary opportunity to merge the best of all traditions in service to the well-being of the patient.

At the same time, yesterday's science fiction is rapidly becoming today's science fact. Breakthroughs in the understanding of nutrition are blurring the boundaries between food and medicine, opening an entire new terrain of "nutraceuticals" for health and healing. Mounting scientific data on herbal medicines show documented efficacy confirming ancient folk traditions. Perhaps insights into the nature of quantum physics and complexity theory may one day provide a matrix for explaining the potency of the infinitesimal doses of homeopathic remedies. Research is proving placebos to be an unimaginably powerful healing force, dissolving distinctions between mind and body. Biological revelations about the natural world illustrate that health is more akin to an intricate ecology of interdependent relationships than to the rigid mechanics of a machine.

Humility is the constant companion of empiricism, and outcomes are ultimately what matter in medicine.

Departing the clinic for the last time, I shared a taxi back to the border with an older couple. They were polite but reserved. Respecting their privacy, I sat silently until the taxi stopped short at the last turnaround before the U.S. border. The man asked the driver for directions to walk to a nearby shopping area on the Mexican side. As we got out of the cab, he turned to me and smiled broadly. He had just gotten a clean bill of health at the clinic. After five years on the tonic, he was cancer-free and heading for his first margarita in a very long time.[9] I wished him well and set off on foot to merge with the flow of humanity funneling through U.S. customs to cross that philosophical border.

Epilogue

Does the Hoxsey tonic really work? That is the big question, after all. Realistically, only scientific research can finally provide a definitive answer, but I have come to some personal conclusions.

When Judge William Atwell did finally rule in federal court on the efficacy of the Hoxsey therapy, he estimated its effectiveness as "comparable to surgery, radium, and X-ray," but without the destructive effects of those measures. In the end, that is my conclusion, too.[1]

But the confounding variable is that the vast majority of patients coming to Hoxsey are terminal and have undergone the immune-damaging effects of radiation or chemotherapy, which sabotage the very rationale of the tonic. Harry Hoxsey claimed, as Mildred does, to cure 80 percent of people who have not had these prior treatments. Who knows?

However, Judge Atwell had earlier commented that he also believed Hoxsey healed his patients "like Jesus Christ," a therapeutic wild card that deepens the enigma. As Norman Cousins, the late author of *Anatomy of an Illness*, noted, we know a little about how disease works but almost nothing about how healing happens. Medicine has been almost solely focused on disease mechanisms rather than the healing response in all its complexity.

The curative powers of love, hope, and faith—of mind and spirit—remain mysterious, elusive, and potent. Perhaps Harry Hoxsey had it right when he strode into a glum waiting room in his Dallas clinic to cheer his patients. "I believe love is here to stay—what do you think about it? There's too much love in this world for it to ever sink!" It's also spirit that conjures cures, though of course the herbs and the medicines help.

In the end the debate returns to a familiar conflict of medical opinion. The allopaths have long believed the cause of disease to be entirely knowable, explainable by a theory and traceable to a single mechanism. To the contrary, the empirics have suggested that one can know symptoms and therapeutic effects but seldom the "cause" of disease. Considering the vast intricacies and relational interdependencies of biology—not to mention the mysteries of the human spirit—some questions in medicine may forever persist as starry enigmas. The real issue is the outcome. Getting well is finally the point.

There are just too many people using Hoxsey who got well when they weren't supposed to for it to be accidental or rampant good luck. The Hoxsey herbs are now documented as possessing abundant anticancer properties, and surely they constitute a credible and compelling basis for further investigation. There is no debate that the Hoxsey external escharotics work, only questions about their proper place in medical practice.

In 1999 the long-awaited preliminary government review of Hoxsey patient records was completed by Mary Ann Richardson and her team. Intended as a feasibility study, the limited number of cases and inability to track down a significant proportion of the patients prevented any definitive judgment or comparison with conventional treatment outcomes. Of 149 cancer patients, 17 were alive, 68 dead, and 64 lost to follow-up. In particular, the report notes the seven-year survival of a melanoma patient, an extreme rarity, who was treated solely with the Hoxsey tonic and escharotics.

The report concludes, referring to Hoxsey, "A best-case series or more systematic prospective monitoring of patients is justified not only because of the public health issue to justify the large number of patients who seek treatment at this clinic, but also because of the several *noteworthy cases of survival.*"[2]

In other words, a "noteworthy" number of terminal patients got well when they weren't supposed to. The call for a formal scientific investigation now bears the imprimatur of the federal government.

Why was Hoxsey not investigated in the first place seventy-five years ago? The overarching truth is that the Hoxsey treatment has been politically railroaded instead of medically tested. The civil war has distorted cancer from a medical question into a political issue. The many courageous practitioners and doctors thrust involuntarily into the front lines of the cancer wars would surely prefer to settle the question in a clinic or laboratory, not a courtroom. Meanwhile, cancer patients remain trapped in the crossfire, fighting for their lives and for their very right to survive using harmless treatments in a victimless crime.

In medicine the goal is supposed to be the well-being of the patient. As Mildred Nelson told our camera eye, "Surely to goodness, we're going to have enough heart and compassion for people, that the day has to come that everybody's going to be concerned about everybody else, and in some manner help to take care of 'em. What were we put here for except to help each other?"

Perhaps there is another kind of heroic medicine, a heroism from the heart of healing, a devotion to inspired service. There is a deep healing unfolding today within medicine. It's something about simple caring, about respect for another person's unique path, about the healing forces of nature and the spirit. It's also something about taking the greed out of medicine.

The end of the Hoxsey story is yet to be written. Nurse Mildred Nelson and her patients hang in the balance while a potentially valuable cancer treatment is poised on the border of extinction.

Afterword

In January 1999, after the substantial completion of this book, Mildred Nelson suffered a stroke in her bed in Tijuana and died shortly after. She was just shy of eighty years old.[1]

She was buried next to her mother and father at the family grave in Jacksboro, Texas. There wasn't a flower left to be had for miles around.

Notes

INTRODUCTION

[1] "Cough Medicine for Cancer," *Journal of the American Medical Association* (*JAMA*), Vol. 155, No. 7, June 12, 1954, pp. 667–668.

[2] Media General/Associated Press poll, *San Diego Tribune*, 11.11.85.

[3] "Snake Oil," *Townsend Letter for Doctors & Patients*, February/March 1999, p. 16; "Fish Oil for Cancer Patients," *Townsend Letter for Doctors & Patients*, 12.98, p. 52.

[4] Morris Fishbein, *Quacks and Quackeries of the Healing Cults* (Girard, Kan: Haldeman-Junius Publications, 1927), p. 24.

[5] SEER (Surveillance, Epidemiology and End Results) Cancer Statistics Review, National Cancer Institute.

[6] American Cancer Society, *Cancer Facts and Figures*, 1998 (New York, 1998).

[7] Robert N. Proctor, *Cancer Wars: How Politics Shapes What We Know and Don't Know About Cancer* (New York: BasicBooks, 1995), p. 1.

[8] Dr. Samuel Epstein, "Winning the War Against Cancer?. . . Are They Even Fighting It," *Ecologist*, Vol. 28, No. 2, March/April 1998, pp. 69–80, citing American Hospital Association report.

[9] J.C. Bailar and H.L. Gornik, "Cancer Undefeated," *New England Journal of Medicine*, Vol. 336, pp. 1569–74, 1997.

[10] Mary Ann Richardson, Nancy C. Russell, Tina Ramirez, Robert Barrett, Catherine Salveson, John F. Annegers, "Assessment of Outcomes of Alternative Medicine Cancer Clinics: A Feasibility Study," Center for Alternative Medicine Research (UTCAM) and the University of Texas, Houston Health Science Center School of Public Health, scheduled for publication in 2000.

CHAPTER 1
Riding the Cancer Underground

[1] Harry Hoxsey, *You Don't Have to Die*, (New York: Milestone Books, 1956).

[2] Mildred Nelson, personal interview, 1984 [Interviews with Mildred were conducted 1984–87 and in 1998].

[3] US vs. Hoxsey Cancer Clinic, Civil No. 4144, District Court of the US, N.D.

Texas, Dallas Division, 12/21/50; US Court of Appeals, Fifth Circuit, No. 13645, US vs. Hoxsey Cancer Clinic, Appeal from the US District Court for Northern District of Texas, 7.31.52.

[4] Following Hoxsey's judgment against Fishbein, No. 31011-B in the District Court, 44th Judicial District, Dallas County, Texas, on 8.9.52, the AMA and FDA ceased calling Hoxsey's external remedies worthless and publicly condemning them.

[5] "Court Eliminates Hoxsey Treatment," *New York Times*, 9.17.60.

[6] Personal interview.

[7] Peter Barry Chowka, "Herbal Healing: A Cancer Alternative With a Record," *New Age*, Vol. 6, No. 6, 12.80, pp. 46–50; Chowka, "Does Mildred Nelson Have an Herbal Cure for Cancer?" *Whole Life Times*, No. 32, Jan/Feb 1984.

[8] *Regarding other sources for this book*:

The AMA private library and FDA files provided copious materials. FDA files include: AF 27-026, Vol. 1–23, Inj. 232, (Injunction Papers Only: 63A292 + 592; Carton 526; Accession #63A292); Interstate Seizure #4-052M. [Several folders and volumes were missing or absent. We had to file twice through FOLA to retrieve a number of those we finally did examine.] Also useful were the collection at the National Health Federation in Monrovia, CA; the Gerald Winrod archive in Wichita, KS; Dallas County Medical Society records; Morris Fishbein Papers, Dept. of Special Collections, University of Chicago; National Library of Medicine, including film archives. Also worth reading is: James Harvey Young, *Medical Messiahs: A Social History of Health Quackery in Twentieth-Century America* (Princeton, NJ: Princeton University Press), which draws principally on the files of the AMA and FDA. However, it portrays what amounts to an "official story" reflecting closely the views of these two institutions.

[9] The book contains an extensive and unique oral history from personal interviews with participants including: Mildred Nelson, Della Mae Nelson, James Wakefield Burke, James Martin, Robert Heath, Dr. Harry M. Spence, Oliver Field, William Grigg, Hoxsey's son and daughter, and Jimmy Kerr.

CHAPTER 2
"People Who Got Well When They Weren't Supposed To"

[1] Personal interviews with all patients. Medical Records for the film were reviewed in 1987 by Hugh, Riordan, MD, and for the book by Gar and Christeene Hildenbrand, including a reassessment of all the cases from the film as well as new ones for this book.

[2] Gar and Christeene Hildenbrand provided me with coded documents verifying diagnosis and assessing every aspect of the condition, prognosis and relevant aspects from the original doctors' notes or comments.

[3] Gwen Scott, *Hoxsey Connection* newsletter, 2/276 Westminster St., Christchurch, NZ.

[4] Dr. Eva Hill, *Cancer and Cure: A Doctor's Story*, (London, Bachman and Turner, 1976).

[5] Jane E. Brody, "Detecting Colon Cancer When It Is Curable," *New York Times*, 9.28.99.

CHAPTER 3
A Formula for Conflict

[1] The print of Hoxsey's film had no titles or credits, and its condition tended to accord with Mildred Nelson's assertion that Hoxsey was unable to obtain the negative, only a rough work print. It may have been the only print, and we dubbed it onto videotape as well as making a dupe negative.

[2] The early years are mainly described in Hoxsey's book *You Don't Have to Die*. Court depositions also contain numerous accounts of the same events.

[3] Hoxsey, ibid., pp. 67–68.

[4] Hoxsey, ibid., p. 69.

[5] Hoxsey, ibid., p. 71.

[6] Hoxsey, ibid., p. 72.

[7] Hoxsey, ibid., p. 73.

[8] Hoxsey, ibid., pp. 73–74.

[9] Hoxsey, ibid., p. 77.

[10] Hoxsey, ibid., p. 79; Hoxsey deposition, Harry M. Hoxsey vs. Morris Fishbein, William Engle, W.R. Hearst Jr., The American Weekly Inc., Hearst Consolidated Publications Inc., and The American Medical Association, A Corporation, No. 3203 Civil, in the District Court of the US for the Northern District of Texas, Dallas Division, 11.15–16.48, pp. 15–19.

[11] "'Hoxsey Day' Wednesday, A Success," *Girard Gazette*, 7.18.29.

[12] Hoxsey deposition, Hoxsey vs. Fishbein et al., No. 3203, 11.15–16.48, p. 23.

[13] "Many Cures Are Credited to New Cancer Treatment," *Mattoon Illinois Journal Gazette*, 12.23.24. Note: The AMA files contain voluminous press clippings from this era. Many appeared in the Taylorville *Daily Breeze* and *Daily Courier*.

[14] Hoxsey Deposition, Harry M. Hoxsey vs. Morris Fishbein et al., No. 3203 Civil, 11.15–16.48, p. 31; Hoxsey, op. cit., p. 90.

[15] US vs. Norman Baker, Federal Court, Davenport, IA, 1932, *Federal Reporter*, 2nd Series, 1932; *Federal Supplement*, 1932; Thomas Mannix, direct examination, transcript, p. 1625.

[16] Harry Hoxsey Deposition, Hoxsey vs. Fishbein et al., No. 3203 Civil, 11.15–16.48, p. 33.

[17] Other documentation verifies the existence of Mannix as a cancer patient at Alexian Brothers: AMA Bureau of Investigation Western Union Telegram to

Celestine J. Sullivan, 10.1.24; Oliver Field, internal AMA memo, 1949; Loesch, Scofield & Burke letter to Dwight Simmons, 2.22.49.

[18] Hoxsey Deposition, Hoxsey vs. Fishbein et al., No. 3203 Civil, pp. 38–39.

[19] Ibid., p. 39.

[20] Hoxsey, *You Don't Have to Die* (henceforth: Hoxsey, op. cit., unless otherwise noted), p. 100.

[21] Hoxsey Deposition, Hoxsey vs. Fishbein et al., No. 3203 Civil, pp. 39–40.

[22] Various: Mannix Deposition, US vs. Baker; Arthur J. Cramp letter to Philip Stern, 11.28.33; Loesch, Scofield & Burke letter to Dwight Simmons, 2.22.49.

[23] For detailed discussions of the AMA's origins and history: Paul Starr, *The Social Transformation of American Medicine* (New York: Basic Books, 1982); Harris L. Coulter, *Divided Legacy: The Conflict Between Homeopathy and the American Medical Association* (Berkeley: North Atlantic Books, 1973).

[24] Coulter, ibid., pp. 419–23.

[25] Starr, op. cit., p. 5.

[26] American Medical Association public information packet: "AMA's Bureau of Investigation," no date, c. 1920; "Home of the American Medical Association," no date, c. 1920.

[27] "Home of the American Medical Association," pamphlet, c. 1920, under section titled: "Inspection of the Building, Fifth Floor, Propaganda Department Room," cites both quotation as well as "card index files containing over 10,000 cards. . . . "

[28] "The AMA Becomes an Autocracy," *Illinois Medical Journal*, 12.22.

[29] Milton Mayer, "The Rise and Fall of Dr. Fishbein," *Harper's* magazine, Vol. 199, No. 1194, 11/49, pp. 76–85, p. 78.

[30] Morris Bealle, *Medical Mussolini* (Washington, D.C., Columbia Publishing, c. 1939) appendix, reproduction of ads; *TNT: The Naked Truth* magazine, "The Medical Trust Exposed," 6.30; citing *Jim Jam Jems* magazine, "An Ethical Quack," 3.13.

[31] George H. Simmons, letter to Ethical Relations Committee, Chicago Medical Society, University of Chicago Library, 4.29.09.

[32] Bealle, op. cit., p. 31; *TNT* magazine, op. cit.

CHAPTER 4
Quacking Around

[1] National Cancer Research Institute and Clinic brochure, No. 6, Chicago, 5.29.24, AMA files; *JAMA*, Vol. 86, No. 1, 1.2.26.

[2] *JAMA*, ibid., p. 25; "Hoxide Will Be 'Mayo Bros.' to Taylorville," Taylorville *Daily Courier*, 4.17.25.

[3] Letter from Homer Keeney to *JAMA*, 2.2.26, AMA files.

[4] "Dr. Keeney Wins Approval of State Medical Board," Taylorville *Daily Breeze*, 12.19.26.

[5] Dr. Homer I. Keeney, letter to Board of Medical Examiners, 12.30.25, AMA files.

[6] "The Hoxide Cancer Cure," *JAMA*, Vol. 86, No. 1, 1.2.26, pp. 55–57.

[7] Samuel B. Herdman, letter to Dr. Arthur J. Cramp, 10.9.24, AMA files.

[8] Hoxsey, op. cit., p. 134.

[9] Conflicting accounts suggest that Hoxsey was principally treating external cancers using the yellow powder, but there are occasional, oblique references to some kind of internal treatment as well. At times he appears to have used the yellow powder internally. Whether any of these references are to the herbal tonic is unclear. A 4.17.26 letter from Dr. R.L. Morris to the AMA about a bladder cancer case referred to "the only treatment she received was some medicine internally." Another letter from Hilda George of Espanola, New Mexico about her mother's breast cancer treatment by Hoxsey says, "They treat mostly external cases," but goes on to say, "We take some kind of internal medicine." Numerous other references indicate otherwise. A 9.15.24 letter from G.W. Nott to the AMA said, "They stated they had not tried it on internal cancer." Letters from the Hoxide Institute itself variously suggest, "We have not as yet been properly equipped to cope with the situation of internal cancers, although we have administered our preparation in large doses and relieved several...diagnosed as cancer of the stomach (Dr. Washburn, 12.20.25); "Although most of our work has been external cancers, we have administered the same treatment internally and relieved cases..." (Dr. Washburn, 12.20.25); "We do not claim to be able to cure internal cancer, though we may reach that point later on." (H.T. Morphy, Hoxide Inst. 4.17.25, Taylorville *Daily Courier*.) Hoxsey himself said otherwise: "We have treated every type and style of cancer" (letter to Mrs. Peris, 12.14.25). "The internal medication is just as important as the external especially in the metastacized cases." (Hoxsey deposition, Hoxsey vs. Fishbein No. 3203); by the time Hoxsey worked with Norman Baker, he definitely used an internal tonic, as reported in newspapers. A letter from Dr. Arthur J. Cramp at the Bureau of Investigation to Dr. A. Compton Broders re Frank Anderson's lung cancer further corroborated that Hoxsey used only "an internal medicine compounded by Mr. Hoxsey." (12.2.33). Dr. Joseph Durkee, an osteopath who worked with Hoxsey from 1946 to 1952, reported in interviews with the FDA that he believed Hoxsey did not start with an internal formula, but got it from a naturopath around 1936, as reported by Inspector W.L. Prillmayer in "Hoxsey Medicines" (FDA memorandum, 8.6.56). The same memo, however, acknowledged that "while [Dr. Durkee] may not be considered a friend of Hoxsey, he is a loyal adherent of the Hoxsey Cancer Treatment." Durkee had left the clinic in 1952, followed by a hostile lawsuit he lost to gain control of all patient records. Moreover, the generally prejudicial stance of the FDA and its prosecutorial threats may have distorted or misrepresented Dr. Durkee's stance.

[10] T.L. Hussleton, manager Chamber of Commerce of Atlantic City, letter to Dr. Arthur J. Cramp, 12.19.32.

[11] "Darrow Is Not Employed, He States," *International News Service*, 4.8.26; "Hoxide Suit Won't Come to Trial Soon," Taylorville *Daily Courier*, 3.16.26.

[12] Hoxsey, op. cit., pp. 137–40; Hoxsey vs. Fishbein No. 3203, pp. 44–46.

[13] James R. Hoxsey, Noah D. Hoxsey et al., vs. the Hoxide Institute, Harry Hoxsey and William H. Hoxsey, in the Circuit Court, Christian County, IL, 3.27; "$500,000 Lawsuit Over Disposition of Cancer Formula," *East St. Louis Illinois Journal*, 3.4.27.

[14] Hoxsey, op. cit., pp. 141–53; *East St. Louis Illinois Journal*, "$500,000 Lawsuit Over Disposition of Cancer Formulas," 3.4.27; State of Illinois, Christian County, Circuit Court, March, 1927, Various vs. Hoxide Institute; Hoxsey depositions, Hoxsey vs. Fishbein, No. 3203, pp. 49–53.

[15] Hoxsey deposition, Hoxsey vs. Fishbein, No. 3203, pp. 236–40.

[16] Hoxsey, op. cit., pp. 154–55.

[17] "'Hoxsey Day' Wednesday, A Success," *Girard Gazette*, 7.18.29.

[18] Ibid.

[19] Ibid.

[20] Ibid.

[21] *JAMA*, 8.3.29, pp. 400–02.

[22] Several sources provide versions of the Baker story: Hoxsey, op. cit., pp. 156–61; trial record, US vs. Norman Baker, Davenport, IA, 1932; Hoxsey testimony, US vs. Norman Baker et al., US District Court for the Eastern District of Arkansas, Western Division, Vol. 1, 1940; Alvin Winston, *Doctors, Dynamiters and Gunmen: The Life Story of Norman Baker* (Muscatine, IA: TNT Press, 1931); Nat Morris, *The Cancer Blackout* (Los Angeles, Regent House, 1977), p. 96; *TNT* magazines, AMA files; Hoxsey deposition, Hoxsey vs. Fishbein et al., No. 3203, pp. 69–77, pp. 145–54, pp. 230–35, pp. 244–52.

[23] Hoxsey deposition, trial record, US vs. Norman Baker, Davenport, IA, 1932.

[24] Ibid.

[25] Ibid.

[26] Hoxsey, op. cit., pp. 159–60; Hoxsey vs. Fishbein et al., No. 3203, pp. 71–77.

[27] Hoxsey deposition, US vs. Norman Baker, 9.5.30.

[28] Hoxsey deposition, US vs. Norman Baker, 9.5.30; Hoxsey testimony, US vs. Baker et al., 1940.

[29] *JAMA*, Vol. 94, No. 15, 4.12.30; numerous other *JAMA* references to Baker include: "The Baker Ballyhoo," Vol. 94, No. 17, 4.26.30, pp. 1340–41; "A Baker Institute 'Diagnosis'," 7.26.30, p. 285; "Medicolegal: Injunction to Prevent Unlawful Practice," 1.9.32, p. 168; "Norman Baker vs.. the American Medical Association: The Jury Declares the Association Not Guilty of Libeling Baker, Vol. 98, No. 12, 3.19.32, pp. 1012–16; "Norman Baker's Radio Station KTNT," Vol. 96, No. 14; "Current Comment: Norman Baker Convicted," Vol. 114, No. 5, 2.3.40, p. 416; "The Baker Hospital and J.L. Statler, M.D.," Vol. 114, No. 9,

3.2.40; also Arthur J. Cramp, "Norman Baker vs. the American Medical Association, *Hygeia*, 5.32, p. 432.

[30] Hoxsey vs. Fishbein, No. 3203, trial record, pp. 1181–90.

[31] Nat Morris, *The Cancer Blackout* (Los Angeles: Regent House, 1977) p. 96.

[32] *TNT* magazine, July, 1930.

[33] Hoxsey deposition, Hoxsey vs. Fishbein et al., No. 3203, pp. 230–35.

[34] *JAMA*, Vol. 98, No. 12, 3.19.32.

[35] Hoxsey deposition, US vs. Norman Baker, 9.5.30.

[36] Hoxsey, op. cit., p. 161.

[37] Ibid, p. 155.

[38] The Detroit episode is chronicled in: Hoxsey, op. cit., pp. 161–68; Hoxsey deposition, Hoxsey vs. Fishbein No. 3203, pp. 77–86; reports of Harry J. Kloppenberg to Dr. Fishbein, "Hoxsey vs. American Weekly," 2.7.49, 2.10.49, 2.16.49; Report of James E. Bowden, 2.11.49, Hoxsey vs. American Weekly; numerous newspaper clippings in AMA files; numerous letters from Wayne County Medical Society, AMA files.

[39] Hoxsey deposition, Hoxsey vs. Fishbein et al., No. 3203, p. 82.

[40] Ibid, p. 90; "Cases Decided in the Supreme Court of Michigan," *Michigan Reports*, Vol. 260, p. 648, "People vs. Hoxsey, Michigan 245 NW 543; 260 Michigan 648, Physicians 6(1)," (Criminal Law, Physicians and Surgeons, Licenses, Unlawful Practice of Medicine), Appeal from Recorder's Court of Detroit; Skillman (W. McKay), J., submitted 10.13.32, Docket No. 195, Calendar No. 36,344), Decided 12.6.32: Harry M. Hoxsey was convicted of practicing medicine without a license, verdict then reversed and defendant discharged.

[41] Hoxsey, op. cit., p. 163.

[42] Dr. G.E. Phahler, letter to Dr. Arthur J. Cramp, 12.11.33, AMA files.

[43] Sources for West Virginia episode include: Hoxsey, op. cit., pp. 169–70; Hoxsey deposition, Hoxsey vs. Fishbein et al., No. 3203, pp. 94–99; reports of Harry J. Kloppenberg to Dr. Fishbein, "Hoxsey vs. American Weekly," 2.7.49, 2.10.49, 2.16.49; assorted newspaper clippings, AMA files; H.C. Gerber, letter to Dr. Arthur J. Cramp, 9.10.32; Dr. Russell Bond, Ohio County Medical Society, letter to Dr. Arthur J. Cramp, 8.25.32; Office Memorandum, US Government, Clyde H. Russell, Cincinnati District, 4.11.56.

[44] Sources for the Atlantic City episode include: Hoxsey, op. cit., pp. 170–71; Hoxsey deposition, Hoxsey vs. Fishbein et al., No. 3203, pp. 99–108; reports of Harry J. Kloppenberg to Dr. Fishbein, "Hoxsey vs. American Weekly," 2.7.49, 2.10.49, 2.16.49; assorted documents, AMA files, especially correspondence to and from Dr. Arthur J. Cramp.

[45] Seymour S. Preston, letter to AMA Bureau of Investigation, 6.2.34.

[46] Dr. Arthur J. Cramp, letter to Preston, 6.6.34.

[47] Harry J. Kloppenburg, report to Dr. Fishbein, "Hoxsey vs. American Weekly," 2.7.49, pp. 4–5.

[48] Hoxsey letter to Fishbein, 12.21.35., AMA files.

[49] James Wakefield Burke, personal interview.

[50] Sources for the Philadelphia and Dr. Clarence Cook Little episodes include: Hoxsey, op. cit., pp. 172–79; Hoxsey deposition, Hoxsey vs. Fishbein et al., No. 3203, pp. 109–34; AMA files; FDA files; Report of Harry J. Kloppenburg re Hoxsey vs. Fishbein, 2.7.49, 2.10.49, 2.16.49, re Hoxsey vs. Fishbein, No. 3203; Hoxsey deposition, Hoxsey vs. Fishbein et al., no. 3203, pp. 109–33; extensive correspondence, AMA files; correspondence, FDA files; Office Memorandum, US government, William H. Phillips, Inspector, Chief Philadelphia Station, 4.18.46; "Written Interrogatories," Clarence Cook Little, Witness, by Harry J. Kloppenberg, 1.17.49, AMA files; letter from Herbert G. Brower to Dr. C.C. Little, 1.3.49, AMA files.

[51] Letter from Maurice Lichtman, Business Manager, to a doctor, no date, AMA files.

[52] "Office Memorandum," US government, William H. Phillips, Inspector, Chief Philadelphia Station, 4.18.46 [Numerous FDA documents are henceforth noted as Office Memorandum.]

[53] Hoxsey deposition, Hoxsey vs. Fishbein et al., No. 3203, 1948, p. 126.

[54] Ibid, p. 126.

[55] Letter from Dr. Clarence Cook Little to Herbert G. Brower, 1.5.49, AMA files.

[56] Letter from Dr. Clarence Cook Little to Herbert G. Brower, 1.19.34, AMA files.

[57] Ibid.

[58] Ibid.

[59] Written Interrogatories, Clarence Cook Little, Witness, by Harry J. Kloppenberg, 1.17.49, AMA files, p. 10.

[60] *JAMA*, Vol. 104, No. 20, 5.18.35, p. 1815.

[61] Letter from Dr. Clarence Cook Little to Oliver Field, AMA Bureau of Investigation, 1.28.48, AMA files.

[62] Letter from Herbert G. Brower to Dr. Clarence Cook Little, 1.3.49, AMA files.

[63] Hoxsey deposition, Hoxsey vs. Fishbein, No. 3203, 11/15-15.48, p. 132.

[64] Office Memorandum, US government, William H. Phillips, Inspector, Chief Philadelphia Station, 4.18.46.

[65] Ibid.

[66] Quoted in Dr. Morris Fishbein, "History of Cancer Quackery," *Perspectives in Biology and Medicine*, vol. 8, pp. 139–66, 1965.

[67] Patricia Spain Ward, "History of BCG," contract report to Office of Technology Assessment (OTA), 6.88, pp. 5–6; George Crile Jr., "Factors Influencing the Spread of Cancer," *Surgery, Gynecology and Obsetetrics*, Vol, 103, pp. 342–52, 9.56.

[68] Hoxsey, op. cit., p. 179.

CHAPTER 5
Gone To Texas—The Medical Wild West

[1] Personal interview.

[2] Sources for this chapter and for the Texas episodes include personal interviews conducted for the *Hoxsey* film from 1984 to 1987 with Robert Heath, James Wakefield Burke, Mildred Nelson, Dr. Harry M. Spence, Hoxsey's son, daughter and third wife; Hoxsey, op. cit., pp. 180–200; Hoxsey deposition, Hoxsey vs. Fishbein et al., N. 3203, pp. 163–76; Dallas County Medical Association files; AMA files; FDA files; numerous public and trial records; miscellaneous sources.

[3] Hoxsey deposition, Hoxsey vs. Fishbein et al., pp. 134–35.

[4] Ibid, p. 134.

[5] Letter from Dr. T. J. Crowe to Council on Medical Education and Hospitals, 4.8.36, AMA files; Spann brochure, 1936, AMA files.

[6] Spann brochure, 1936.

[7] Ibid.

[8] Letter from Mrs. J.B. Whitehead to Dr. R.L. Spann, 4.11.36, AMA files; same for following quotes; FDA report by Inspectors W.F. Breaux and W.B. Robertson, 7.25.47 re Whitehead testimonial, FDA files.

[9] Additional testimony in "Excerpts from Sworn Testimony from Court and U.S. Senator Hearing," Hoxsey Cancer Clinic brochure, c. 1950, pp. 34–37.

[10] Hoxsey, op. cit., pp. 180–81; FDA report by Inspectors W.F. Breaux and W.B. Robertson, 7.25.47 re Whitehead testimonial, FDA files.

[11] Hoxsey, op. cit. p. 181; Bryan & Peak Cancer Clinic brochure, 1936, AMA files.

[12] Hoxsey, op. cit., pp. 181–84.

[13] Ibid, p. 185.

[14] Hoxsey, op. cit., pp. 185–88; story confirmed by interviews with Mildred Nelson and James Martin regarding Templeton's switch to Hoxsey's lawyer.

[15] "Templeton Quits as Patton's Aide, " *Dallas Times Herald*, 3.11.40.

[16] On 3.13.40, the *Dallas Times-Herald* cited Frank Ivey as a prosecutor against Hoxsey ("Cancer Clinic Man Fined $25, Costs"); in July, 1941, both Ivey and Templeton are cited as Hoxsey's attorneys in the *Dallas Morning News* ("Lacks License to be Doctor, State Charges").

[17] "D.A. (Al.) Templeton, Former Judge, Dies," *Dallas Morning News*, 12.8.59.

[18] Hoxsey, op. cit, pp. 191–92, reproduced p. 304.

[19] "Blast by Adoue Stirs Interest in Council Race," *Dallas Morning News*, 3.31.51.

[20] Personal interview.

[21] Hoxsey, op. cit, p. 190–91; Hoxsey deposition, Hoxsey vs. Fishbein et al., No. 3203, p. 184; original cancer pathologies on file from No. 3203, National Archives, Fort Worth, Texas; "Doctor Tells Damage Suit Jury of Prescribing Hoxsey Method," *Dallas Times-Herald*, 5.26.48.

[22] "Cancer Clinic Wins Round in Doctor's Suit," *Dallas Morning News*, 1.4.40.

[23] Hoxsey, op. cit., pp. 194–95.

[24] Ibid, p. 196.

[25] Hoxsey deposition, Hoxsey vs. Fishbein et al., No. 3203, pp. 192–95.

[26] Letter from Hoxsey to Dr. W.W. Fowler, 3.18.41, "Copies of Letters Showing Our Request for Investigation of Our Clinic. Why Don't They Answer or Accept this Challenge?," AMA files.

[27] "Guarded Formula Offered Clinical Association Free," *Dallas Morning News*, 3.13.40.

[28] "Convicted Operator of Clinic Says He'll Run for Governor," *Dallas Morning News*, 11.30.41; "Hoxsey Faces Charges under Medical Act," *Dallas Morning News*, 12.17.41.

[29] Personal interview.

[30] Hoxsey, op. cit, pp. 196–200.

[31] Personal interview.

[32] Cited by Morris Bealle, *Medical Mussolini*, pp. 52–53.

[33] Milton Mayer, "The Rise and Fall of Dr. Fishbein," p. 79.

[34] Ibid, p. 82; Morris Bealle, op. cit., pp. 48–49; ad for *American Home Medical Adviser, American Weekly*, 2.13.49.

[35] Dr. Morris Fishbein, "Quacks and Quackery," speech before Medical Society of the State of New York, 4.29.36.

[36] Milton Mayer, op. cit, p. 76.

[37] Milton Mayer, "The Dogged Retreat of the Doctors," *Harper's Magazine*, Vol. 199, No. 1195, 12.49, pp. 25–37, p. 27); "AMA's Fund Program Shunned by Doctors," *Dallas Times-Herald*, 2.13.49.

[38] Milton Mayer, "The Rise and Fall of Dr. Fishbein," p. 82; Howard Wolinsky and Tom Brune, *The Serpent and the Staff: The Unhealthy Politics of the American Medical Association*, (New York, Jeremy P. Tarcher, Putnam, 1994), pp. 23–24.

[39] Dr. Morris Fishbein, "Quacks and Quackery," *Vital Speeches of the Day*, 6.1.36, pp. 562–64, speech before Medical Society of the State of New York on 4.29.36, University of Chicago Fishbein Papers.

[40] Howard Wolinsky and Tom Brune, op. cit., citing Frank D. Campion, *The AMA and US Health Policy Since 1940* (Chicago: Chicago Review Press, 1984), quoting Wilbur J. Cohen, p. 268.

[41] Morris Fishbein, *The Medical Follies* (New York, Boni and Liveright, 1925) pp. 61 and 98.

[42] Kenny Ausubel and Catherine Salveson, *Hoxsey How Healing Becomes A Crime*, film 1987.

[43] *Conquering of Cancer*, March of Time, Vol. 3, issue 6, 1937; *Men of Medicine*, March of Time, Vol. 4, Issue 11, 1943; *Your Life Is Their Toy*, Warner Bros., 1938, unreleased; *Miracle Money*," MGM, 1938.

[44] *Conquering of Cancer*, 1937.

[45] *Illinois Medical Society Journal*, op. cit.

[46] Mayer, "The Rise and Fall of Dr. Fishbein, pp. 77–78; Bealle, *Medical Mussolini*, pp. 69–71; Morris Bealle, *The Drug Story* (Utah: Hornet's Nest, 1949), pp. 178–79.

[47] Mayer, "The Rise and Fall of Dr. Fishbein," pp. 77–78.

[48] Bealle, *Medical Mussolini*, pp. 80–89.

[49] Ibid, pp. 89–91.

[50] This episide is recounted in: Wolinsky and Brune, op. cit., pp. 144–47; Bealle, *Medical Mussolini*, pp. 92–95.

[51] Bealle, *Medical Mussolini*, p. 93.

[52] "Deaths Following Elixir of Sulfanilamide-Massengill—II," editorial, *JAMA*, Vol. 109, No. 18, 10.30.37, p. 1456.

[53] Wolinsky and Brune, op. cit., p. 159.

[54] Bealle, *Medical Mussolini*, pp. 96–97.

[55] *Conquering of Cancer*, 1937.

CHAPTER 6

Hoxsey vs. the AMA—"Thrice Is He Armed Who Hath His Quarrel Just"

[1] Hoxsey, op. cit., pp. 201–08; "Chronological Data on Harry M. Hoxsey," AMA memo, 2.21.49; letters from R.R. Spencer to Morris Fishbein, 11.19.45, 11.22.45, AMA files.

[2] Ibid (all).

[3] Letters from R.R. Spencer to Morris Fishbein, 10.19,45 and 10.22.45, AMA files.

[4] Letter from Morris Fishbein to R.R. Spencer, 10.24.45, AMA files.

[5] Letter from R.R. Spencer to Hoxsey, 11.14.45; letter from R.W. Braund, USPHS Tumor Clinic, to R.R. Spencer; 12.18.45.

[6] Letter from Marvin Bell to R.R. Braund, USPHS, 12.5.45, AMA files; letter from R.R. Braund to R.R. Spencer, op. cit.; biopsy reports, National Archives, Fort Worth Branch, TX (Hoxsey vs. Fishbein et al., No. 3203).

[7] Letter from Carl Voegtlin, NCI Chief, to W.W. Fowler, Dallas County Medical Society, 7.1.41; Letters from Wilbert Breaux, Inspector FDA Dallas Substation to AMA Bureau of Investigation, 12.11.45 and 12.14.45.

[8] *Dictionary of American Biography*, Supplement Seven, 1961-65; *Biographical Directory of the American Congress*, pp. 1261–62.

[9] Hoxsey, op. cit., pp. 208–12; "Excerpts from Sworn Testimony from Court and U.S. Senator Hearing," Hoxsey Cancer Clinic brochure, c. 1950, pp. 17–58, AMA files; "Excerpts from Transcript of Proceedings Held in Dallas, Texas on Sunday February 2, 1947 at the Hoxsey Cancer Clinic," c. 1948, pp. 13–44; Chapman testimony, p. 42–44, AMA files.

[10] "Excerpts from Transcript of Proceedings Held in Dallas, Texas on Sunday February 2, 1947 at the Hoxsey Cancer Clinic," c. 1948, p. 42.

[11] Ibid.

[12] "Excerpts of Transcripts of Proceedings Held in Dallas, Texas, 2.2.17," In Hoxsey Cancer Clinic brochure, (another edition) c. 1950, p. 41.

[13] "US Officials Asked to Study Reputed 'Cure,'" *Lawton Constitution*, 2.3.47.

[14] "Chronological Data on Harry M. Hoxsey," 2.21.49, AMA files.

[15] Letter from Elmer Thomas to Hoxsey, 6.2.47, AMA files; letter from Elmer Thomas to Surgeon General Thomas Parran, 2.25.47; "Thomas Asks Full Cancer Cure Inquiry," *Tulsa Daily World*, 3.24.47; *Dallas Morning News*, c. 4.47.

[16] Hoxsey, op. cit., pp. 212–13.

[17] Hoxsey, op. cit., pp. 213–16; "Solons Hear Hoxsey Back Cancer Cure Claims," "Solons Flay Medics Over Cancer Probe," *Tulsa Daily World*, no date, c. 1947.

[18] Hoxsey, op. cit., pp. 215–16.

[19] Ibid, p. 216, citing Pauls's speech in the Oklahoma legislature on 4.15.47.

[20] Personal interview.

[21] Hoxsey deposition, Hoxsey vs. Fishbein et al., No. 3203, p. 114 and p. 90.

[22] Personal interview.

[23] W.R. Moses, "Cancer Remedies," FDA Office Memorandum, FDA files, 9.30.47.

[24] Story corroborated in "SWMC Doctor Testifies at Hoxsey Trial," *Dallas Times-Herald*, 5.21.48.

[25] Personal interview.

[26] Hoxsey promotional film, 1957.

[27] *JAMA*, Vol. 133, No. 11, 3.15.47, pp. 774–75.

[28] 44th District Court of Texas, 6.4.48; numerous newspaper clippings including *Dallas Morning News* and *Dallas Times-Herald.*

[29] "Jury Rules Doctor Finds Cancer Cure," *Dallas Morning News*, 6.6.48.

[30] "Jury Favors Hoxsey, Awards No Damages," *Dallas Times-Herald*, 6.4.48.

[31] Personal interview.

[32] Notarized statement of Mrs. Victor A. Gerstenkorn, 8.26.43 AMA files; Richards vs. Hoxsey, 44th District Court of Dallas County, No. 13241-B, 6.4.48.

[33] Morris Fishbein, M.D. and William Engle, "Blood Money," "Medical Hucksters" series, *The American Weekly*, 2.15.48, pp. 22–23.

[34] Hoxsey deposition, Hoxsey vs. Fishbein et al., No. 3203, pp. 243–44.

[35] Hoxsey vs. Morris Fishbein,William Engle, W.R. Hearst Jr., The American Weekly Inc., Hearst Consolidated Publications, Inc. and the American Medical Association, A Coporation, No. 3203, Civil, District Court of the US for the Northern District of Texas, Dallas Division, 1948.

[36] "Angry Voice," *Time* Magazine, 6.16.47.

[37] "Harry M. Hoxsey Is Taking Dr. Fishbein into Courts," *El Sereno News*, 2.29.48.

[38] Mayer, "The Rise and Fall of Dr. Fishbein," pp. 76–84.

[39] Promotional literature for *The Drug Story* and *Medical Mussolini* by Morris Bealle, 1940s.

[40] Letter from William Rankin, *Warner Bros.*, to Morris Fishbein, 1.13.38, University of Chicago Fishbein Papers.

[41] Mayer, "The Rise and Fall of Dr. Fishbein," pp. 83–84; also, "The Dogged Retreat of the Doctors."

[42] American Medical Association vs. United States, 110 F 2d, 703 (1937); American Medical Association vs. United States, 317 US 519 (1943).

[43] "Remedy for Fishbein," *Time*, 7.15.46; Mayer, "The Rise and Fall of Dr. Fishbein," p. 76; "Angry Voice," *Time*, 6.16.47.

[44] Letter from Roy Topper to Walter Howey, editor, *American Weekly*, 12.15.48.

[45] "Notes on an Interview by Pat McGrady Sr. with Harry M. Hoxsey," 8.17.48, AMA files.

[46] Ibid.

[47] Ibid.

[48] *Journal of the National Medical Society*, July-September, 1947.

[49] Wilbur L. Matthews, *San Antonio Lawyer: Memoranda of Cases and Clients* (San Antonio, TX: Corona Publishing, 1983), p. 119.

[50] Hoxsey vs. Fishbein et al., No. 3203, for following sequence.

[51] "Witnesses Say Hoxsey Cured Them," *Dallas Morning News*, 3.17.49.

[52] Hoxsey vs. Fishbein et al., No. 3203; "Hoxsey Ordered to Reveal Secret," *Dallas Times-Herald*, 1.4.49; "Hoxsey Told to Disclose Secret Cure," *Dallas Morning News*, 1.4.49.

[53] Also in Federal Supplement, Vol. 83, pp. 282–84.

[54] Personal interview.

[55] Rupert Sheldrake, "How Widely Is Blind Assessment Used in Scientific Research?" *Alternative Therapies in Health and Medicine Journal*, Vol. 5, No. 3, 5.99, pp. 88–91.

[56] Personal interview.

[57] "Hoxsey Takes Stand in Trial," *Dallas Times-Herald*, 3.17.49; "Witnesses Say Hoxsey Cured Them," *Dallas Morning News*, 3.17.49; testimony also in Hoxsey Cancer Clinic brochure, c. 1950, pp. 50–52.

[58] Personal interview.

[59] AMA files contain numerous documents, including: critiques of all alleged cured cases; interviews with Dr. Mason, Dr. Cutler, Dr. Simmons, Dr. Grollman; analyisis of Hoxsey formulas.

[60] Personal interview.

[61] "Hoxsey Cancer Treatment," Central District, FDA memorandum, 6.21.48; "Re: Dr. C.E. Von Hoover," 65381-3-E, Chief New Orleans Station, FDA memo, 8.29.43.

[62] "Certified Copy of a Record of Death," AMA files; letter from R.H. Woodruff to Oliver Field, 9.16.48, AMA files; letter from G.E. Hill to Arthur J. Cramp, 12.21.25; memo from Oliver Field, 9.7.48; "No. 18, John Hoxsey, AMA files; "John C. Hoxsey," AMA files.

[63] "The Hoxide Cancer 'Cure'," *JAMA*, Vol. 86, No. 1. p. 55.

[64] Hoxsey, op. cit., pp. 234–35; letter from Hoxsey to Oliver Field, 6.6.53; letter from Wilmer A. Rowen, Texas State Board of Medical Examiners, to Olin West, AMA, 2.26.37; letter from G.E. Hill to Arthur J. Cramp, 12.21.25.

[65] Hoxsey deposition, Hoxsey vs. Fishbein et al., No. 3203, pp. 221–28.

[66] Personal interviews, Mildred Nelson and Hoxsey's son; "Hoxsey Given $2 Damages in Libel Lawsuit," *Dallas Morning News*, 3.19.49.

[67] Letter from Morris Fishbein to Dr. Ed Cary, 11.12.48, Dallas County Medical Society files.

[68] Hoxsey vs. Fishbein et al., No. 3203; Hoxsey, op. cit., pp. 235–36.

[69] Personal interview.

[70] Hoxsey, op. cit., p. 236–37.

[71] Hoxsey vs. Fishbein et al., No. 3203, verdict 3.18.49; Federal Supplement, Vol. 83, pp. 282–84.

[72] Inspector Frank McKinlay, "Appearance of Harry M. Hoxsey on Television (KCOP) Program," FDA memorandum, 7.14.57, p. 3; W.L. Prillmayer, "Hoxsey Cancer Treatment," FDA memorandum, 6.18.58.

[73] Mayer, "The Rise and Fall of Dr. Fishbein," pp. 76–77.

[74] Harry Hoxsey vs. Morris Fishbein, No. 31011-B in the District Court 44th Judicial District, Dallas County, Texas, 4.52; Judgement, 7.21.52; Hoxsey, op. cit., pp. 238–43. For technical reasons, Hoxsey attached Millard Heath, secretary of the Dallas County Medical Association (Robert Heath's father), to the complaint, even though he had no part in "Blood Money," and exulted in turning the tables on his sworn local enemy.

[75] Personal interview.

[76] K.L. Milstead, "Hoxsey Medications," FDA memorandum, St. Louis District, 9.24.56.

[77] Letter from Hoxsey to FDA Commissioner George C. Larrick, 5.4.56; *Defender*, 8.56.

[78] Hoxsey, op. cit., p. 240; *Defender* 8.56.

[79] Hoxsey, op. cit., p. 241; Hoxsey vs. Fishbein et al., No. 3203; testimony reproduced in "New Cures for Old Ailments, *Defender Publications*, c. 1953, pp. 117–22; Bealle, *Medical Mussolini*, p. 61; Bealle, *The Drug Story*, p. 172; letter from George H. Simmons to Morris Fishbein hiring him as assistant editorial staff, 8.21.13, University of Chicago Fishbein Papers.

[80] Harry Hoxsey vs. Morris Fishbein, No. 31011-B in the District Court 44th Judicial District, Dallas County, Texas, 4.52; Judgement, 7.21.52.

[81] Ibid (Judgement); Hoxsey, op. cit., pp. 241–42; "Rules Fishbein Libeled Cancer Clinic Operator," *Chicago Tribune*, 8.10.52; reproduced in "New Cures for Old Ailments," *Defender Publications*, pp. 122–23.

[82] Personal interview.

[83] "The Great Humiliation," *Time*, 8.9.54; "Texas Quackdown," *Time*, 12.16.57; "Things Get Hotter for Hoxsey," *Life*, 4.16.56; "Hoxsey and His 'Cure'," *Life*, 4.23.56.

[84] "Former Editor Dr. Morris Fishbein Dies," *JAMA* Vol. 236, No. 16, 10.18.76.

[85] Mayer, "The Rise and Fall of Dr. Fishbein," p. 77.

[86] Ibid, p. 81.

CHAPTER 7
Uncle Sam's Quackdown—"A Conspiracy Against the Health of the Nation"

[1] Letter from Hoxsey to J.R. Heller, Director NCI, 6.6.50.

[2] "Summation by Harry M. Hoxsey of Pathologies Submitted by Him to the

National Cancer Institute; with Discussion of the Essential Evidence," 11.2.50, pp. 5–6, AMA files.

[3] Letters from: G.A. Granger, Acting Medical Director FDA, to R.R. Spencer, NCI Chief, 8.18.47; Leonard Scheele, NCI Director, to G.A. Granger, FDA, 8.22.47; Leonard Scheele, NCI, to Harry Hoxsey, 8.22.47; G.A. Granger, FDA, to Oliver Field, AMA; Inspector W.F. Breaux, Dallas FDA substation, "Hoxsey Cancer Treatment," 7.7.50.

[4] Letters including: J.R. Heller, NCI Director, to Harry M. Hoxsey, 8.14.50, 10.13.50, 11.1.50, FDA files.

[5] Gilcin F. Meadors, Chief of Technical Services, NCI, "List of Patients Treated at the Hoxsey Clinic," US Public Health Service memorandum to Gilbert S. Goldhammer, FDA, 7.20.50.

[6] US vs. Hoxsey Cancer Clinic et al., Civ. No. 4144, District Court of the US, Northern District of Texas, Dallas Division, 12.21.50; Hoxsey, op. cit, pp. 246–56.

[7] Letter from Surgeon General Leonard Scheele to Harry Hoxsey, 11.24.50, FDA files.

[8] John L. Harvey, "Cancer Cure," Division of Regulatory Management, Kansas City, New Orleans, St. Louis, Chicago and Denver Districts, 4.4.50.

[9] Inspector W.F. Breaux to G.S. Goldhammer, FDA memorandum, 7.7.50.

[10] "Abstracts of 'Tests' and 'Cures'," Committee on Cancer Diagnosis and Therapy, National Research Council, 2.1.51: "Hoxsey 'Cure' for Cancer," pp. 1–2.

[11] Letter from G.A. Granger, Acting Medical Director FDA, to Dr. Clarence Cook Little, 7.5.50, FDA files.

[12] Richard Carter, *The Gentle Legions* (Garden City, NY: Doubleday, 1961) pp. 151–59; Ralph Moss, *The Cancer Industry* (Brooklyn, NY: Equinox Press, 1996), pp. 401–02.

[13] Trial record, US vs. Hoxsey Cancer Clinic et al., Civ. No. 4144, District Court of the US, Northern District of Texas, Dallas Division, 12.21.50; "Summation by Harry M. Hoxsey of Pathologies Submitted by Him to the National Cancer Institute; with Discussion of the Essential Evidence," 11.2.50, pp. 4–5 AMA files; "Dr. Hoxsey Answers 'Time'," *Defender*, 9.54.

[14] "An Examination of the Claims of the Hoxsey Cancer Clinic," *The Review and Herald*, Vol. 133, Nos. 50, 51, 12.13.56 and 12.20.56, pp. 2–3.

[15] US vs. Hoxsey Cancer Clinic, Civ. No. 4144, Judgement, 12.21.50; Federal Supplement, Vol. 94, pp. 464–68; "Judge Atwell Upholds Hoxsey Cancer Remedy," *Dallas Morning News*, 12.22.50.

[16] "Comment on Court Opinion that Internal Cancer Can Be Cured with Medicine," *JAMA*, Vol. 145, No. 4, 1.27.51.

[17] US vs. Hoxsey Cancer Clinic et al., No. 13645, US Court of Appeals, Fifth Circuit, 7.31.52; Federal Reporter (Second Series), Vol. 198, pp. 273–81; Hoxsey, op. cit., pp. 258–60.

[18] "Atwell Told To Change His Decree," *Dallas Morning News*, 10.28.53.

[19] Robert G. Houston, *Repression and Reform in the Evaluation of Alternative Cancer Therapies* (Washington DC: Project Cure, Inc. 1987), pp. 53–54, p. 56.

[20] US vs. Hoxsey Cancer Clinic and Harry M. Hoxsey, In the District Court of the US for the Northern District of Texas, Dallas Division, No. 4144 Civil, 6.29.53.

[21] In the US Court of Appeals for the Fifth Circuit, No. 14690, Petition for a Writ of Mandamus, 10.22.53.

[22] "Atwell Told To Change His Decree," *Dallas Morning News*, 10.28.53.

[23] Hoxsey Cancer Clinic vs. USA, US Court of Appeals, Fifth Circuit, No 14870, 5.14.54; Federal Reporter (2nd Series), Vol. 212, p. 439.

[24] Letter from J.R. Heller, NCI Director, to C.W. Crawford, FDA Commissioner, 11.5.53, FDA files.

[25] Hoxsey, op. cit, pp. 258–64.

[26] "Factory Inspection Report," E.C. Boudreaux, FDA Chief New Orleans District, Inspector W.L Prillmayer, Gordon A. Granger, Division of Regulatory Management, 3.1.54.

[27] Dwight L. Simmons, "Memorandum re: Hoxsey vs. Fishbein," 12.21.48, pp. 2 and 5; "The Amazing Story of the Hoxsey War against Cancer," *Defender*, 11.53 (*Tiempo* article published in Mexico 9.7.53); "Luncheon Program," Adolphus Hotel Palm Garden, Junior Chamber of Commerce invitation re Dr. Durkee, including work with National Medical College in Mexico City, 7.28.48; letter from Hospital Superintendent, Hospital Nuevo Laredo, Mexico, to Hoxsey Cancer Foundation, 2.20.48, AMA files; Bealle, *The Drug Story*, pp. 96–97; Hoxsey deposition, Hoxsey vs. Fishbein et al., No. 3203, p. 181.

[28] "Factory Inspection Report," E.C. Boudreaux, FDA Chief New Orleans District, Inspector W.L Prillmayer, Gordon A. Granger, Division of Regulatory Management, 3.1.54.

[29] "Mr. Hoxsey Has A Setback," *JAMA*, Vol. 150, No. 1, 9.6.52.

[30] S. Res. 142, 5.22.51, 82nd Congress; S. Res. 186, 8.6.51, 82nd Congress.

[31] "Abstracts of 'Tests' and 'Cures'," Committee on Cancer Diagnosis and Therapy, National Research Council, 2.1.51; letter from L.T. Coggeshall to John H. Teeter, American Cancer Society, 2.15.49.

[32] *Krebiozen: Thirteen Years of Conflict*, David Wolper Productions, TV movie 1963; Herbert Bailey, *A Matter of Life and Death* (New York: MacFadden Books, 1964); Herbert Bailey, *K*Krebiozen—Key to Cancer?* (New York: Hermitage House, 1955).

[33] Oliver Field, AMA Bureau of Investigation memo to Dr. Fishbein and Dr. Smith, 10.14.48, AMA files.

[34] Dr. Andrew Ivy, "Notes: On a Visit to the Hoxsey 'Cancer Clinic' at Dallas, Texas, Thursday, February 10, 1949," in "Abstracts of 'Tests' and 'Cures'," Committee on Cancer Diagnosis and Therapy, National Research Council, 2.1.51.

[35] Ibid.

[36] Letter from L.T. Coggeshall to John H. Teeter, American Cancer Society, 2.15.49; "Abstracts of 'Tests' and 'Cures'," Committee on Cancer Diagnosis and Therapy, National Research Council, 2.1.51.

[37] For in-depth history of Krebiozen: "Krebiozen: Thirteen Years of Conflict," David Wolper Productions/TIMEX, TV movie 1963; Herbert Bailey, *A Matter of Life and Death* (New York: MacFadden Books, 1964); Herbert Bailey, *K* Krebiozen—Key to Cancer?*, (New York: Hermitage House, 1955; Nat Morris, *The Cancer Blackout*, (Los Angeles: Regent House, 1977), pp. 156–82; A.C. Ivy, John S. Pick and W.F.P Phillips, *Observations on Krebiozen in the Management of Cancer* (Chicago: Henry Regnery Company, 1956).

[38] Nat Morris, op. cit., pp. 168–69.

[39] "Ivy, Koch and Lincoln," *Defender*, 4.52.

[40] *Krebiozen: Thirteen Years of Conflict*, op. cit.

[41] Council on Pharmacy and Chemistry, "A Status Report on Krebiozen," *JAMA*, Vol. 147, No. 9, 10.27.51, pp. 864–73.

[42] Nat Morris, op. cit. p. 173.

[43] "Krebiozen: Thirteen Years of Conflict," op. cit.

[44] Personal interview.

[45] For in-depth history and explanation of the Koch treatment: Morris, op. cit, pp. 73–86.; William F. Koch, *The Survival Factor in Neoplastic and Viral Diseases: An Introduction to Carbonyl and Free Radical Therapy*, (Detroit: Vanderkloot Press); William F. Koch, *The Functional Carbonyl Group in Pathogenesis and Its Reversal*, (Solana Beach: International Association of Cancer Victims and Friends, 1967); William F. Koch, *Neoplastic and Vial Parasitism*, (Rio de Janeiro, Brazil: self-published c. 1962); William F. Koch, *Cancer and Allied Diseases* (Detroit: self-published, 1933); Albert L. Wahl, Bessie L. Rehwinkel, Lawrence Reilly, *The Birth of a Science* (Detroit: Lutheran Research Society, 1949); Gerald F. Winrod, *The Koch Treatment* (Wichita: Defenders of the Christian Faith, no date, c. 1951).

[46] Morris, op. cit. pp. 78–81; also see Otto Warburg, *The Prime Cause and Prevention of Cancer*, (Wurtzburg, Germany: Konrad Triltsch, 1969), English Edition by Dean Burk, National Cancer Institute, revised lecture at the meeting of the Nobel Laureates on 6.30.66 at Lindau, Lake Constance, Germany.

[47] Reilly, op. cit.

[48] "The Koch Treatment," *Defender*, 6.48.

[49] Bealle, *The Drug Story*, pp. 43–44 and 93–94; "Ivy, Koch and Lincoln," *Defender*, 4.52.

[50] Wallace F. Janssen, "Cancer Quackery—The Past in the Present," reprint from FDA, 1979.

[51] Wahl, Rehwinkel and Reilly, *The Birth of a Science*, title page; *Journal of the American Association of Physicians*, Vol. 1, No. 2, 8.15.51, p. 6.

[52] Wahl et al., *The Birth of a Science;* "Program of the Christian Medical Research League Anoounced," *Defender,* 9.50; "Dr. Swain's Keynote Address," *Defender,* 11.51; "Annual Convention of Koch Doctors," *Defender,* 8.50; "Medical League Convention a Success," *Defender,* 10.50.

[53] "Program of the Christian Medical Research League Announced," *Defender,* 9.50.

[54] Houston, op. cit., p. 19; Albert Szent-Gyorgyi, *Electronic Biology and Cancer* (New York: Marcel Dekker, 1976), p. 95.

[55] Personal interview, 1984.

[56] Nat Morris, op. cit. pp. 103–13; "Ivy, Koch and Lincoln," *Defender,* 4.52.

[57] Morris, op. cit. p. 111.

[58] Ibid, p. 109.

[59] Ibid, p. 109.

[60] Charles Tobey Jr., "Charles Tobey Jr. Reports on Cancer and the Venal Medical Conspiracy," as reported in *Exposé* magazine, 5.53, and reprinted variously also as "Charles Tobey Jr. on Cancer" and "Is Cancer Curable?" (California: Health Research c. 1954).

[61] "FitzGerald Well Fitted to Investigate Issues," *Union Press-Courier,* 7.8.54; "'Bloodshed' Predicted By Haluska," *Portage Dispatch,* 7.1.54; "Memorandum of Telephone Conversation," between Senator Walker, Idaho, and Gordon Granger, FDA, 7.27.55, FDA files; Hoxsey, op. cit., pp. 293–98.

[62] Benedict FitzGerald, "A Report by Special Counsel for a US Senate Investigating Committee Making a Fact-Finding Study of a Conspiracy against the Health of the American People," aka, "A Report to the Senate Interstate Commerce Committee on the Need for Investigation of Cancer Research Organizations," *Congressional Record,* Vol 99, Part 12, pp. 4045–52, 83rd Congress, 1st Session, 7.2.53-8.28.53.

[63] Letter from Benedict FitzGerald to Senator William Langer, 9.21.53, reprinted as "Benedict FitzGerald's Second Senate Report," *Defender,* 10.53; William Kullgren, "Is Cancer Curable? FitzGerald Report Plus," 1954, report and letter from FitzGerald to Senator Bricker, 8.11.53; Charles Tobey Jr., "Charles Tobey Jr. Reports on Cancer and the Venal Medical Conspiracy," as reported in *Exposé* magazine, 5.53, and reprinted variously also as "Charles Tobey Jr. on Cancer" and "Is Cancer Curable?" (California: Health Research c. 1954); Hoxsey, op. cit., pp. 293–98;"Dr. Hoxsey's Closing Chapter," *Defender,* 3.56.

[64] Letter from Oliver Field, AMA, to Dr, Carl A. Phetteplace, 11.15.54, AMA files.

[65] Letter from Benedict FitzGerald to Senator William Langer, 9.21.53, reprinted as "Benedict FitzGerald's Second Senate Report," *Defender,*10.53.

[66] Ibid.

[67] Tobey Jr., "Charles Tobey Jr. Reports on Cancer and the Venal Medical Conspiracy."

[68] Alex Jack, "The War on Cancer: Another Vietnam?" reprinted in *Cancer Control Journal*, Vol. 5, No. 3/4, p. 117.

[69] Letter fom Oliver Field to Dr. Carl A. Phetterplace, 11.15.54, AMA files; "Tragedy in Maine," pamphlet, c. 1954; "FitzGerald Well Fitted to Investigate Issues," *Union Press-Courier*, 7.8.54.

[70] "The American Medical Association: Power, Purpose, and Politics in Organized Medicine," *The Yale Law Journal*, Vol. 63, No. 7, 5.54, pp. 938–1022.

CHAPTER 8
Twelve Thousand Patients in Dallas—"You Couldn't Run Me Out of Here with a Gatling Gun"

[1] "Ten Doctors Declare 'Quack' Cures Cancer," Hoxsey press release, 4.12.54.

[2] Inspector A.E. Ledder, "Hoxsey Medicines," FDA memorandum, 6.21.55; memo from R.M.S., AMA, in Oliver Field's AMA files, 8.18.54.

[3] Allen Bernard, "*Man's Magazine* Investigates a Cure for Cancer," *Man's Magazine*, 8.55; Bernard, "I Conquered Cancer," *Man's Magazine*, 8.54, includes introduction re 15,000 letters; "An Important Message," *Man's Magazine*, 10.54; "Latest on the Hoxsey Cancer Clinic," *Man's Magazine*, 12.54.

[4] Harry M. Hoxsey, "I Cure Cancer," *Male* magazine, 12.53; *Sir* magazine, no date, c. 1953.

[5] "The Great Humiliation," *Time*, 8.9.54.

[6] Personal interview (all following).

[7] Personal interview.

[8] "Investigator's Report on Harry M. Hoxsey's Cancer Clinic," attached to letter from Joseph E. Blum, Executive Director Washington Division American Cancer Society, to Mefford R. Runyon, American Cancer Society New York, 4.9.49, AMA files.

[9] W.L. Prillmayer, "Confidential" FDA memorandum to Chief, New Orleans District, 4.13.54.

[10] Personal interview.

[11] "Findings of the Ten Doctors Who Investigated the Facilities, Procedure and Treatment at the Hoxsey Cancer Clinic," Press Release, 4.10-11.54; individual letters from each doctor attached to letter from Oliver Field, AMA, to Dr. John Repasky, who sent them to the Bureau of Investigation, 8.26.54, AMA files.

[12] Letter from Oliver Field, AMA to Delos Smith, Science Editor, United Press Associations, 4.15.54.

[13] Letter from Delos Smith to John Bach, AMA, 4.13.54.

[14] Letter from Oliver Field, AMA, to Delos Smith, Science Editor, United Press Associations, 4.15.54.

[15] Unattributed editorial in the "Current Comments" column, "Accuracy in Medical News," *JAMA*. Vol. 114, No. 3, 1.20.40, p. 252.

[16] Tom Duggan show, KCOP-TV, 8.3.56; Paul Coates, *Confidential File*, TV show, including letter from Albert Holland Jr., Medical Director, Bureau of Medicine, to American Cancer Society re reviewing from "factual viewpoint"; letter from Oliver Field to Clifton R. Read, American Cancer Society, 3.14.58 re Coates show; letter from George Lull to Dr. Lafe Ludwig re Oliver Field's efforts to block Hoxsey on TV, 7.21.57; memo from Oliver Field re multiple calls to Los Angeles TV stations Channel 13 and KCOP to prevent Hoxsey's appearances, 7.18.57.

[17] Irwin B. Berch, Acting Chief, FDA Los Angeles District, memorandum, 7.17.57.

[18] Letter from Oliver Field, AMA, to Delos Smith, Science Editor, United Press Associations, 4.23.54.

[19] The *Defender* archives yielded extensive documentation including complete back issues of *Defender* magazine, radio broadcast audiotapes, and numerous books, pamphlets and miscellaneous flyers and other publications. Also, see G.H. Montogomery, *Gerald Burton Winrod* (Wichita: Mertmont Publishers,, 1965); *Amazing History of the Defenders of the Christian Faith*, (Wichita: Defenders of the Christian Faith, 1966).

[20] Gerald Winrod, *Defenders of the Christian Faith* radio broadcast, c. 1955 (featured in *Hoxsey* film).

[21] "Hoxsey Cancer Treatment," Inspector Frank McKinlay, Los Angeles District, FDA memorandum, transcript of XERB radio broadcast by Gerald Winrod, 10.21.57.

[22] Hon. John D. Dingell, "Statement About the Hoxsey Cancer Treatment," in the House of Representatives, 3.7.57, *Congressional Record*, Appendix, 3.7.57, A1857.

[23] Will Chasan and Victor Riesel, "Keep Them Out! The Reverend Gerald B. Winrod," *The Nation*, 7.4.43; Roy Tozier, "Mr. Dies Kills an Investigation," *The New Republic*, 4.22.40; "Gerald Winrod Dies; Called 'Kansas Hitler,'" *NY World Telegram and Sun*, 11.12.57.

[24] *Defender*, no date, c. 1954.

[25] *Defender*, 7.50.

[26] Inspector Frank McKinlay, "Hoxsey Cancer Clinic (Public Offer to Prospective Patients per Radio XERB)," transcript of Winrod radio broadcasts, FDA memo, 10.21.57.

[27] W.L. Prillmayer, "Hoxsey," FDA memorandum, 4.13.54; Eugene Spivak, Dallas Inspector, "Inj. 32-A," excerpts from Hoxsey deposition, Texas State Board of Medical Examiners vs. Harry M. Hoxsey et al., in the District Court, Dallas County, Texas, 134th judicial District, file no. 22,873-G, 6.5.57, 6.26.57, p. 33; Inspector Eugene Spivak, "Inj.232-A" abstracted from depositions of Harry M. Hoxsey et al., 6.26.57, p. 33; Wallace F. Janssen, "Facts, Fancy, and Corruption

in the Interpretation of Science to the Public," Linsly R. Williams Memorial Lecture in the 24th Series, Lectures to the Laity, delivered to New York Academy of Medicine, NY, NY, 11.5.58, reprinted as article by FDA.

[28] W.L. Prillmayer, "Inj. 232," confidential FDA memorandum, 5.12.54.

[29] Janssen, "Cancer Quackery—The Past in the Present," p. 530.

[30] "Report on Background of Harry M. Hoxsey and Hoxsey Cancer Clinic," FDA, 8.52; G.S Goldhammer, "Inj. 311," FDA memorandum, 5.7.57.

[31] Letter from George Larrick to Congressman Minshall's office, 7.15.57.

[32] Letter from James A. Powell to Honorable Porter Hardy Jr., 5.20.57, FDA files.

[33] Ibid.

[34] Letter from George P. Larrick to Congressman Porter, 5.31.57.

[35] Personal interview.

[36] Numerous references including: G.S. Goldhammer, Division of Regulatory Management, "Inj. 231," FDA memorandum, 5.7.57; Eugene Spivak, Dallas Resident Inspector, "Inj. 232-A," FDA memorandum, 7.23.57.

[37] Allen Bernard, "I Conquered Cancer," *Man's Magazine*, 8.54.

[38] "Hospital Battle Traced to Senator's Sister," *The Pittsburgh Press*, 6.28.54; "Story Haluska Told Legislature About Sister Called Untrue," *Pittsburgh Post-Gazette*, 10.19.56; "Haluska Claim of Cancer Cure for Sister Hit," *Johnstown Tribune-Democrat*, 10.19.56.

[39] Senator John J. Haluska, "As I see It," *Union Press-Courier*, 8.12.54; "Haluska and Hoxsey to Inspect County Clinic Sites," "Portage to get Hoxsey Clinic," *Union Press-Courier*, 11.11.54.

[40] Letter from Cambria County Medical Society to Senator William F. Langer, printed in *Union Press-Courier*, 2.25.54.

[41] Senator John J. Haluska, "Doctors Back Investigation; Will Make Trip to Texas," *Union Press-Courier*, 4.8.54; Allen Bernard, "I Conquered Cancer," *Man's Magazine*, offers to pay for doctors's trip for investigation.

[42] "Dr. Hoxsey's Closing Chapter," *Defender*, 3.56.

[43] "Harry Hoxsey and His Cancer Clinic," *Time*, 8.9.54.

[44] "Senator Haluska's Great Speech," *Defender*, edited from *Legislative Journal of the Commonwealth of Pennsylvania*, 2.7.55.

[45] Ibid.

[46] "Haluska Severs All Connections with Hospital," *Cleveland Plain Dealer*, 7.23.54; "Cash Price Set for Haluska to Quit, Doctors Say," *Cleveland Plain Dealer*, c. 7.54; "US Agents Raid Hoxsey Cancer Clinic," *Pittsburgh Post-Gazette*, 3.26.55.

[47] "Announce Dr. Newton C. Allen Will Direct Hoxsey Clinic in this County," "Portage to Get Hoxsey Clinic," *Portage Dispatch*, 11.11.54.

[48] "Hoxsey Cheered as Hero in Cambria Towns," *The Pittsburgh Press*, 6.30.54; photos in *Portage Dispatch*, 6.10.54.

[49] "Hoxsey in Person—Exclusive Interview," *Portage Dispatch*, 6.10.54.

[50] Ibid. FDA letter to Larry B. Johnson, 8.10.56, showing Hoxsey licensed as a naturopath in Texas in 1949; Paul Coates, *Confidential File* TV show, transcript, p. 6.

[51] "Hoxsey in Person—Exclusive Interview," *Portage Dispatch*, 6.10.54.

[52] "Defends Naturopaths," re Benedict FitzGerald, news release 9.10.57, reprinted in *Defender*, no date; "Naturopathic Physicians Persecuted in South Carolina," *Defender*, 9.55; "Texas Quackdown," *Time*, 12.16.57.

[53] Harry M. Hoxsey, "Medical Dictatorship in This Country," pamphlet, c. 1957.

[54] "'Cancer Clinic' Director Lacks Medical License," *Pittsburgh Press*, 3.6.55.

[55] "US Raids Hoxsey Cancer Clinic," *Pittsburgh Post-Gazette*, 3.26.55.

[56] US vs. Hoxsey Cancer Clinic, Federal District Court in Pittsburgh, Civil No. 13251.

[57] "The Hoxsey Clinic Raid," editorial, *Union Press-Courier*, 3.31.55.

[58] Inspector Carl. R. Baeuerlen, "Drugs," FDA memorandum, 3.30.55.

[59] Ibid.

[60] "Hoxsey Clinic's Doctor Arrested," *Pittsburgh Sun-Telegraph*, 4.2.55; "Cancer Clinic Set to Open as Usual," "Clinic Chief Lacks MD License," local Pennsylvania clippings from AMA files, no citation or date, c. 4.2.55; John J. Haluska, "Senator Haluska's Statement," *Defender*, 6.55.

[61] FDA memo from FDA Commissioner George Larrick, "Harry Hoxsey's Worthless Cancer Cure—Public Warning against Use," 1954; "Public Warning," widely published, e.g. *Today's Health*, 7.56; Wallace F. Janssen, "Facts, Fancy and Corruption in the Interpretation of Science to the Public," speech/article delivered to the New York Academy of Medicine, NY, NY 11.5.58, pp. 7–8; Janssen, "Enhancement of Public Protection Through Public Information," speech/article, to Central Atlantic States Association of Food and Drug Officials, NY, NY 5.24.62; Gordon G. Thompson, FDA memo 8.10.57; Thomas Brown, "Hoxsey Warning Posters," FDA memo, 7.9.57; "US Hits Hoxsey on Cancer Clinic," *New York Times*, 4.5.56.

[62] Personal interview.

[63] National Consumers Committee for Research and Education, "Consumer Activists: They Made a Difference," Consumers Union Foundation, Mount Vernon, NY, c. 1.83.

[64] FDA Public Warning poster, 1.57, under section 705(b) of the Federal Food, Drug and Cosmetic Act, 21 USCA, 375(b).

[65] *F-D-C Reports, Drugs and Cosmetics*, 8.27.56.

[66] Letter from Gordon Granger, FDA, to Oliver Field, AMA, 1.24.57.

[67] Leo E. Brown "Food and Drug Administration," FDA memorandum, 3.29.57.

[68] Letter from Janssen to Fishbein, 10.20.63.

[69] Wallace F. Janssen, "Enhancement of Public Protection Through Public Information," reprint of speech to Central Atlantic States Association of Food and Drug Officials, 5.24.62.

[70] Telegram from Janssen to Ausubel, 3.27.86.

[71] W.L. Prillmayer, "Warning Release," FDA memorandum, 4.6.56.

[72] W.L. Prillmayer, "Warning Release," FDA memorandum, 4.6.56; letter from Hoxsey to George Larrick, FDA Commissioner, 5.4.56.

[73] "US Hits Hoxsey on Cancer Clinic," *New York Times*, 4.5.56.

[74] Inspector Frank McKinlay, "Appearance of Harry M. Hoxsey on Television (KCOP) Program," FDA memorandum, 7.14.57, report on Dan Lundberg TV program where Hoxsey claimed 12,000 patients.

[75] Inspector Frank McKinlay, "Appearance of Harry M. Hoxsey on Television (KCOP) Program," FDA memorandum, 7.14.57, p. 2; Hoxsey promotional film, 1957.

[76] Personal interview.

[77] Inspector Frank McKinlay, Chief Los Angeles Division, "Hoxsey Cancer Treatment (New Outlet in Los Angeles)," FDA memorandum, 10.14.57; "A Call to Prayer," *Defender*, 8.55.

[78] "Mrs. Smith Writes Her Congressman," *Defender*, 5.8.57; "Petition Crusade Gathers Force," *Defender*, 1956; "The Hoxsey petition Crusade," *Defender*, 1956; "Letters to Larrick," *Defender*, 7.56.

[79] Hoxsey Cancer Clinic vs. Marion B. Folsom, Secretary, Department of Health Eduction and Welfare and George P. Larrick, Commissioner, FDA, Civil Action No, 1688–57, US District Court, District of Columbia, 10.11.57; Federal Supplement, Vol. 155, pp. 376–78; Federal Judge Alexander Holstzhoff, 10.11.57; Letter from Wallace Janssen to Morris Fishbein, 10.20.61.

[80] Personal interview.

[81] "Hoxsey Set to Run for Governor," *Dallas Morning News*, 4.10.56; "Hoxsey Eying Governor Bid," *Dallas Times-Herald*, 4.10.56.

[82] Mildred Nelson, personal interview; also, documentation in AMA and FDA files on Hoxsey clinics in: Arkansas, California (2), Colorado, Kansas, Louisiana, Michigan, Missouri, New Mexico, Oklahoma, Pennsylvania, Texas.

CHAPTER 9
Endgame—The Government "Liquidates" Hoxsey

[1] William Goodrich, court record, John J. Haluska, "Haluska Charges FDA Agents and Attorneys as Publicity Hounds," 8.22.57, FDA files.

[2] Letter from Dr. C.L. Palmer, Chairman of The Medical Society of the State of Pennsylvania to Oliver Field, AMA Bureau *of Investigation*, 11.8.56; "Case Against Hoxsey Cancer Clinic Opened," *Chicago Daily Tribune*, 10.10.56.

[3] "Expert Says Hoxsey Pills Only Laxative," *Johnstown Tribune-Democrat*, 10.13.56; *The Pittsburgh Trial*, (Wichita: Defender Publications, 1956).

[4] "Expert Says Hoxsey Pills Only Laxative," *Johnstown Tribune-Democrat*, 10.13.56; "Posing Patient Tells of Clinic," *Johnstown Tribune-Democrat*, 10.16.56; "Hoxsey Cancer Diagnosis Told by US Agent," *Chicago Daily Tribune*, 10.12.56; "Masquerading Agent Tells of 'Cancer Cure'," *Johnstown Tribune-Democrat*, 10.12.56; Dr. Harry M. Spence, personal interview; Judge Miller, "Opinion and Order," US vs. Hoxsey Cancer Clinic, Civil No. 13251, FDC No. 37908, 5.28.57.

[5] Letter, from John H. Teeter, Damon Runyon Memorial Fund, to Oliver Field, AMA, 4.1057; Memo from John H. Teeter, 5.23.57, FDA files; FDA memo from Goldhammer to William Prillmayer, 10.24.57.

[6] *The Pittsburgh Trial*, Dr. Harry K. Hill, testimony, pp. 72–76 and Dr. Eva Esther Hill, pp. 77–81.

[7] Dr. Harry M. Spence, personal interview; *The Pittsburgh Trial*; Inspector W.L. Prillmayer, "Inj. 232-A," FDA memorandum, 12.29.56, pp. 4–5.

[8] Original testimony in "Cancer Research," Hearings before a Subcommittee of the Committee on Foreign Relations, US Senate, 79th Congress, Second Session on S. 1875, Senator Claude Pepper, 7.1-3.46, pp. 116–20.

[9] Judge Miller, "Opinion and Order," US vs. Hoxsey Cancer Clinic, Civil No. 13251, FDC No. 37908, 5.28.57.

[10] Inspector Louis E. Buckley, Chief Buffalo District, "Visit to Dr. George Miley," FDA memorandum, 5.31.56.

[11] Trial record, US vs. Hoxsey Cancer Clinic, Federal District Court in Pittsburgh, Civil No. 13251; *The Pittsburgh Trial*, p. 19–36 including reproduction of Riemann testimony.

[12] Inspector Louis E. Buckley, Chief Buffalo District, "Visit to Dr. George Miley," FDA memorandum, 5.31.56.

[13] Reprint of letter from Senator Claude Pepper to Dr. Riemann, government exhibit 152, p. 117 trial record, *The Pittsburgh Trial*, Defender publications, 12.56, p. 35.

[14] Judge John L. Miller, Oral Charge of the Court, 11.15.56, trial record, op. cit., reprinted in *The Pittsburgh Trial*, pp. 37–57.

[15] *The Charlatan*, General Electric Theater, CBS TV; *The Pittsburgh Trial*, pp. 9–10; *TV Guide*, 11.11.56.

[16] US vs. Hoxsey Cancer Clinic, Civil No. 13251, 11.15.56; George Larrick, FDA Commissioner, "Report on Legal Actions Against the Hoxsey Cancer Treatment," FDA, US Dept of Health, Education and Welfare; "Facts Regarding the Hoxsey Cancer Treatment," FDA, Dept of Health, Education and Welfare, 3.12.57.

[17] "Federal Government Puts Restriction on Haluska," *Johnstown Tribune-Democrat*, 7.14.54; "Hoxsey Cancer Clinic, Inc., Portage Pennsylvania, Facts and Policy," *Johnstown Tribune-Democrat*, 10.8.57.

[18] Supplemental Consent Decree, US vs. Hoxsey Cancer Clinic, John J. Haluska et al., Civil Action No. 15807, in the Western District Court for the Western District of Pennsylvania, 10.30.58; "Consent Decree Puts Clinic Out of Business," *Johnstown Tribune-Democrat*, 10.30.58; "Haluska to Close Clinic in Portage," *Johnstown Tribune-Democrat*, 10.30.58; "Decree Brings End for Hoxsey Clinic," *Johnstown Tribune-Democrat*, 10.31.58.

[19] Inspector Eugene Spivak, "Inj. 232-A," Excepts of Depositions of Hoxsey et al., Texas State Board of Medical Examiners vs. Harry M. Hoxsey et al., District Court, Dallas County, Texas, 134th Judicial District, File No. 22, 873-G (6.5.57), 6.26.57, p. 35; "Transcript of Meeting Held in Dr. Leard R. Altamus' Office in Johnstown, Pennsylvania, 4.6.54" with letter from Lester Perry, Executive Secretary of the Medical Society of Pennsylvania to AMA, re Allen Bernard et al., 4.29.54, pp. 6–7.

[20] Hoxsey, op. cit., pp. 264–65.

[21] Hoxsey movie, 1957.

[22] Personal interview.

[23] Inspector Frank McKinlay, "Hoxsey Cancer Treatment," FDA memorandum, 6.17.58, p. 3; Inspector William L. Prillmayer, "Harry M. Hoxsey," FDA memorandum, 5.13.58.

[24] *New Cures for Old Ailments* (Wichita: Defender publications, c. 1958), p. 113.

[25] Inspector Frank McKinlay, Chief LA District, "Hoxsey Cancer Treatment (Sources of Drugs and Supplies,)" FDA memorandum, 11.14.57; Inspector Frank McKinlay, "Hoxsey Cancer Treatment," FDA memorandum, 11.25.57; Inspector Henry B. Packscher, "Surveillance in Fremont College Area," FDA memorandum, 10.28.57; Inspector Frank McKinlay, "Hoxsey Cancer Treatment (New Outlet in LA)," 10.29.57; Inspector Frank McKinlay, "Hoxsey Cancer Treatment (New Outlet in LA)," FDA memorandum,10.31.57; Inspector Eugene Spivak, Chief New Orleans District, "Inj. 232-A," FDA memorandum, 8.2.57; Inspector Eugene Spivak, Chief New Orleans District, "Inj. 232-A," FDA memorandum, 9.9.57.

[26] Letter from Oliver Field, AMA, to Paul Coates, Confidential Telepictures, 8.14.56; "Television Appearance by Harry M. Hoxsey," LA District, FDA confidential memorandum, 7.17.57; Inspector Frank McKinlay, "Appearance of Harry M. Hoxsey on Television (KCOP) Program," FDA memorandum, 7.14.57; K.L. Milstead, Chief LA District, FDA memorandum, 7.31.57; Inspector Frank McKinlay, "Hoxsey Promotion Meetings and Television Appearance," FDA memorandum, 7.11.57.

[27] "Texas Quackdown," *Time*, 12.16.57; "Hoxsey and His 'Cure'," *Newsweek*, 4.23.56; "Things Get Hotter for Hoxsey," *Life*, 4.16.56; Walter Winchell, "Walter Winchell on Broadway," 10.22.57.

[28] Inspector Frank McKinlay, "Radio Talk by Harry M. Hoxsey, Station XERB, 6.4.58 (p.m.)," FDA memorandum, 6.4.58.

[29] Inspector Frank McKinlay, "Hoxsey Cancer Treatment," FDA memorandum re XERB radio broadcasts, 6.17.58.

[30] Inspector W.L. Prillmayer, "Hoxsey Cancer Treatment (Possible Use of Laetrile by Hoxsey Cancer Clinic)," FDA memorandum, 2.26.53.

[31] Personal interview.

[32] Texas State Board of Medical Examiners vs. Harry M. Hoxsey et al., District Court, Dallas County, Texas, 134th Judicial District, File No. 22, 873–G, (6.5.57) 6.26.57.

[33] "Judge Thornton Disqualifies Self in Case of 7 Clinic Doctors," *Dallas Morning News*, 2.3.56.

[34] Dr. Donald Watt, D.O., vs. Texas State Board of Medical Examiners, No. 15240, court of Civil Appeals of Texas, 5.31.57; Southwestern Reporter (2nd Series) (Texas cases only), Vol. 303, pp. 884–88; "Jury Finds Dr. Watt Innocent," *Dallas Morning News*, 5.3.56.

[35] Texas Medical Practice Act, Section 12 of Article 4505, Vernon's Annotated Civil Statutes re: "permitting or allowing another to use his license or certificate to practice medicine in this State for the purpose of treating or offering to treat sick, injured or afflicted human beings."

[36] "Five of Staff at Hoxsey's Disqualified," *Dallas Morning News*, 7.18.56; "7th Hoxsey Doctor Loses Permit," *Dallas Times Herald*," 8.21.56; "Hoxsey Ban Continued by Court," *Dallas Morning News*, 12.21.57; Dr. Donald O. Watt, D.O. Appellant, vs. Texas State Board of Medical Examiners, No. 15240, Civil Court of Appeals, Dallas, 5.31.57, Rehearing Denied 6.28.57; "Revocation of License for Associating in the Practice of Medicine with an Unlicensed Person," Law Department, *JAMA*, Vol. 165, No. 11, p. 1489, 11.16.57; "Dr. Watt's Trial," *Defender*, 6.56; "How Dr. Hoxsey Wins and Loses His Cases," *Defender*, 8.56; "Judge Long's Amazing Decision," *Defender*, 10.56 (including "Judge Long's Letter").

[37] "Defends Naturopaths," *Defender*, citing release by Benedict FitzGerald, 9.10.57; ruling by Texas State Attorney General that existing legislation permitting the practice of naturopathy was illegal; "Texas Quackdown," *Time*, 12.16.57.

[38] Letter from Harry M. Hoxsey to "Friend," 5.1.57; Depositions of Hoxsey and Dr. Taylor, Texas State Board of Medical Examiners vs. Harry M. Hoxsey et al., District Court, Dallas, Texas, 134th Judicial District, File No. 22, 873–G, 6.5.57, pp. 42–50.

[39] Inspector Eugene Spivak, FDA memo, 6.26.57, reproducing Hoxsey Deposition, Texas State Board of Medical Examiners vs. Harry M. Hoxsey et al., 6.5.57, pp. 31–32.

[40] Eugene Spivak, "Inj. 232-A," Dallas Inspector, FDA memorandum, 7.23.57.

[41] Letter from William Goodrich, FDA Assistant General Counsel, to Jerome

Gerber, Deputy Attorney General, Pennsylvania, 9.17.57; Inspector Eugene Spivak, "Inj. 232-A," FDA memorandum, 7.23.57.

[42] "Gerald Winrod Dies, Called 'Kansas Hitler'," *NY World Telegram*, 11.12.57; Inspector Henry B. Packscher, "Surveillance of Fremont College Area," FDA memorandum, 10.28.57; "Hoxsey Cancer Treatment to be Administered in California," *Defender*, 10.57; "Hoxsey Victory at Santa Ana," *Defender*, 11.56; "Fremont Christian Clinic," *Defender*, 1.58.

[43] Inspector W.L. Prillmayer, LA District, "Hoxsey Cancer Treatment," FDA memorandum, 6.18.58; Paul V. Coates, "Confidential File: New Study of Hatred and Its High Priest," *LA Mirror News*, 6.17.58; "Will Russia Invade America?" *Defender*, no date, c. 1957.

[44] W.L. Prillmayer, "Hoxsey Cancer Treatment," FDA memorandum, 6.18.58.

[45] "Consent Decree Ends Hoxsey Cure—We Hope," Better Business Bureau of Los Angeles, 11.9.60; "News Release," California Medical Association, 8.1.57.

[46] AB2359, presented by Assemblyman Casper W. Weinberger; "Bill Regulating 'Cancer Quacks' Safely Over First Hurdle in State Legislature Today," *Humboldt Standard*, Eureka, California, 3.20.57; "State Senate President Claims Cancer Quack Bill 'Down Drain'," *Humboldt Standard*, 4.22.57; "'Cancer Quacks' Bill on Way to State Senate After Strong Vote in House," *Humboldt Standard*, 11.30.57.

[47] Inspector Frank McKinlay, "Hoxsey Cancer Treatment," FDA memorandum, 6.17.58; Morris, op. cit., p. 6 and pp. 1–17.

[48] Morris, op. cit., pp. 1–17 and pp. 159–60.

[49] Senate Resolution 194, 6.5.59; "California Outlaws the Cancer Quack," *Today's Health*, 8.59; "Crusade on Quacks: Federal, State, Private Agencies Step Up Fight Against False 'Cures'," *Wall Street Journal*, 6.22.60.

[50] "Medical Team from Canada to Study Hoxsey Treatment," *Dallas Morning News*, 7.20.57; "Cancer Cure Probe Spurs Controversy," *The Vancouver Sun*, 1.28.58; letter from Dr. Lynn Gunn, Registar, College of Physicians and Surgeons, B.C., to Oliver Field, 4.4.56 and 4.9.56.

[51] K.L Milstead, "Memorandum of Conference with Committee from British Columbia to Investigate Hoxsey Cancer Treatment," FDA, 7.30.57.

[52] "Report of a Committee of Faculty members of the University of British Columbia Concerning the Hoxsey Cancer Treatment for Cancer," 1957; "B.C. Probers Blast Hoxsey Cancer Claims," *Daily Colonist*, 1.28.58; "B.C. Probers Condemn Hoxsey's Cancer Cure," *The Vancouver Sun*, 1.27.58.

[53] *Unproven Methods of Cancer Management*, American Cancer Society pamphlet, various editions.

[54] Permanent Injunction 382, 9.60; "Consent Decree Ends Hoxsey Cancer Cure—We Hope," Better Business Bureau of Los Angeles, 11.9.60.

[55] Hoxsey deposition, Texas State Board of Medical Examiners vs. Harry Hoxsey et al., No. 22, 873-G, 6.5.57.

[56] "Court Eliminates Hoxsey Treatment," *Dallas Morning News*, 9.17.60; "Consent Decree Ends Hoxsey Cancer Cure—We Hope," Better Business Bureau of Los Angeles, 11.9.60.

[57] "US Seizes Cancer Drug from Clinic," *Dallas Morning News*, 12.30.60; "FDA seizes 'Cancer' Capsules," *Dallas Morning News*, 3.18.61; "Marshals to Seize Misbranded Drugs," *Dallas Morning News*, 1.24.63.

[58] Personal interview.

CHAPTER 10
Mexican Standoff

[1] Personal interview.

[2] Harold R. Southworth, "Cancer Cure," St. Louis District, FDA memorandum, to Division of Regulatory Management, 11.8.61; Roy S. Pruit, "Cancer Cure," St. Louis District, FDA memorandum to Division of Regulatory Management, 10.26.61.

[3] FDA memorandum from E.C. Harkins to Director LA District, "Follow-up on Mail Cover," 5.10.61 re "distributing medicines from Taylor Clinic"; Dr. Durkee treated Mrs. Margaret Griffin, whose story is told in Chapter 2.

[4] Personal interview.

[5] Letter from Mildred Cates to Mrs. Brock, undated, c. 1960–61; FDA memorandum from G.S. Goldhammer, Division of Regulatory Management, to Directors, Atlanta et al., "Injunctions 232(a) and 382," 5.5.61; FDA memorandum from Gordon R. Wood, LA District, to Administration, "Hoxsey Treatment," 2.21.61.

[6] FDA memorandum from Inspector Frank McKinlay, Director LA District, re "State Cooperation," "Inj. 382 and Hoxsey Cancer Treatment," 2.17.61.

[7] "Hoxsey Cancer Treatment," FDA memorandum from G.S. Goldhammer, Division of Regulatory Management, 5.25.62.

[8] "Injunctions 232(a) and 382," FDA memorandum from G.S. Goldhammer, Division of Regulatory Management, to Directors, Atlanta et al., 5.5.61; "Harry Hoxsey, Mildred Cates, Homer Cate, D.O., et al.," FDA memorandum from Samuel Alfend, Denver District, to Division of Regulatory Management, Att. Mr. Brandenburg, 8.28.62; "Hoxsey Cancer Treatment," FDA memorandum from Inspector Keith S. Shostrom, SLG, to Director, Denver District, 6.14.62.

[9] Letter from Dr. Homer D. Cate, D.O., to Gordon Thompson, 6.5.62; "DOC 22-271 T—Tape Recording of Interview with John J. Cates," FDA memorandum from Inspector Harry E. Butts to Chief Inspector John J. Cox, 8.17.62.

[10] "Hoxsey Cancer Treatment," FDA memorandum from Inspector Keith S. Shostrom, Salt Lake City (SLC), to Director Denver District, 6.14.62.

[11] Ibid.

[12] "Hoxsey Cancer Treatment," FDA memorandum from Inspector Keith S. Shostrom, SLC, to Director, Denver District, 6.8.62; FDA memorandum from Inspector Keith S. Shostrom, SLC, to Director, Denver District, "Hoxsey Cancer Treatment," 6.5.62; "Hoxsey Cancer Treatment," FDA memorandum from Inspector Keith S. Shostrom, SLC, to Director, Denver District, 6.7.62; "Hoxsey Cancer Treatment," FDA memorandum from Inspector Keith S. Shostrom, SLC, to Director, Denver District, 6.5.62; "Hoxsey Cancer Treatment," FDA memorandum from Inspector Keith S. Shostrom, SLC, to Director, Denver District, 6.2.62.

[13] "Hoxsey Cancer Treatment," FDA memorandum from Inspector Keith S. Shostrom, SLC, to Director, Denver District, 6.8.62; "Hoxsey Cancer Treatment," FDA memorandum from Inspector Keith S. Shostrom, SLC, to Director, Denver District, 6.7.62; "Hoxsey Cancer Treatment," FDA memorandum from Inspector Keith S. Shostrom, SLC, to Director, Denver District, 6.1.62.

[14] "Hoxsey Cancer Treatment," FDA memorandum from Inspector Harry E. Butts to Director, Denver District, 7.10.62.

[15] Personal interview.

[16] "Marshals to Seize Misbranded Drugs," Dallas Morning News, 1.31.63.

[17] Personal interview.

[18] "Hoxsey Cancer Treatment," FDA memorandum from Supervisory Inspector Eugene Spivak to Director, LA District, 3.22.65; "Hoxsey Cancer Treatment," FDA memorandum from Gordon R. Wood, Dallas District, to Director, LA District, 4.23.64.

[19] "Hoxsey Cancer Treatment," FDA memorandum from Inspector Harvey E. Shevling to Director, LA District, 4.5.65; "Hoxsey Cancer Treatment," FDA memorandum from Supervisory Inspector Eugene Spivak to Director, LA District, 3.22.65; "2 Couples Face Arraignment in Drug Case," *San Diego Union*, 4.3.65; "4 Arrested in Cancer Fraud Case," *San Diego Union*, 4.1.65.

[20] "Hoxsey Cancer Treatment," FDA memorandum from Supervisory Inspector Eugene Spivak to Director, LA District, 3.22.65.

[21] Judith Ramsey, "Cancer Victims Go 'Underground' To Mexico," *Medical World News*, 12.1.67.

[22] "Former Editor Dr. Morris Fishbein Dies," *JAMA*, Vol. 236, No. 16, 10.18.76.

[23] Wallace F. Janssen, "Cancer Quackery—The Past in the Present," FDA reprint, Dept. of Health, Education and Welfare, 1979; Bailey, op. cit.

[24] Report of Director, National Cancer Institute, to Secretary, Dept. of Health, Education and Welfare, concerning decision not to undertake clinical testing of Krebiozen, released 10.16.63; FDA Records, 539.1.P.X.

[25] FDA Notices of Judgment, No. 121, FDA Papers, 6.68, p. 43.

[26] "Krebiozen Trial Ends—All Not Guilty," *Chicago's American*, 1.31.66.

[27] Janssen, "Cancer Quackery—The Past in the Present."

[28] Ibid.

[29] "Dr. Ivy Relates History of His Research on Cancer," *Ivy Cancer News*, Vol. 3, No. 3, 12.65, p. 2.

[30] Ibid., p. 2.

[31] Ibid., p. 5.

[32] "Progress Report: Krebiozen Injunction Suit," The Judicial Review Foundation, 2.5.66.

[33] Personal interview.

[34] Personal interview.

[35] Personal interview, 1986; death certificate on file in Dallas, Texas, Registrar's File No. 8789, recorded 12.26.74, "Carcinoma, prostate," Paul A. Greenberg, M.D., death on 12.23.74.

[36] Personal interview; letter from James W. Burke to Colston E. Warren, 6.21.56, reprinted in *Defender*, no date, c. 1956.

CHAPTER 11
Tempest in A Tonic Bottle: "A Bunch of Weeds?"

[1] *Fraud Fighters*, op. cit.

[2] Morris Fishbein, *The New Medical Follies*, (New York: Boni and Liveright, 1927), p. 148.

[3] "Cough Medicine for Cancer," *JAMA*, Vol. 155, No. 7, 6.12.54, pp. 667–68.

[4] Anne Raver, "A Man with a Garden That's a Medicine Cabinet," *New York Times*, 10.15.98.

[5] Principal sources for this chapter include: NAPRALERT; Father Nature's Farmacy database (USDA) founded by James Duke, Ph.D. (http://www.ars-grin.gov/~ngrlsb/); Dr. Duke's private database; research conducted by Francis Brinker and published as "The Hoxsey Treatment: Cancer quackery or effective physiological adjuvant?" *Journal of Naturopathic Medicine*, Vol. 6, No. 1, 8.15.96, pp. 9–23; Patricia Spain Ward, "History of the Hoxsey Treatment," contract report to the Office of Technology Assessment," 1987, republished in *Townsend Letter for Doctors & Patients*, 5.97, pp. 68–72; *Unconventional Cancer Treatments*, OTA report to Congress, 1990, (GPO #052-003-01203-3), pp. 75–80; personal interviews with Duke, Brinker, and Ward during 1984–86 and 1998–99. For an expanded list of key medical/scientific citations for the Hoxsey herbs, see the appendix.

[6] NAPRALERT(SM) is currently maintained by the Program for Collaborative Research in the Pharmaceutical Sciences within the Department of Medicinal Chemistry and Pharmacognosy in the College of Pharmacy of the University of Illinois at Chicago, 833 South Wood Street (m/c 877), Chicago, IL 60612, N.R. Farnsworth—Director and Editor-in-Chief.

[7] Ralph W. Moss, *Herbs Against Cancer* (Brooklyn: Equinox Press, 1998), p. 277.

[8] Jonathan L. Hartwell, *Plants Used Against Cancer* (Lawrence, MA: Quartermain Publications, 1982); originally published in eleven installments in *Lloydia*, 1970–1971).

[9] James Duke, "The Herbal Shotgun Shell," *HerbalGram*, No. 18/19, Fall 1988/Winter 1989, pp. 12–13.

[10] Francis Brinker, N.D., "The Hoxsey Treatment: Cancer quackery or effective physiological adjuvant?" *Journal of Naturopathic Medicine*, Vol. 6, No. 1, 8.15.96, pp. 9 23.

[11] Hoxsey, op. cit., pp. 45–46.

[12] That formula listed alfalfa, buckthorn bark, cascara sagrada, prickly, ash, red clover, potassium iodide, and honey drip cane syrup.

[13] Here cascara sagrada was replaced by cascara amarga, a very different plant.

[14] Hoxsey vs. Fishbein et al., No. 3203 Civil, pp. 26, 27, 139, 143, 197–98; Dr. Delmar M. Randall, William Prillmayer, Lloyd Rhode, Dr. G.A. Granger, "Memorandum of Interview," FDA memorandum, 6.16.55; Inspector W.L. Prillmayer, "Hoxsey Method..." FDA memorandum, 8.6.56; letter from Julius Keller Jr. to John Teeter, Damon Runyon Cancer Fund, 12.22.52, AMA files; Inspector W.L. Prillmayer, "Hoxsey Cancer Treatment (Possible Use of Laetrile by Hoxsey Cancer Clinic)," FDA memorandum, 2.26.53; Inspector Eugene Spivak, "Inj. 232-A," excerpts from depositions of Harry M. Hoxsey et al., Texas State Board of Medical Examiners vs. Harry M. Hoxsey et al., "File No. 22, 873-C," 6.5.57, FDA memorandum, 6.26.57, p. 30.

[15] For people with stomach sensitivity or ulcers, there is another "pink" tonic with lactate of pepsin and without the laxative herbs burdock, cascara sagrada, and prickly ash.

[16] Francis Brinker, "The Role of Botanical Medicine in 100 Years of Naturopathy," *HerbalGram*, No. 42, spring, 1998, pp. 49–59; "Where Does Eclectic Come From?" Eclectic Institute, Inc. promotional literature, Sandy Oregon, 1998.

[17] Brinker went on to publish several peer-reviewed articles in the field of botanical medicine, as well as editing a series of old Eclectic reprints for a naturopathic herb company, the Eclectic Institute, and its publishing affiliate, Eclectic Medical Publications (Eclectic Institute, 36350 Industrial Way, Sandy, OR 97055: (800) 865-1487). Today he also works as a facilitator in botanical medicine for Dr. Andrew Weil's Program in Integrative Medicine at the University of Arizona.

[18] Public advertisements, Parke, Davis and Co.; *Organic Materia Medica*, Parke, Davis and Co., Second Edition (Detroit, MI: 1890), 1904; *National Formulary*, Fifth Edition, American Pharmaceutical Association, 1926; *National Formulary*, Sixth Edition, 1935.

[19] *King's American Dispensatory*, Felter and Lloyd, 1898–1900, p. 1996.

[20] Brinker goes on: "These organs include the kidneys, liver, skin, and lungs. While the lungs expel gaseous waste from the blood, the sweat glands of the skin

excrete some water-soluble substances. The kidneys excrete much of the soluble waste from the blood. However, it is necessary for many compounds to be processed by the liver before they can be excreted. If the liver does not adequately metabolize physiologic or foreign substances, these compounds accumulate and produce toxic symptoms. The liver excretes some of these metabolites along with bile into the intestines where they are hopefully eliminated through the colon along with the waste from undigested food.

"Maintaining optimal blood purification especially requires efficient elimination from the bowels. In cases of constipation, the reabsorption of waste compounds from the colon contaminates the blood. Toxins produced by intestinal bacteria from the breakdown of undigested protein can also be absorbed. An increased burden of waste excretion then falls on the skin, lungs, and kidneys as toxins accumulate in the blood."

[21] Brinker: "They are taken to mean an increase in digestive secretions (barberry, prickly ash), increased bile secretion (barberry), laxative effect (cascara, buckthorn), or immunomodulating activity (licorice, barberry, poke, prickly ash). Other influences include competitive estrogen inhibition (red clover, licorice), thyroid stimulation (potassium iodide), antimicrobial activity (burdock, barberry), and anti-inflammatory effects (licorice). These combined effects could help improve cellular nutrition and metabolism and enhance elimination of waste, relieve inflammatory conditions, and improve resistance against infections, as was claimed for the Trifolium Compound alterative formulas. These formulas have been applied to treat a variety of mainly chronic conditions."

[22] Conventional laboratory testing methodologies have relied heavily on two main protocols. One uses live human tissue-cell cultures in a petri dish which are exposed to various agents to ascertain anticancer or other effects. The second employs live mice, sometimes genetically engineered for specific attributes, which are also subjected to certain agents and observed for effects.

[23] Father Nature's Farmacy, http://www.ars-grin.gov/~ngrlsb/; also, http://www.inform.umd.edu/PBIO/MEDICAL_BOTANY/index.html.

[24] Duke's principal references for red clover and all the following Hoxsey herbs are the Father Nature's Farmacy database and his own database as listed in previous citation, as well as his own books, especially the *CRC Handbook of Medicinal Herbs* (Boca Raton, FL: CRC Press, 1985).

[25] Along with genistein, it contains daidzein, hormonal neuton, and Biochanin A, all of which are estrogenic and fungicidal. Kaufman P.B., Duke J.A., et al., "A Comparative survey of leguminous plants as sources of the isoflavones, genistein and daidzen: implications for human nutrition and health," *The Journal of Alternative and Complementary Medicine*, Vol. 3, No. 1, 1997, pp. 7–12; Kennedy A., "The Evidence for soybean products as cancer preventive agents," *Journal of Nutrition*, 1995, pp. 125, 733.

[26] Kennedy A., ibid, pp. 125, 733.

[27] Stephen Barnes, "Evolution of the health benefits of soy isoflavones," *Proceedings of the Society for Experimental Biology and Medicine*, Vol. 217, 1998, pp. 386–92.

[28] Zava D.T., Dollbaum C.M., et al., "Estrogen and progestin bioactivity of foods, herbs and spices," *Proceedings of the Society for Experimental Biology and Medicine*, Vol. 217, 1998, pp. 369–78.

[29] Kathy Fackelman, "Blocking Breast Cancer: Do Faulty Estrogen Receptors Make a Meaner, Tougher Tumor?" *Science News*, Vol. 137, No. 19, 5.12.90, pp. 296–97. Genistein may discourage tumor growth by blocking off estrogen receptors.

[30] Dr. Samuel Epstein, *The Politics of Cancer Revisited* (Fremont Center, NY: East Ridge Press) 1998, pp. 484–89.

[31] Gina Kolata, "A Cautious Awe Greets Drugs that Eradicate Tumors in Mice," *New York Times*, 5.3.98; Christine Gorman, "The Hope and the Hype," *Time*, special report, 5.18.98, pp. 39–51; Sharon Begley and Claudia Kalb, "One Man's Quest to Cure Cancer," *Newsweek*, 5.18.98, pp. 55–62.

[32] Nicholas Wade, "Progress Reported in Attacking Tumor Blood Supply," *New York Times*, 3.16.99; Wade, "Scientists Develop a Mouse That Resists Some Tumors," *New York Times*, 10.14.99.

[33] Jethro Kloss, *Back to Eden* (Santa Barbara, CA: Woodbridge Press Publishing Company, 1972; original copyright 1939); James Duke, *CRC Handbook of Medicinal Herbs* (Boca Raton, FL: CRC Press, 1985).

[34] Brinker, "The Hoxsey Treatment," op. cit., p. 13; personal interview. Brinker adds that water-soluble polysaccharides (long-chained sugars insoluble in ethanol) extracted from the plant have shown antitumor activity as well as immune-stimulating properties in laboratory tests with mice. Belkin M., Hardy W.G., Perrault A., Sato H., "Swelling and vacuolization induced in ascites tumor cells by polysaccharides from higher plants," *Cancer Research*. Vol. 19, 1959, pp. 1050–62.

[35] Brinker further reported: "Two chemical lignins contained in burdock have shown anticancer activity in tumor cell-culture laboratory tests. Burdock also has polysaccharides in significant quantities which show strong immuno-modulating properties. A tumor growth-inhibiting mixture was isolated by extraction from burdock root. Several independent studies were positive (and several negative) for antitumor activity in animal systems." Personal interview; studies include: Belkin et al., op. cit.; Morita K., Kada T., Namiki M., "A desmutagenic factor isolated from burdock (*Arctium lappa* Linne)," *Mutation Research*. Vol. 129, 1984, pp. 25–31; Morita K., Nishijima Y., Kada T., "Chemical nature of a desmutagenic factor from burdock (*Arctium lappa* Linne)," *Agric. Biol. Chem.* Vol. 49, No. 4, pp. 925–32, 1985; Dombradi C.A., Földeák S., "Screening report on the antitumor activity of purified *Arctium lappa* extracts," *Tumori*, Vol. 52, 1966, pp. 173–76; Földeák S., Dombradi C.A., "Tumor-growth inhibiting substances of plant origin. I. Isolation of the active principle of *Arctium lappa*," *Acta Univ. Szeged, Acta Phys. Chem.* Vol. 10, 1964, pp. 91–93, (*C.A.* Vol. 62, p. 6339c); OTA, *Unconventional Cancer Treatments*, Chap. 4, "Herbal Treatments," pp. 69–87, Congress of the United States, Washington, D.C., 1990.

[36] Dombradi C.A., and Földeák S., "Screening report on the antitumor activity of purified *Arctium lappa* extracts," *Tumor*, Vol. 52, 1966, p. 173.

[37] Kupchan M.S., "Recent Advances in the Chemistry of Tumor Inhibitors of Plant Origin," Swain, Tony (ed.), *Plants in the Development of Modern Medicine* (Cambridge, MA, and London: Harvard University Press, 1972), pp. 261–78.

[38] Morita K., Kada T., and Namiki M., "A desmutagenic factor isolated from burdock (*Arctium lappa* Linne), *Mutation Research*, Vol. 129, 1984, pp. 25–31.

According to Brinker, op. cit.: Along with cancer, burdock has been used to treat a wide variety of maladies including tumors and hardened spots in the breast, glands, intestine, knee, lip, liver, sinus, stomach, tongue, and uterus. The root decoction (water extraction) is said to alleviate ulcerated, glandular, and white tumors. The root is an alterative, mucosal tonic, and remedy for many skin diseases, as well as for treating syphilis and other venereal diseases.

[39] There are several books on Essiac, but the most objective critical analysis is contained in *Herbs Against Cancer* by Ralph Moss, pp. 108–35.

[40] Moss, *Herbs Against Cancer*, p. 45. Jones found poke root especially beneficial in cancers of the breast, throat, and uterus, particularly in patients past middle age. Lymphomas were also said to be cured by poke root. Eli Jones, *Definite Medication*, 1910, reprinted by (New Delhi, India: Jain Publishing Co., no date); Eli G. Jones, *Cancer: Its Causes, Symptoms and Treatment*, (Boston: Therapeutic Publishing Co., Inc., 1911).

[41] Uckun et al., "Pokeweed antiviral protein as a potent inhibitor of human immunodeficiency virus," *Antimicrobial Agents and Chemotherapy*, Vol. 42, No. 2, 1998, pp. 383–88; also see "Editorial: Phytolacca in Carcinoma," *Eclectic Medical Journal*, Vol. LVI, No. 1, 1896.

[42] It is important to note that this modified antiviral poke protein is derived mainly from the plant's leaves, though similar or equivalent factors have been isolated from the root as well.

[43] As Ward cites in her OTA report:"Between 1964 and 1968, four articles appeared in the journals *Lancet*, *Pediatrics*, and *Nature*, describing the mitogenic activity of pokeweed, which triggers the immune system." According to Ward, the orthodox medical literature even during Hoxsey's era "contained at least one suggestive article based on empirical observation by a regular orthodox practitioner. In 1896, in the *Medical and Surgical Reporter* (Philadelphia), a surgeon described the action of poke root as retarding growth of some cancers and increasing the patient's survival time, if it was given before ulceration became extensive. Despite bibliographic tools that make it easy to search the medical literature back through the nineteenth century and beyond, this article had apparently escaped the attention of the AMA, the FDA, and the NCI." Farnes P., Barker B.E., Brownhill L.E., et al., "Mitogenic activity in *Phytolacca americana* (pokeweed), *Lancet*, Vol. 2, 11.21.64, pp. 1100–01; Barker B.E., Farnes P., Fanger H. "Mitogenic activity in *Phytolacca americana* (pokeweed)," *Lancet*, Vol. 1, 1.16.65, p. 170; Barker B.E., Farnes P., and LaMarche P.H., "Peripheral blood plasmacytosis following systemic exposure to *Phytolacca americana* (pokeweed)," *Pediatrics*, Vol. 38, 1966, pp. 490–93; Downing H.J., Kemp G.C.M., Denborough M.A., "Plant agglutinins and mitosis," *Nature*, Vol. 2317, 1968, pp. 654–55.

[44] Brinker, "Periscope: Phytolacca," *The Eclectic Medical Journals*, Vol. II, no. 5, Oct/Nov., 1996, p. 2–4; W.H. Davis, M.D., "Art. XLVIII. – On the effects of Phytolacca Decandra on the glands," *Eclectic Medical Journal*, Vol. 36, 1876, pp. 259–60; "Phytolacca in Carcinoma," *Eclectic Medical Journal*, editorial, 1896, pp. 335–36; F.R. Millard M.D., "Some of the Uses of Phytolacca Decandra," *Medical Surgical Reporter*, Vol. LXXV, 10.3.1896, pp. 420–22.

[45] Poke is conventionally used as a screening procedure for immune competence.

[46] Hoshi A., Ikekawa T., Ikeda Y., et al., "Antitumor activity of Berberrubine derivatives," *Gann*, Vol. 67, 1976, pp. 321–25; Owen, Tsung-Yao W., Show Yin C., Su-Yin, et al., "A new antitumor substance—Lycobetaine," *K'o Hsueh Tung Pao*, Vol. 21, No. 6, 1976, pp. 285–87; Wolf S., Mack M., "Experimental study of the action of bitters on the stomach of a fistulous human subject," *Drug Standards*, Vol.24, No.3, 1956, pp. 98–101; lkram M., "A review on the chemical and pharmacological aspects of genus *Berberis*," *Planta Medica*, Vol. 28, 1975, pp. 353–58; Suess T.R., Stermitz F.R., "Alkaloids of *Mahonia repens* with a brief review of previous work in the genus *Mahonia*," *Journal of Natural Products*, Vol. 44, 1981, pp. 680–87; Velluda C.C., Goina T., Ticsa I., Petcu P., Pop S., Csutak W., "Effect of *Berberis vulgaris* extract and of the berberine, berbamine, and oxyacanthine alkaloids on liver and bile function," *Luci. Prez. Conf. Nau. Farm., Bucharest, 1958*, pp. 351–54, (contained in *Chemical Abstracts [C.A. henceforth]* Vol. 53, p. 15345a); Turova A.D., Konovalov M.N., Leskov A.L., "Berberine, an effective cholagogue," *Med. Prom. SSSR* Vol. 18, No. 6, 1964, pp. 59–60 (*C.A.* Vol. 61, p. 15242f); Amin A.H., Subbaiah T.V., Abrasi K.M., "Berberine sulfate: antimicrobial activity, bioassay, and mode of action," *Cancer Journal of Microbiology*, Vol. 15, 1969, pp. 1067–76; Kumazawa Y., ltagaki A., Fukumoto M., Fujisawa H., Nishimura C., "Activation of peritoneal macrophages by berberine-type alkaloids in terms of induction of cytostatic activity," *International Journal of. Immunopharmacology*, Vol. 6, No. 6, 1984, pp. 587–92; Schmitz H., "The influence of berberine on cellular metabolism," *Z. Krebsforsch.* Vol. 57, 1950, pp. 137–41, (*C.A.*, Vol. 46, p. 4680i); Shvarev I.F., Tsetlin A.L., "Antiblastic properties of berberine and its derivatives," *Mater. Vses. Konf. Issled. Lek. Rast. Perspekt. Ikh Ispol'z. Proizvod. Lek. Prep.*, 1972, p. 245, (*C.A.*, Vol. 83, p. 674m); Taylor A., KcKenna G.F., Burlage H.M., "Anticancer activity of plant extracts," *Texas Reports in Biological Medicine*, Vol. 14, 1956, pp. 538–56; *Unconventional Cancer Treatments*, op. cit.

Barberry has traditionally been used for cancers or tumors of the liver, neck and stomach. The bark of the stem is considered cleansing and toning to organs of digestion and elimination. It contains numerous protoberberine alkaloids, such as berberine sulfate, which has shown activity in a number of tumor systems. It also contains the alkaloid oxyacanthine, which is active against at least one tumor system. Brinker, op. cit.

The species of barberry which Hoxsey cited is *Berberis vulgaris*, which grows in the Midwest. According to Ward: respective 1976 Japanese and Chinese studies established the presence of antitumor substances in this variety of barberry. Testing tumor size in mice, Hoshi and his co-workers found "strong antitumor activity" in berberrubine, an alkaloid isolated from *Berberis vulgaris*. (op. cit.) Also in 1976, Owen et al.. derived from berberine a new antitumor substance which they have named Lycobetaine (op. cit.).

[47] Berberine is also present in another popular herb, goldenseal, which has strong antibacterial and antifungal properties. Bark of the two species of northern prickly ash *Z. americanum* and *Z. clava-herculis* contains the alkaloids chelerythrine and nitidine. Nitidine exhibits cytotoxicity and has shown high activity in leukemia test systems. Chelerythrine was cytotoxic to tumor cells in test tubes. Studies include: Rao K.V., Davies R., "The ichthyotoxic principles of *Zanthoxylum clava-herculis*," *Journal of Natural Products*, Vol. 49, No. 2, 1986, pp. 340–42; Jacobson M., "The structure of echinacein, the insecticidal component of American cone-flower roots," *Journal of Organic Chemistry*, Vol. 32, 1967, pp. 1646–47; Fish F., Waterman P.G., "Alkaloids in the bark of *Zanthoxylum clava-herculis*," *Journal of Pharmacy and Pharmacology*, Vol. 25 (Supplement), 1973, pp. 115P–16P; Fish F., Gray A.L., Waterman P.G., Donachie F., "Alkaloids and coumarins from North American *Zanthoxylum* species," *Lloydia*, Vol. 38, 1975, pp. 268–70.

Cordell G.A., Farnsworth N.R., "Experimental antitumor agents from plants, 1974-76," *Lloydia*, Vol. 40, No. 1, 1977, p. 1–44; Stermitz F.R., Larson K.A., Kim D.K., "Some structural relationships among cytotoxic and antitumor benzophenanthridine alkaloid derivatives," *Journal of Medical Chemistry*, Vol. 40, No. 8, 1973, pp. 939–40.

[48] Buckthorn was also traditionally used for hard spots on the liver and spleen.

[49] Kupchan S.M., Karim A., "Tumor inhibitors. 114. Aloe emodin: antileukemic principle isolated from *Rhamnus frangulus* L.," *Lloydia*, Vol. 39, No. 4, 1976, pp. 223–24.

[50] Ibid. For other studies, see the appendix.

[51] Kupchan M.S., and Karim A., op. cit., 1976, pp. 223–24.

[52] Taylor A., KcKenna G.F., Burlage H.M., "Anticancer activity of plant extracts," *Texas Reports in Biological Medicine*, Vol. 14, 1956, pp. 538–56. Other studies include: Fairbairn J.W., "The active constituents of the vegetable purgatives containing anthracene derivatives," *Journal of Pharmacy and Pharmacology*, Vol. 1, 1949, pp. 683–92; Hoerhammer L., Wagner H., Hoerhammer H.P., "New methods in pharmacognostical education. XIII. Thin-layer chromatography of components of *Rhamnus* cortical drugs and their preparation," *Deut. Apoth.-Ztg.*, Vol. 107, No. 17, 1967, pp. 563–66, (*C.A.*, Vol. 67, p. 84920u); Mary N.Y., Christensen B.V., Beal J.L., "A paper chromatographic study of aloe, aloin and of cascara sagrada," *Journal of the American Pharmaceutical Association*, Vol. 45, 1956, pp. 229–32; Lish P.M., Dungan K.W., "Peristaltic-stimulating and fecal-hydrating properties of dioctyl sodium sulfosuccinate, danthron, and cascara extracts in the mouse and rat," *Journal of the American Pharmaceutical Association*, Vol. 47, 1958, pp. 371–75; Tyson R.M., Shrader E.A., Perlman H.H., "Drugs transmitted through breast milk," *Journal of Pediatrics*, Vol. 11, 1937, pp. 824–32; Dwivedi S.P.D., Pandey V.B., Shah A.H., Rao Y.B., "Chemical constituents of *Rhamnus procumbens* and pharmacological actions of emodin," *Phytotherapy Research*, Vol. 2, No. 1, 1988, pp. 51–53; Kupchan M.S., Karim A., op. cit., 1976.

[53] Eli Jones, *Cancer: Its Causes, Symptoms and Treatment* (Boston: Therapeutic Publishing Co., Inc., 1911).

[54] McKenna G.F., Taylor A., "Screening plant extracts for anticancer activity," *Texas Reports in Biological Medicine*, Vol. 20, 1962, pp. 214–20.

[55] Adolf W., and Hecker E., "New irritant diterpene-esters from roots of *Stillingia sylvatica* L. *(Euphorbiaceae)*," *Tetrahedron Letters*, Vol. 21, 1980, p. 2887. Stillingia has long been used for respiratory infections and syphilitic symptoms.

[56] Brinker, op. cit.; Gibson M.R., "Glycyrrhiza in old and new perspectives. *Lloydia*, Vol. 41, No. 4, 1978), pp. 349–54.

Doll R., Hill I.D., Hutton C., Underwood K.J. II, "Clinical trial of a triterpenoid liquorice compound in gastric and duodenal ulcer," *Lancet*, 10.20.62, pp. 793–96; Tangri K.K., Seth P.K., Parmar S.S., Bhargava K.P., "Biochemical study of anti-inflammatory and anti-arthritic properties of glycyrrhetic acid," *Biochemical Pharmacology*, Vol. 14, 1965, pp. 1277–81; Tamura Y., Nishikawa T., Yamada K., Yamamoto M., Kumagai A., "Effects of glycyrrhetinic acid and its derivatives on D4-5a- and 5b-reductase in rat liver," *Arzneimittel Forschung*, Vol. 29, 1979, pp. 647–49; Bannister B., Ginsburg R., Shneerson J., "Cardiac arrest due to liquorice-induced hypokalaemia," *British Medical Journal*, 9.17.77; Wash L.K., Bernard J.D., "Licorice-induced pseudoaldosteronism," *American Journal of Hospital Pharmacy*, Vol. 32, No.1, 1975, pp. 73–74; Abe N., Ebina T., Ishida N., "Interferon induction by glycyrrhizin and glycyrrhetinic acid in mice," *Microbiology and Immunology*, Vol. 26, No. 6, 1982, pp. 535–39.

[57] Licorice's pharmacological activity is ascribed to the saponin constituent glycyrrizin and its derivative, glycerrhetic acid. Glycyrrizin has been shown to induce interferon production in living mice, which can lead to enhanced immune response. (Abe et al., op. cit.)

[58] Nishino H., Kitagawa K., Iwashima A., "Antitumor-promoting activity of glycyrrhetic acid in mouse skin tumor formatian induced by 7,12-dimethylbenz[a]anthracene," *Carcinogenesis*, Vol. 5, No. 11, 1984, pp. 1529–30; Kitagawa K., Nishino H., Iwashima A., "Inhibition of the specific binding of 12-O-tetradeconoylphorbol-13-acetate to mouse epidermal membrane fractions by glycyrrhetic acid," *Oncology*, Vol. 43, 1986, pp. 127–30; Kumagai A., Nishino K., Shimomura A., Kin T., Yamamura Y., "Effect of glycyrrhizin on estrogen action," *Endocrinologica Japonica*, Vol. 14, No. 1, 1967, pp. 344–48; Reiners W., "7-Hydroxy-4'-methoxy-isoflavon (formononetin) aus sussholzwurzel. Uber inhaltsstoffe der sussholzwurzel," II. *Experientia*, Vol. 22, 1966, p. 359; Taylor A., KcKenna G.F., Burlage H.M., "Anticancer activity of plant extracts," *Texas Reports in Biological Medicine*, Vol. 14, 1956, pp. 538–56.

[59] Arase Y.K., Ikeda N., et al., "The Long term efficacy of Glycyrhizin in chronic hepatitis C patients," *Cancer*, Vol. 79, 1997, pp. 1494–1500.

[60] Because alfalfa has not been listed in the Hoxscy formula since 1949, I have not presented data on it here. It too has a strong anticancer profile, including the anti-angiogenic genistein. See Father Nature's Farmacy and appendix.

[61] The Eclectics used potassium iodide as a treatment for syphilis, rheumatism, and scrofula (an erosive infection of the lymph nodes of the neck). Brinker, op. cit.

[62] Letter from Dr. G.M. Anderson, *Defender*, 4.56. Conventional doctors employed it extensively earlier in the century to promote the absorption of broken-down tissues and dissolve fibrous lesions after pneumonia, bronchitis, pleurisy, syphilis and other diseases.

[63] Arthur Bryan, "Clinical Observations in Treatment of Chronic Swellings with Topical Injections of Potassium Iodide," *The North American Veterinarian*, Vol. 7, No. 11, 11.26, pp. 23–24; Bryan, "Therapeutic Indications for Potassium Iodide," *Veterinary Medicine*, Vol. XXV, No. 4, 4.30, pp. 144–51.

These studies carefully documented potassium iodide as "one of the few specific cures" for actinomycosis [lumpy jaw], inflammatory fungal swellings in horses, cows, and other animals. It was used both orally and by injections. Its practical results were unmistakable. The administration of potassium iodide caused the resolution and repair of these large lumps and inflammations. It was able to dispel pumpkin-sized, hard swellings "resembling a bloody sponge bleeding copiously," within two weeks, in one case. In another instance, it eliminated a cauliflower-size growth on an animal's hoof. In the 1926 study, the author concluded, "I unhesitatingly recommend potassium iodide injection for all growths chronic in character," as well as cysts, warts, collar tumors, and other similar maladies.

Bryan's follow-up 1930 publication documented an even broader range of astonishing cures including cancer. One case was "an ugly, inoperable neoplasm, diffuse hemorrhagic and with an offensive odor located around the vulva of a Holstein cow. I used a saturated solution of potassium iodide and it resulted in extensive necrosis [tumor death] all around the original tumified area. Due to the laboratory diagnosis of malignant carcinomatosis [cancer], the owner refused to keep the cow, and she was slaughtered two weeks later. A microscopic examination of sections taken at this time revealed almost no cancer cells. The potassium iodide evidently destroyed and disintegrated the tissues which it penetrated to, bringing about cell shrinkage or necrosis with resorption of the detritus and broken down tissue structures." (Bryan concluded that he believed it to be only a temporary treatment, however, since the spread of the cancer might theoretically continue afterward.)

[64] Letter from Arthur Bryan to AMA Bureau of Investigation, 3.11.51.

[65] Letter from Edmund M. Burke to Oliver Field, AMA Bureau of Investigation, 6.11.51.

[66] Letter from Dr. Gordon A. Granger, FDA, to R.M. Davenport, with list of medical citations, including testimony of Dr. Maxamillian A Goldzieher from Hoxsey trials; "Four Doctors Blast Claims of Hoxsey," *Johnstown Tribune-Democrat*, 10.17.56.

Bryan also wrote Hoxsey in 1951, eager to draw attention to his exciting findings. Dr. Durkee replied, noting "We have felt that the iodides, especially potassium iodide, reacted as a catalyst at the time the medications were prepared, and that the end result of this was what gave us the reaction." Letters from Arthur Bryan to Hoxsey Cancer Clinic, 2.19.51 and from J.B. Durkee, D.O., Medical Director, to Bryan, 3.28.51.

During Dr. Ivy's visit to the clinic, Dr. Durkee reported to him that he thought that "the mixing of the ingredients in the internal solution produced a new anticancer substance. This they said was indicated because the solution got cold and this occurred when the KI was added." "Abstracts of 'Tests' and 'Cures'," Committee on Cancer Diagnosis and Therapy, National Research Council, 2.1.51, containing Dr. Ivy's "Notes: On a Visit to the Hoxsey 'Cancer Clinic'," 2.10.49.

67 Houston, op. cit., p. 7 (quoting Schweitzer, 1962).

68 Dr. Max Gerson, *A Cancer Therapy: Results of 50 Cases and the Cure of Advanced Cancer by Diet Therapy* (Bonita, CA: The Gerson Institute in association with Station Hill Press, fifth edition, 1990; first edition copyright 1958); "Cancer Research: Hearings before a Subcommittee of the Committee on Foreign Relations," US Senate, 79th Congress, Second Session on S. 1875, US Government Printing Office, 7.1-3.46, pp. 98–123. According to Gar Hildenbrand, former director of the Gerson Institute, Dr. Gerson said he found a severe imbalance in cancer patients of the ratio of sodium and potassium, with a deficiency of the latter. He was convinced by laboratory findings of the time that potassium iodide would better supply iodine to replenish deficiencies and enhance metabolism quickly. Dr. Gerson believed, as subsequent research has shown, that iodine helps increase cell metabolism by stimulating the thyroid gland's production of hormones, in turn retarding and inhibiting tumor growth.

69 David West, M.D., who headed the Hoxsey Research Foundation, contended that potassium iodide "inhibits glycolosis" (the anaerobic metabolism of sugars), which he characterized as causing the specific biochemical lesion of the malignant cell. He agreed with Dr. Max Gerson that malignant tissues are impoverished of potassium and iodine and correctual it with potassium iodide. Dr. West and many naturopathic physcians explicitly considered it an alterative. Dr. David West, "Answering Commissioner Larrick, *Defender*, c. 1953, pp. 7–8; also, E. Edgar Bond, B.L.M.D., "What's in the Hoxsey Treatment?" National Health Federation Reprint 4H, c. 1953; "2 Hoxsey Witnesses, Both Doctors, Bared as Crime Violators," *Pittsburgh Post-Gazette*, 10.30.56; "Potassium Iodide Claimed Beneficial," *Johnstown Tribune-Democrat*, 10.30.56; Dr. David West, "Answering Commissioner Larrick," *Defender*, 6.56; West, "Hoxsey Chemotherapy," *Defender*, no date; Physicians of the period commonly employed potassium iodide for a wide range of diseases including pneumonia, bronchitis, pleurisy, and syphilis. It was believed to promote the absorption of deposits of broken-down tissues, while stimulating the thyroid and other glands which enable blood cells to combat infectious processes.

70 Letter to the editor from Alan Morris, "For a Clear KI Policy," *New York Times*, 11.21.88; "Report on the Accident at Chernobyl Nuclear Power Station," US Nuclear Regulatory Commission, NUREG-1250; "States Will Now Receive Drug for Public Use in Nuclear Mishaps," *New York Times*, 8.22.98; "Atom Agency Tries to Avoid Financing Fallout Drug," *New York Times*, 4.24.99.

Potassium iodide is also used by conventional medicine to protect against radiation. It is administered in tandem with the diagnostic usage of radioactive iodide. Studies further show that it is an effective antioxidant for its free-radical scavenging properties. It is used to treat a disease called Sweet's syndrome which is associated with cancer but is not cancer. Mouse tests have shown both pro- and anti-cancer effects. Medline on the world wide web at a public site has numerous references on potassium iodide from which this is drawn: http://www.ncbi.nlm.nih.gov/PubMed.

71 Cited in *Unconventional Cancer Treatments* (OTA).

[72] Letter from Dr. Richard Early to Martin Murphy, President and CEO, Hipple Cancer Institute, Dayton, Ohio, personally provided to author.

[73] Steve Austin, Ellen Baumgartner Dale and Sharon DeKadt, "Long term follow-up of cancer patients using Contreras, Hoxsey and Gerson therapies," *Journal of Naturopathic Medicine*, Vol. 5, No. 1, 1994, pp. 74–76.

[74] Ward, "History of the Hoxsey Treatment," op. cit., p. 70.

CHAPTER 12
Hoxsey's Eclectic Approach to Cancer

[1] "Comment on Court Opinion that Internal Cancer Can Be Cured with Medicine," *JAMA*, Vol. 145, No. 4, 1.27.51, pp. 252–53.

[2] Hoxsey, op. cit., pp. 44–45.

[3] Ibid, p. 45.

[4] Eli G. Jones, *Definite Medication*, 1910, reprinted by Jain Publishing Co., New Dehli, India; also by Jones: *Cancer: Tumors and Malignant Growths Both External and Internal Permanently Cured without a Surgical Operation* (New Brunswick, 1905), and *Cancer: Its Causes, Symptoms and Treatment* (Boston: Therapeutic Publishing Company, 1911).

[5] Cascara sagrada is a northwestern plant, and the original cascara amarga is a tropical species also known as Honduras bark. Nor is licorice native to the Illinois region.

[6] Brinker, "The Role of Botanical Medicine in 100 years of American Naturopathy," *HerbalGram*, No. 42, Spring 1998, pp. 49–59.

[7] H.W., Felter, J.U. Lloyd, *King's American Dispensatory*, 18th ed., 3rd rev., 1898, reprinted by Eclectic Medical Publications, Portland, Ore., 1983. It was developed by John King, a teacher at the Eclectic Medical Institute in Cincinnati, the mother ship of Eclectic medicine. King, who taught obstetrics and gynecology, was widely regarded as a brilliant scholar and compiler of botanical medicine, and he developed technologies for plant extraction which are still utilized. The edition published in 1898 continues to be used today and is viewed by herbalists as a treasure trove of empirical information on botanical medicines.

[8] A.M. Kapuler and S. Gurusiddiah, "Carrots, Peas, Apios and Others," Vol. IV of "The Twenty Protein Amino Acids Are Primary Human Food: A Food System with Nonviolent Roots," *Peace Seeds Journal*, Vol. 7, 1994, pp. 66–74; earlier analysis of commercial alcohol-based Hoxsey imitation formula: Kapuler and Gurusiddiah, "More Results of Free Amino Acids in Vegetables and Medicinal Herbs," Volume III of above, *Peace Seeds Research Journal*, Vol. 6, 1991, pp. 9–17. Oregon Hoxsey patient Alan Kapuler, a seed collector formerly trained in molecular biology, conducted laboratory amino acid assays of the water-based Tijuana Hoxsey tonic and compared them against an imitation commercial Hoxsey formula using an alcohol extraction process and base. The test showed distinctive differences between the two products.

According to Francis Brinker, most of the active compounds in the Hoxsey herbs are generally water-soluble, and most plant remedies were traditionally prepared that way. Although the potency of stillingia and buckthorn appears to be augmented in alcohol, both are effective as water extracts. The potassium iodide may also serve as a natural preservative in place of alcohol, and itself is a potent antioxidant. (Brinker, "The Role of Botanical Medicine.")

⁹ As naturopathic medicine progressed, it became more disposed toward pharmaceutical-grade botanical extracts over the more inconsistent plant preparations of the nineteenth century. Only in the early 1800s did early laboratory experimenters succeed in isolating and purifying "active" ingredients such as morphine and quinine from complex plants. The variability of plants was a serious problem which was part of the basis for attempts at standardization by the emergent pharmaceutical industry.

¹⁰ Letter from Thompson. Knight, Wright, Weisberg & Simmons to Edward M. Burke, 1.29.49; letter from Dr. Max Cutler to Edward M. Burke, 2.15.49, AMA files.

¹¹ Morris Fishbein, *The New Medical Follies*, p. 140.

¹² Norman R. Farnsworth and R.W. Morris, "Higher Plants: The Sleeping Giant of Drug Development," *American Journal of Pharmacy*, Vol. 147, 1976, pp. 46–52; Edward O. Wilson, *The Diversity of Life* (Cambridge, MA: Harvard University Press, 1992), pp. 282–85.

¹³ *King's American Dispensatory*. The formula was also was prized by the Eclectics for its effects on the liver.

¹⁴ Moss, *Herbs Against Cancer*, pp. 160, 273.

¹⁵ Barbara Griggs, *Green Pharmacy: The History and Evolution of Western Herbal Medicine*, (Rochester, VT: Healing Arts Press, 1981), p. xi.

¹⁶ John Noble Wilford, "Lessons in Iceman's Pehistoric Medicine Kit," *New York Times*, 12.8.98.

¹⁷ Farsnworth N.R., Akerele O., Bingel A.S., Soejarto D.D., and Gua Z.G., "Medicinal Plants in Therapy," *Bulletin of the WHO*, No. 63, 1985, pp. 83–97.

¹⁸ Richard W. Spjut and Robert E,. Perdue Jr., "Plant Folklore: A Tool for Predicting Sources of Antitumor Activity?" *Cancer Treatment Reports*, Vol. 60, No. 8, 1976, pp. 979–85.

¹⁹ Ryan J. Huxtable, "The Pharmacology of Extinction," *Journal of Ethnopharmacology*, Vol. 37, 1992, p. 1.

²⁰ Letter from Robert G. Houston to Senator Charles Grassley, citing this failure, 12.7.88.

²¹ Letter from Oliver Field, AMA Bureau of Investigation, to Noah Sarlat, Editor of *Male* magazine, 6.26.52, AMA files; personal interview.

²² Brinker notes that alfalfa, in the original reputed formula, would have been available too.

23 "African Chimps Found to Practice Herbal Medicine," *Los Angeles Times*, 12.27.85; Ralph Moss, *Herbs Against Cancer*, pp. 24–25.

24 Jonathan L. Hartwell, "Plant Remedies for Cancer," *Cancer Chemotherapy Reports*, Vol. 7, 1960, pp. 19–24.

25 Moss, *Herbs Against Cancer*, p. 40.

26 Norman R. Farnsworth and R.W. Morris, "Higher Plants: The Sleeping Giant of Drug Development," *American Journal of Pharmacy*, Vol. 147, 1976, pp. 46–52.

27 Jonathan L. Hartwell, "Plant Remedies for Cancer," *Cancer Chemotherapy Reports*, Vol. 7, 1960, p. 24.

CHAPTER 13
The Hoxsey Escharotics: "Like a Pit from a Peach"

1 Formula published in *You Don't Have To Die* and in court records.

2 Father Nature's Farmacy database; Ingrid Naiman, *Cancer Salves: A Botanical Approach to Treatment* (Santa Fe, NM: Seventh Ray Press and Berkeley, CA; North Atlantic Books, 1998), p. 172–73.

3 Bloodroot contains sanguinarine and chelerythrine, alkaloids which have shown antitumor activity in reducing the growth of certain carcinoma and sarcoma cancers in laboratory mice. (Hartwell J.L., "Plant remedies for cancer," *Cancer Chemotherapy Reports*, Vol. 7, 1960, pp. 19–24.) The root contains another alkaloid, sanguidimerine, that was active in one laboratory cancer cell culture, though it was inactive against another in rats.(Tin-Wa M., Fong H.H.S., Abraham D.J., Trojanek J., Farnsworth N.R., "Structure of sanguidimerine, a new major alkaloid from *Sanguinaria candendensis (Papaveraceae)*," *Journal of Pharmacological Science*, Vol. 61, No. 11, 1972, p. 1846–47; Tin-Wa M., Farnnsworth N.R., Fong H.H.S., Trojanek J., "Biological and phytochemical evaluation of plants. VII. Isolation of a new alkaloid from *Sanguinaria candendensis*," *Lloydia*, Vol. 33, No. 2, 1970, p. 267–69). Sanguinarine and chelerythrine have demonstrated antimicrobial activity in cell cultures against various disease-causing bacteria and yeast. (Mitscher L.A., Park Y.H., Clark D., Clark G.W.III, "Antimicrobial agents from higher plants. An investigation of *Hunnemannia fumariaefolia* pseudoalcoholates of sanguineriane and chelerythrine," *Lloydia*, Vol. 41, 1978, pp. 145–49.)

4 Father Nature's Farmacy database; personal correspondence with James Duke; Brinker, "The Hoxsey Treatment."

5 Kalish R.S., Wood J.A., Siegel D.M., Kaye V.N. and Brooks N.A., "Experimental rationale for treatment of high-risk human melanoma with zinc chloride fixative paste," *Dermatology and Surgery*, Vol. 24, No. 9, 9.98, pp. 1021–25.

6 Naiman, op. cit., pp. 11–15; Morris, op. cit., pp. 29–39.

7 C. Singer, "The Dawn of Microscopical Discovery," *Journal of the Royal Microscopical Society*, Transaction VI, 1915, p. 337; Naiman, op. cit, pp. 1–5.

[8] Jones, *Cancer: Its Causes, Symptoms and Treatment*, p. 87.

[9] Dr. Frederic E. Mohs, "Chemosurgery: A microscopically controlled method of cancer excision," *Archives of Surgery*, Vol. 42, 1941, pp. 279–95; "The chemosurgical method," he wrote, "for the treatment of cancer involves the chemical fixation of tissues so that they may be excised [removed surgically] in stages and systematically studied under the microscope as a guide to treatment. The microscopic control thus obtained makes possible the extirpation of any accessible neoplasm with unprecedented reliability and with a minimum destruction of adjacent normal tissue."

[10] Mohs, "Chemosurgical treatment of cancer of the skin," *JAMA*, Vol. 138, No. 8, 10.23.48, pp. 564–69. Basal and squamous cell carcinomas are both skin cancers. Basal cell is the most common type of skin cancer, slow-growing, and rarely metastasizes but can invade and destroy tissues locally. It is as easily treated as a typical wart. Squamous cell is a surface malignancy of flat, rapidly infiltrating neoplastic cells. It metastasizes relentlessly and is quickly resistant to treatment.

[11] Some other Mohs publications include: *Chemosurgery: Microscopically Controlled Surgery for Skin Cancer*, (Springfield, IL: Charles C. Thomas, 1978); "Chemosurgery for Facial Neoplasms," *Archives of Otolaryngitis* Vol. 95, 1 72; "Chemosurgery: microscopically controlled surgery for skin cancer – past, present and future," *Archives of Dermatology*, Vol. 4, 1978, pp. 41–54; also, Phelan J.T., Milgrom, Halina, Stoll, Howard, et al., "The use of Mohs' chemosurgery technique in the management of superficial cancers," *Surgery, Gynecology and Obstetrics*, Vol. 114, 1962, pp. 25–30; Phelan J.T. and Juardo J, "Chemosurgical management of carcinoma of the nose," *Surgery*, Vol. 53, 1963a (March), pp. 310–14; Phelan J.T., and Juardo J., "Chemosurgical management of carcinoma of the external ear," *Surgery, Gynecology and Obstetrics*, Vol. 117, 1963b (Aug.) , pp. 244–46.

[12] Moss, *Herbs Against Cancer*, p. 105.

[13] "Abstracts of 'Tests' and 'Cures'," Committee on Cancer Diagnosis and Therapy, National Research Council, 2.1.51, with Dr. Andrew Ivy's "Notes on a Visit to the Hoxsey Cancer Clinic, 2.10.49."

[14] Letter from Edward M. Burke to W.T. Mathews, 2.26.49; Notes of defendants' deposition interviews for Hoxsey vs. Fishbein et al., No. 3203, citing Dr. Max Cutler's planned testimony denying that any escharotic could have a selective effect, and that "Mohs' work is purely experimental and is not accepted by the medical profession, although we are watching it with interest." no date, c. 1948, AMA files.

[15] Such as the lips, mouth, nasal cavity, salivary glands, penis, vulva, and anus.

[16] Based on multiple, generally very obscure sources, it appears that Hoxsey did indeed change the formula for the yellow powder around 1930, thereafter claiming to have rendered it nontoxic. His account was corroborated by Dr. Ira Drew, a reputable osteopath, among others. Sources include: "Memorandum of Authorities in Behalf of the Defendants," Hoxsey vs. Fishbein et al., No. 3203, p. 3, where Hoxsey claimed the "aresenic sulphide is burned and baked and cooked into arsenic oxide, and that by this process its poisonous properties are removed.";

letter from Seymour Preston to AMA Bureau of Investigation, c. 1931 stating "Hoxsey claims he has changed his [powder] formula within the past year."; letter from Seymour Preston to Morris Fishbein, 10.24.33, stating "Hoxsey claims to have changed the formula and that today it only affects foreign or diseased tissue and has no effect on healthy tissue." Inspector William H. Phillips, "Cancer Cure," FDA memorandum, 4.18.46, where Dr. Drew is reported as saying: "In which ever way Mr. Hoxsey made it, he rendered the arsenic non-poisonous."; Dr. J.B. Durkee, "Theory and Application of the Hoxsey Method of Treating Cancer," speech to National Medical Society, 10.17.47, asserting that the yellow powder is "selective." However, a letter from Hoxsey to Dr. Harold Camp on 12.20.25 already claimed that the powder worked "without injury to the healthy tissue."

Francis Brinker speculates on how Hoxsey may have transmuted the toxicity. "Arsenic trisulphide occurs in nature as the mineral orpiment. It is also known as 'arsenic yellow,' which may be 'yellow precipitate.' Arsenic trioxide, or white arsenic, was also used as an escharotic mixed with various substances in the form of a paste to be applied to cancers. This seems to be the form that was widely condemned as poisonous. Hoxsey's arsenic sulphide is apparently the same as arsenic trisulphide. Arsenic trisulphide is made from arsenic trioxide and four or five parts sulphur. Maybe the presence of sulphur in Hoxsey's yellow powder keeps it from reverting to the more toxic white arsenic form. That's my guess."

[17] Moss, *Herbs Against Cancer*, p. 28.

[18] Ibid, p. 28.

[19] Cited in Moss, *Herbs Against Cancer*, p. 103: William Halsted, *Annals of Surgery*, 7.07.

[20] Clarence Wilbur Taber, *Taber's Cyclopedic Medical Dictionary*, edition 17, (F.A Davis Company), 1993, p. 1229.

[21] Naiman, op. cit.

[22] Dr. Perry Nichols, *The Value of Escharotic Medicines* (East Aurora, NY: Roycroft Shops, 1929); Naiman, op. cit., pp. 18–19. Other similar escharotic traditions include the use of taro root in Japan, and in Chinese medicine the application of mashed tulip bulbs, which contain colchicine, a toxic agent.

[23] "Skin Cancer Rise," *Time*, 7.7.97, p. 10.

CHAPTER 14
Nutrition with Attitude

[1] Harry M. Hoxsey, "Hoxsey Science for Treating Cancer Explained," *Defender*, 10.55.

[2] Transcript of "Hoxsey Program Notes II," Paul Coates TV show, 1957, p. 7.

[3] Inspector Frank McKinlay, "Hoxsey Cancer Treatment," FDA memorandum, 2.17.58, p. 4.

[4] Ralph Moss, *Cancer Therapy* (New York: Equinox, 1992), pp. 187–88.

[5] Some of the literature: Hildenbrand G.L., Hildenbrand L.C., Bradford K., Rogers D.E., Straus C.G., and Cavin S., "The role of follow-up and retrospective data analysis in alternative cancer management: the Gerson experience." *Journal of Naturopathic Medicine*, Vol. 6, No.1, 1996, pp. 49–56. Tannenbaum A., "The initiation and growth of tumors I: effects of underfeeding." *The American Journal of Cancer*, Vol. XXXVIII No. 3, 1940, pp. 335–50. Tannenbaum A., "The genesis and growth of tumors: effects of a high-fat diet." *Cancer Research* Vol. 2, 1942, pp. 468–75. Tannenbaum A., "The genesis and growth of tumors II: effects of caloric restriction per se." *Cancer Research*, Vo. 2 1942, pp. 460–67. Tannenbaum A., "The dependence of tumor formation on the degree of caloric restriction." *Cancer Research*, Vol. 5 No. 2, 1945, pp. 609–15. Silverstone H., Tannenbaum A., "Influence of thyroid hormone on the formation of induced skin tumors in mice." *Cancer Research*, Vol. 9, 1949, pp. 684–88. Wilson J.D., Foster D.W., *Textbook of Endocrinology* (Philadelphia, PA: W.B. Saunders Co., 1985). Guyton A.C., *Textbook of Medical Physiology* (Philadelphia, PA: W.B. Saunders Co., 1986). Basu K.P., De H.N., "Role of vitamins in the metabolism of calcium, magnesium and phosphorous in human subjects," *Ann. Biochem. Exp. Med.* Vol 8, No. 3–4, 1948, pp. 127–36. *Alternative Medicine: Expanding Medical Horizons*, NIH publication No. 94–006: (*US Government Printing Office*, 12.94), see "Diet and Nutrition in the Prevention and Treatment of Chronic Disease," pp. 207–70.

[6] For comprehensive data, among other sources: Samuel Epstein, *The Politics of Cancer Revisited*, (Fremont Center, NY: East Ridge Press, 1998).

[7] Craig W.J., "Phytochemicals: guardians of our health," *Journal of the American Dietetic Association*, Vol. 97 (supplement 2), 1997, pp. S199–S204.

[8] Knekt P., Jarvinen R., Seppanen R., Heliovaara M., Teppo L., Pukkala E. and Aromaa A., "Dietary flavanoids and the risk of lung cancer and other malignant neoplasms," *American Journal of Epidemiology*, Vol. 143, No. 3, 1997, pp. 223–30.

[9] Dorant E., Van den Brandt P.A., Goldbohm R.A. and Sturmans F., "Consumption of onions and a reduced risk of stomach carcinoma," *Gastroenterology*, Vol. 110, 1996, pp. 12–20.

[10] Dr. Harvey Arbesman, presentation at American Academy of Dermatology, 2.27.98.

[11] Harold Foster, "Lifestyle Changes and the 'Spontaneous' Regression of Cancer," *International Journal of Biosocial Research*, Vol. 10, No. 1, 1988, pp. 17–33.

[12] Original testimony in "Cancer Research," Hearings before a Subcommittee of the Committee on Foreign Relations, US Senate, 79th Congress, Second Session on S. 1875, Senator Claude Pepper, 7.1-3.46, pp. 97–116.

[13] Ibid, pp. 117–23.

[14] "Vitamin E Found to Cut Risk of Prostate Cancer by a Third," *New York Times*, 3.18.98.

[15] "What About Hoxsey," *Prevention*, 6.57. p. 48.

[16] Lamm D. et al., "Megadose vitamins in bladder cancer: a double-blind clinical trial," *Journal of Urology*, Vol. 151, 1994, pp. 21–26.

[17] Jerome Groopman, "Dr. Fair's Tumor," *The New Yorker*, 10.26 and 11.2.98; Dr. William Fair, presentations at Comprehensive Cancer Cancer Conference, 6.98, transcripts available from: http://www.cmbm.org/Conference98/transcripts/ccc_toc.html.

[18] "Mineral May Cut Risk of Advanced Prostate Cancer, Study Says," *New York Times*, 8.19.98.

[19] Hoxsey, op. cit., p. 60.

[20] Hoxsey promotional film, 1957.

[21] George Larrick, "Comments on Congresman Hardy's Letter 5-22.57," FDA memorandum, 5.31.57.

[22] All quotations from Dr. Bernie Siegel, unless otherwise noted, are from personal interviews from the *Hoxsey* film.

[23] Caryle Hirshberg and Marc Barasch, *Remarkable Recovery* (New York: Riverhead Books, 1995).

[24] Ibid, p. 73; Dr. Herbert Benson, presentation at Comprehensive Cancer Care Conference, 6.98, as noted above.

[25] Marcia Angell, "Disease as a Reflection of the Psyche," *New England Journal of Medicine*, Vol. 312, No. 24, 6.13.85, pp. 1570–72.

[26] Norman Sartorius, quoted in Brendan O'Regan and Thomas J. Hurley, "Placebo—The Hidden Asset in Healing," *Investigations* (Research Bulletin of the Institute of Noetic Sciences), Vol. 2, No. 1, 1985, p. 5.

[27] Norman Cousins, *Head First: The Biology of Hope and the Healing Power of the Human Spirit* (New York: Penguin, 1989), p. 122–124; Cousins, *Human Options: An Autobiographical Notebook* (New York: W.W. Norton, 1981), p. 205.

[28] "The Brain's Triumph Over Reality," *New York Times*, 10.13.98.

[29] Marcia Barinaga, "Can Psychotherapy Delay Cancer Deaths?" *Science*, Vol. 246, 10.27.89, p. 448–449; David Spiegel et al., "Effect of psychosocial treatment on survival of patients with metastatic breast cancer," *The Lancet*, Vol. 14, 10.89, p. 888–890; Daniel Goleman, "Cancer Patients Benefit from Therapy Groups," *New York Times*, 11.23.89; Goleman, "Support Groups May do More in Cancer than Relieve the Mind," *New York Times*, 10.18.90.

[30] David Spiegel, "A psychosocial intervention and survival time of patients with metastatic breast cancer," *Advances*, Vol. 7, No. 3, Summer, 1991, p. 15.

[31] Dean Schrock, Raymond F. Palmer and Bonnie Taylor, "Effects of a psychosocial intervention on survival among patients with Stage I breast and prostate cancer: a matched case-control study," *Alternative Therapies*, Vol. 5, No. 3, 5.99, pp. 49–55.

[32] Susan Gilbert, "Optimism's Bright Side: A Healthy, Longer Life," *New York Times*, 6.30.98.

[33] Dr. Bernie Siegel, presentation at Comprehensive Cancer Care Conference, 6.98.

[34] Hirshberg and Barasch, op. cit., p. 85.

[35] Ibid, p. 303.

[36] Ibid, p. 295; Alan H. Roberts, "The Magnitude of Nonspecific Effects," (Paper presented at the Conference on Examining Research Assumptions in Alternative Medical Systems, NIH Office of Alternative Medicine, National Institutes of Health, Bethesda, MD, 7.11-13.92, p. 2.

[37] Sandra Blakeslee, "Enthusiam of Doctor Can Give Pill Extra Kick," *New York Times*, 10.13.98.

[38] Susan Gilbert, "For Cancer Patients, Hope Can Add to Pain," *New York Times*, 7.9.98.

[39] Jan Hoffman, "Cancer Doctor Mindful of Body and Soul," *New York Times*, 5.28.99.

[40] Herbert Benson, Comprehensive Cancer Care Conference, 6.98.

[41] Dossey, *Healing Words: The Power of Prayer and the Practice of Medicine* (San Francsico: HarperCollins, 1993); *Reinventing Medicine* (San Francisco: HarperCollins, 1999).

[42] Dr. Andrew Weil, *Spontaneous Healing* (New York: Ballantine, 1995).

[43] Ron Rosenbaum, "A Journey Through the Cancer Cure Underground," *New West*, 11.17.80.

CHAPTER 15
Conventional Cancer Treatments: "Heroic Medicine"

[1] "Good News from the Front in the War Against Cancer," *New York Times*, 5.26.98.

[2] L.A.G. Ries et al., SEER cancer statistics review, 1973-1991: Tables and Graphs, Bethesda, MD, 1994.

[3] Proctor, *Cancer Wars: How Politics Shapes What We Know & Don't Know About Cancer*, p. 16.

[4] Jane E. Brody, "Cancer Trailblazer Follows the Genetic Fingerprints," *New York Times*, 4.13.99; Robert A. Weinberg, *One Renegade Cell: How Cancer Begins* (New York: Basic Books, 1998); for a discussion of viral involvements in cancer, see David. J. Hess, *Can Bacteria Cause Cancer?* (New York and London: NYU Press, 1997); Judith Hooper, "A New Germ Theory," *Atlantic Monthly*, Vol. 282, No. 2, 2.99, pp. 41–53.

[5] Daniel S. Greenberg, "A Critical Look at Cancer Coverage," *Columbia Journalism Review*, January-February 1975.

[6] For an in-depth critical discussion of chemotherapy and its effects on a variety of cancers: Ralph Moss, *Questioning Chemotherapy* (Brooklyn, NY: Equinox Press, 1995).

[7] Hardin B. Jones, "A Report on Cancer," Speech delivered to the ACS 11th Annual Science Writers' Conference, New Orleans, LA, 3.7.69; Greenberg, "Progress in Cancer Research—Don't Say It Isn't So," *New England Journal of Medicine*, Vol. 292, 1975, pp. 707–08; also, Transcriptions, New York Academy of Sciences, Section II, Vol. 18, No. 4, 1.9.56, pp. 298–333.

[8] Robert Houston and Gary Null, "War on Cancer: A Long Day's Dying," *Our Town*, 10.29.78.

[9] *New York Times*, 3.9.75.

[10] Peter Barry Chowka, "The National Cancer Institute and the Fifty-Year Coverup," *East West*, 1.78, p. 23.

[11] Walter H. Walshe, *The Anatomy, Physiology, Pathology and Treatment of Cancer* (Boston: Ticknor & Co., 1844).

[12] Ralph Moss, *The Cancer Industry*, pp. 43–58 (a comprehensive history of surgery and the related rise of the cancer industry).

[13] Seale Harris, *Woman's Surgeon: The Life Story of J. Marion Sims* (New York: Macmillan Publishing Co., 1950).

[14] Moss, *The Cancer Industry*, p. 41.

[15] Jones, op. cit. (speech).

[16] Ibid, pp. 42–46.

[17] Thomas H. Maugh and Jean L. Marx, *Seeds of Destruction: The* Science *Report on Cancer Research* (New York: Plenum Publishing, 1975).

[18] Pat McGrady Sr., *The Savage Cell*, (New York: Basic Books, 1964).

[19] Phillip Rubin, *Clinical Oncology for Medical Students and Physicians* (New York and Rochester: American Cancer Society and University of Rochester School of Medicine, 1971); Moss, *The Cancer Industry*, pp. 55–56.

[20] Moss, *The Cancer Industry*, pp. 55–56.

[21] Alan R. Cantor, *And a Time to Live* (New York: Harper and Row, 1978).

[22] Personal interview, 1998; unless otherwise noted, Moss quotations from interview.

[23] Herbert Bailey, *Vitamin E: Your Key to a Healthy Heart*, (New York: Arco Books, 1971).

[24] Moss, *The Cancer Industry*, pp. 59–72.

[25] Lucien Israel, *Conquering Cancer* (New York: Random House, 1978), p. 95; Bernard Fisher et al., "Surgical adjuvant chemotherapy in cancer of the breast," *Annals of Surgery*, Vol. 161, 1968, pp. 339–56; "Effectiveness of Lumpectomy Reaffirmed for Localized Tumors," *Santa Cruz Sentinel*, 11.16.94 (reprinted from *New York Times*).

[26] Moss, *The Cancer Industry*, p. 67.

[27] Proctor, op. cit., pp. 174–96.

[28] Ibid, p. 179.

[29] Ibid, p. 178.

[30] "Go Easy on X-Rays," *The American Weekly*, 2.13.49.

[31] Robert N. Proctor, *The Nazi War on Cancer* (Princeton, NJ: Princeton University Press, 1999).

[32] Denise Grady, "A Glow in the Dark, and A Lesson in Scientific Peril," *New York Times*, 10.6.98; Claudia Clark, *Radium Girls* (University of North Carolina Press, 1997).

[33] Proctor, op. cit., p. 176.

[34] Moss, *The Cancer Industry*, pp. 64–67.

[35] Moss, Ibid, p. 65; Eve Curie, *Madame Curie* (Garden City, NY: Doubleday and Co., 1943).

[36] Moss, ibid, pp. 65–67.

[37] Ibid, pp. 66–67.

[38] Proctor, *The Nazi War on Cancer*, pp. 83, 92–93.

[39] "Diet of Radioactive Particles Possible Soon, Says Scientist," *Dallas Morning News*, 2.3.40.

[40] Inspector William C. Hill, "Case of H.J. Myser," FDA memorandum, 3.22.54.

[41] Inspectors N.A. Gillham and W.F. Breaux, "Case of Mrs. Ludie Johnson," FDA memorandum, 7.14.50.

[42] Hoxsey, op. cit., p. 37.

[43] Proctor, *Cancer Wars*, p. 177.

[44] Sharon Batt, *Patient No More* (Charlottetown, PEI, Canada: Gynergy Books, 1994,) p. 86.

[45] John Robbins, *Reclaiming Our Health: Exploding the Medical Myth and Embracing the Source of True Healing"* (Tiburon, CA: HJ Kramer, 1996), p. 231.

[46] *New York Times*, 4.20.79; Moss, *The Cancer Industry*, p. 69; *New York Times*, 10.21.56.

[47] Moss, *The Cancer Industry*, pp. 68–70.

[48] Ibid, p. 73.

[49] Ibid, pp. 71–72.

[50] C.B. Inlander, L.S. Levin and E. Weiner, *Medicine on Trial: The Appalling Story of Medical Ineptitude and the Arrogance That Overlooks It* (New York: Pantheon Books, 1988), p. 106.

[51] John Gofman, *Preventing Breast Cancer* (San Francisco: Committee for Nuclear Responsibility, 1995), p. 6.

[52] Epstein, op. cit., p. 351.

[53] Ibid, p. 469.

[54] "Cancer Cures More Deadly than Disease," *Midnight Globe*, 9.1.75.

[55] Hardin B. Jones, "A Report on Cancer," Speech delivered to the ACS 11th Annual Science Writers' Conference, New Orleans, LA, 3.7.69; Greenberg, "Cancer: Now the Bad News," *Private Practice*, 5.75, p. 67; "Cancer Cures More Deadly than Disease," *Midnight Globe*, 9.1.75; Richard Walters, *Options: The Alternative Cancer Book* (Garden City Park, New York: Avery, 1993), p. 13.

[56] "Bad News on Radiation, *Time*, 8.3.98, p. 80.

[57] Moss, *The Cancer Industry*, p. 72.

[58] Batt, op. cit., p. 81; Robbins, op. cit., p. 397.

[59] G.T. Pack and E.M Livingston, *Treatment of Cancer and Allied Diseases*, by 147 international authors, (New York: Paul B. Hoeber, 1940).

[60] Moss, *Questioning Chemotherapy*, p. 15–16; A. Gilman, "The initial clinical trial of nitrogen mustard," *American Journal of Surgery*, Vol 105, 1963, pp. 574–78.

[61] Robert Harris and Jeremy Paxman, *A Higher Form of Killing: The Secret Story of Chemical and Biological Warfare* (New York: Hill and Wang, 1982), pp. 119–25; Moss, *Questioning Chemotherapy*, pp. 16–18; Israel, op. cit.; for a discussion of the following, see Moss, *Questioning Chemotherapy*, pp. 15–34, and *The Cancer Industry*, pp. 73–94.

[62] *Time*, 6.27.49.

[63] Moss, *The Cancer Industry*, p. 87.

[64] Moss, *Questioning Chemotherapy*, pp. 24–25.

[65] G. Koren, "Bias Against Negative Studies in Newspaper Reports of Medical Research," *JAMA*, Vol. 266, 1991, pp. 1824–26.

[66] Moss, *Questioning Chemotherapy*, p. 27; Chemotherapy has since proven valuable in testicular and ovarian cancers as well.

[67] John Cairns, "The Treatment of Diseases and the War Against Cancer," *Scientific American*, Vol. 253, No. 5, 1985, pp. 51–59.

[68] Greenberg, op. cit.

[69] Cairns, op. cit.

[70] Ulrich Abel, *Chemotherapy of Advanced Epithelial Cancer* (Stuttgart: Hippokrates Verlag, 1990); "A Dull Weapon: Chemotherapy Almost Useless in Treating Advanced Organic Cancer—Provocative Theses at the Hamburg Cancer Congress," *Der Spiegel*, 3.3.90, pp. 174–76; Abel, *Cytostatic Therapy of Advanced Epithelial Tumors: A Critique* (Stuttgart: Hippokrates Verglag, 1990).

[71] D. Black, "The Paradox of Medical Care," J.R. College of Physicians, London, 1979. Drugs or products which are obviously effective, such as aspirin or penicillin, do not require an RCT.

[72] Moss, *Questioning Chemotherapy*, pp. 43–52; Rupert Sheldrake, "How Widely

Is Blind Assessment Used in Scientific Research?" *Alternative Therapies in Health and Medicine Journal*, Vol. 5, No. 3, 5.99, pp. 88–91.

[73] Kefauver-Harris Amendment to the Food, Drug and Cosmetics Act, 1962.

[74] Moss, *Questioning Chemotherapy*, p. 57.

[75] Epstein, op. cit., "Ralph W. Moss: Congressional Testimony on Clinical Trials and Alternative Treatments," p. 554; Maurie Markman, "The Ethical Dilemma of Phase I Clinical Trials," *Ca: A Cancer Journal for Clinicians*, 11.12.86 (cites 2 percent remissions among 1,248 patients in Phase I trials by the NCI).

[76] Moss, *Questioning Chemotherapy*, pp. 64–65.

[77] Ibid, pp. 64–65.

[78] Personal interview.

[79] *NY Daily News*, 1.14.78; cited in Moss, *The Cancer Industry*, p. 27.

[80] W.J. Mackillop et al., "The use of expert surrogates to evaluate clinical trials in non-small cell lung cancer," *Breast Cancer Journal*, Vol. 54, 1986, pp. 661–67.

[81] Anonymous, "Ein Gnadenloses Zuviel an Therapie: Teil Zweifel an Den Chemischen Waffen," *Der Spiegel*, Vol. 26, 1987.

[82] Moss, *Questioning Chemotherapy*, pp. 56–57.

[83] Vincent T. DeVita Jr. et al., [editors], *Cancer: Principles & Practice of Oncology* (Philadelphia: J.B. Lippincott, 1993).

[84] Ibid.

[85] Maugh and Marx, op. cit.

[86] Moss, *Questioning Chemotherapy*, p. 69; K.K. Fields et al., "Maximum-tolerated doses of Ifofamide, Carboplatin and Etoposide given over 6 days followed by autologous stem-cell rescue: toxicity profile," *Journal of Cancer Oncology*, Vol. 13, 1995, pp. 323–32; Epstein, op. cit., "Ralph W. Moss: Congressional Testimony on Clinical Trials and Alternative Treatments," p. 554.

[87] Epstein, op. cit., p. 554.

[88] Moss, *Questioning Chemotherapy*, p. 22.

[89] Moss, *The Cancer Industry*, pp. 73–74.

[90] Moss, *Questioning Chemotherapy*, p. 67.

[91] Ibid pp. 67–68, 71–72.

[92] Jerome F. Frederick, "Effects of Chemotherapeutic Agents As Causes of Embalming Problems," Dodge Institute for Advanced Mortuary Studies, reprinted in *Cancer Control Journal*, Vol. 5, No. 3/4–5/6, 1979, pp. 105–11.

[93] *The Cancer War*, A Pacific Street Film Projects production by Steve Fischler, Jane Praeger and Joel Sucher, 60 minutes, color, 1984.

[94] Letter from Dean Burk to NCI, 4.20.73, cited in "Chemotherapy and Radiation:

Dangers and Side Effects," *Cancer Control Journal*, Vol. 5, No. 3/4–5/6, Cancer Control Society, 1979, p. 125.

[95] Moss, *Questioning Chemotherapy*, pp. 81–82, pp. 81–150; personal interview; Ivan Illich, *Medical Nemesis*, (New York: Bantam Books, 1976), p. 24; H. Oeser, *Krebsbekampfung: Hoffnung und Realitat* (Stuttgart: Thieme, 1974).

[96] Robbins, op. cit., p. 239; Moss, *Questioning Chemotherapy*, p. 73.

[97] Personal interview.

[98] *The Moss Reports*, 144 St. John's Place, Brooklyn, NY 11217: (718) 636-4433 (ph); (718) 636-0186 (fax); also see Resources for Canhelp database service.

[99] Personal interview.

[100] Project Cure, Michael S. Evers, Esq., Executive Director, 16801 Addison Rd., Suite 207, Dallas, TX 75248; (972) 732-7960.

[101] John Bailar and Elaine Smith, "Progress Against Cancer?" *New England Journal of Medicine*, Vol. 314, 5.8.86, pp. 1226–33.

[102] "Cancer Patient Survival: What Progress Has Been Made?" US General Accounting Office, 1987.

[103] Victor Richards, *Cancer, the Wayward Cell: Its Origins, Nature and Treatment* (Berkeley: University of California Press, 1972), Chapter 13: "The Chemotherapy of Cancer," p. 215.

CHAPTER 16
The Hidden Roots of "Heroic" Cancer Treatment

[1] Coulter, op. cit., p. viii; Samuel Hahnemann, *The Organon of Medicine* (Calcutta: Roysingh and Co., 1962, Sixth Edition,) Section 22, Note 12.

[2] Their struggle has been brilliantly documented by medical scholar Harris Coulter in his seminal work *Divided Legacy: The Conflict Between Homeopathy and the American Medical Association*, part of a four-volume opus. Another classic text in the field is *Green Pharmacy*, by Barbara Griggs, which explores the tradition of botanical medicine within the context of allopathic medical history. These two books provide a comprehensive and detailed discussion of much of the subject of this chapter. Also valuable is Starr, op. cit.

[3] Coulter, op. cit, note on p. 49; W. Hooker, "Rational Therapeutics," *Publications of the Massachussetts Medical Society*, Vol. I, 1865, p. 160.

[4] Coulter, Ibid, pp. 5–86.

[5] Ibid, p. 62; Benjamin Rush, *Sixteen Introductory Lectures to the Courses of Lectures Upon the Institutes and Practices of Medicine*, (Philadelphia: Bradford and Inskeep, 1811), p. 9; Rush, *A Course of Lectures on the Theory and Practice of Medicine, 1790* (at the History of Medicine Division of the National Library of Medicine), p. 35.

[6] For a full discussion, Coulter, op. cit., pp. 90–91; Griggs, op. cit., pp. 148–49.

[7] *Reformed Medical Journal*, Vol. I, No. 1, 1832, p. 6.

[8] Wendell Holmes, "Currents and Counter-Currents in Medical Science," an address delivered before the Massuchusetts Medical Society at the Annual Meeting, 5.30.1860, *Medical Essays*, p. 193.

[9] Griggs, op. cit. p. 153.

[10] Ibid, p. 153.

[11] Coulter, op. cit., p. 69, citing: *Western Journal of the Medical and Physical Sciences*, Vol. XI-XII, 1837–1838, p. 71.

[12] Coulter, op. cit., p. 58, citing: Howard D. Kramer, "The Beginnings of the Public Health Movement in the United States," *Bulletin of the History of Medicine*, Vol. XXI, No. 9, 1947, citing a survey conducted in 1856.

[13] Ibid, p. 49.

[14] Ibid, p. 67.

[15] Ibid, p. 30.

[16] Personal interview with Mark Blumenthal, Executive Director, American Botanical Council, 1998.

[17] Rush, *Medical Inquiries and Observations* (Philadelphia: Pritchard and Hall, 1789, 1793), Vol. I, p. 29.

[18] Coulter, op. cit., p. 72, citing, Kramer, "The Beginnings of the Public Health Movement in the Unites States," pp. 366–67.

[19] Ibid (Kramer), p. 366, quoting Higgininson.

[20] Coulter, op. cit., p. 59, citing Peter Porcupine (William Cobbett), *The Rush Light*, (New York: 2.15-8.30, 1800).

[21] Morris Fishbein, *Fads and Quackery in Healing* (New York: Blue Ribbon Books, Inc., 1932), pp. 38–39.

CHAPTER 17
Cancer Scandals in the Capitol—The Hoxsey Film Goes to Washington

[1] This chapter is substantially drawn from this author's article: "Cancer 'Cures'— An Outbreak of Controversy: The Silent Treatments," *New Age Journal*, cover story, 9.10.89, pp. 33–37, 116–18. The article and the *Hoxsey* film were jointly named for the 1990 "Best Censored Stories" journalism award.

For in-depth discussions of related material: Moss, *The Cancer Industry*; pp. 235–72; Houston, *Repression and Reform in the Evaluation of Alternative Cancer Therapies*; Gary Null, "The Vendetta Against Dr. Burton," *Penthouse*, 3.86; IAT Patients Association newsletters and communications, Frank Wiewel, president, 604 East St., Box 10, Otho, IA 50569; "A Hearing on the Immuno-Augmentive Therapy (IAT) of Dr. Lawrence Burton," *Congressional Public Hearing Summary*, 1.15.86; "The Establishment vs. Dr. Burton," *60 Minutes*, 5.18.80; Peter Barry Chowka, "Cancer 1988: Is a Healing Peace in the Government's War on Cancer

Finally at Hand?" *East West*, 12.87; Lloyd J. Old, "Tumor Necrosis Factor," *Scientific American*, 5.88; *Unconventional Cancer Treatments*, OTA report to Congress; Moss, *The Cancer Chronicles*, a newsletter begun in 1989, which reported ongoing events; (now available through Moss website); IAT Patients' Association Board of Directors, "An Open Rebuttal to *JAMA*," *Health Consciousness*, 8.86; numerous newspaper articles and CNN news.

² Gregory A. Curt, Gale Katterhagen and Francis X. Mahaney Jr., "Immunoaugmentive Therapy," *JAMA*, Vol. 255, No. 4, 1.24/31.86.

³ Lawrence Burton and Frank Friedman, "Detection of Tumor-Inducing Factors in Drosophilia," *Science*, Vol. 124, 8.3.56, pp. 220–21; Burton et al., "The purification and action of Tumor Necrosis Factor extracted from mouse and human neoplastic tissue," *Transactions of the New York Academy of Sciences*, 21, 6.59, pp. 700–07; Kassel et al., "Synergistic action of two refined leukemic tissue extracts in oncolysis of spontaneous tumors," *Transactions of the New York Academy of Sciences*, 15, 11.62, pp. 39–44.

⁴ Moss, *The Cancer Industry*, p. 237.

⁵ Cited in Moss, *The Cancer Industry*; Alan Anderson Jr., "The Politics of Cancer: How Do You Get the Medical Establishment to Listen?" *New York*, 7.29.74; Houston, op. cit., pp. 22–28; S.Y. Yasgur, *Modern Medicine*, 1.1.75, pp. 40–45.

⁶ Houston, op. cit., p. 26.

⁷ Gene Bylinsky, "Science Scores a Cancer Breakthrough," *Fortune*, 11.25.85.

⁸ Moss, *The Cancer Industry*, pp. 252–54; Houston, op. cit. p. 26–27; E.A. Carswell, R.L. Kassel et al., *Proceedings of the National Academy of Sciences, USA*, Vol. 72, 1975, pp. 3666–70.

⁹ Houston, op. cit., p. 27.

¹⁰ Ibid, p. 27, citing Moss, 1980.

¹¹ Ibid, p. 27; Barrie Cassileth et al., "Report of a Survey of Patients Receiving Immunoaugmentive Therapy," University of Pennsylvania Cancer Center, 1987; Moss, *The Cancer Industry*, pp. 268–70.

¹² *60 Minutes*, op. cit.

¹³ For in-depth discussion of Burzynski: Moss, *The Cancer Industry*, pp. 287–338; Houston, op. cit., pp. 28–30; Burzynski, numerous documents and communications, 6221 Corporate Drive, Houston, TX 77036; very lengthy list of scientific publications, including: Burzynski and M.C. Liau, "Hypomethylation of nucleic acids: A key to the induction of terminal differentiation," *International Journal of Experimental Chemotherapy*, Vol. 2, No. 4, 1989, pp. 187–99; N. Eriguchi et al., *The Journal of Japan Society for Cancer Therapy*, Vol. XXIII, No. 7, 7.20.88, pp. 1560–65; Lawrence B. Hendry and Thomas G. Muldoon, "Actions of endogenous antitumorigenic agent on mammary tumor development and modeling analysis of its capacity for interacting with DNA," *Journal of Steroid Biochemistry*, Vol. 30, No. 1–6, 1988, pp. 325–28; Patricia Leeson, "Future Trends in Chemotherapy," *Drug News and Perspectives: The International Drug Newsmagazine*, Vol. 1, No. 2, 5.88, pp. 86–89, 125–26.

[14] "S.R. Burzynski: A Brief History of his IND Application to the Food and Drug Administration," Burzynski Research Institute, 1989; Houston, op. cit., p. 30.

[15] Ibid; Avis Lang, "On the Public Record: Cancer Patients Take the US Government to Court," *Patient Rights Legal Action Fund* (NY), p. 2; "Facts Sheet," Burzynski Institute, 1989.

[16] S.R. Burzynski and E. Kubove, *Drugs in Experimental Clinical Research*, Supplement 1, Vol. 12, pp. 47–55.

[17] Letter from Congressman Molinari et al., to John H. Gibbons, OTA director, 6.27.86; "Project Description—Nontraditional Methods of Cancer Management: Science and Policy Issues," OTA, 9.86; for a detailed account, also see Moss, *The Cancer Industry*, "1996 Update" introduction, pp. VII–XXXIX.

[18] "Half of All Americans Would Risk Unorthodox Cures, Poll Indicates," *San Diego Tribune*, 11.11.85.

[19] "Drug Development Costs Have Soared, New Study Says," *The Indianopolis Star*, 5.20.90, citing Tufts University study by the Center for the Study of Drug Development, estimating that it takes twelve years and $231 million "to research, test and get approval for a new drug."

[20] Personal interview.

[21] I conducted personal interviews in 1987-88 with Patricia Spain Ward, Gar Hildenbrand, Hellen Gelband, Grace Powers Monaco, Michael Lerner, and Michael Evers.

[22] Patricia Spain Ward, "Who Will Bell the Cat?" *Bulletin of Medical History*, Vol. 58, 1984, pp. 28–52.

[23] Memorandum from Patricia Spain Ward to John H. Gibbons, Director OTA, 12.2.88.

[24] Personal interview.

[25] Ibid.

[26] Ward, "History of the Hoxsey Treatment," 5.88.

[27] Personal interview.

[28] Ibid.

[29] Personal interview; letter from Julie Ostrowsky to Ward, 12.12.88.

[30] Also cited in memorandum from Ward to Gibbons, 12.2.88.

[31] Personal interview.

[32] Patricia Spain Ward, "History of Gerson Therapy," OTA contract report, 6.88.

[33] Personal interview.

[34] Memorandum from Ward to Gibbons, op. cit.

[35] Memorandum from Hellen Gelband to John H. Gibbons, 10.25.88; letter from Gibbons to Senator Charles E. Grassley, 11.2.88; letter from Gibbons to Ward, 12.28.88; letter from Gelband to Ward, 1.23.89.

[36] Personal interview.

[37] Letter from Gelband to Ward, 1.23.89.

[38] Letter from Ward to Gibbons, 1.12.89; memorandum from Ward to Gibbons, op. cit.

[39] Letter from Ostrowsky to Ward, op. cit.

[40] Memorandum from Gelband to Gibbons, op. cit.; memorandum from Ward to Gibbons, op. cit.

[41] Ibid.

[42] Personal interview.

[43] Personal interview.

[44] Personal interview.

[45] "Project on Unorthodox Cancer Treatments Case Study: Immuno-Augmentive Therapy," OTA release, 6.88; "NCI May Investigate 'Alternative Therapy'," *Science*, 9.9.88, p. 1286.

[46] Greg D. Hanks and Christina J. Hanks vs. Time Insurance Company, Civil No. 24365, in the District Court, Ninth Judicial District, Wyoming, "Transcript of Proceedings," 9.21.87; "Cancer Victor Awarded Medical 'Rights' in Court," *Cancer Victors Journal*, (newsletter of the International Association of Cancer Victors and Friends), Spring, 1988; Billy W. Brown vs. Prudential Life Insurance Company, Civil No. 81–31687, in the District Court of Harris County, Texas, 151st judicial District, "Final Judgement," 1.26.89; "Judge Orders Insurer to Pay for Disputed Treatment," *Houston Post*, 5.24.90 (re case of Cynthia Grider).

[47] Vincent Canby, "'Hoxsey' and Cancer," *New York Times*, 2.3.88; Harry E. Bishop, "Cancer 'Conspiracy' on Film," *Wall Street Journal*, 2.2.88; HBO/Cinemax, 10.2.88; personal communication from HBO to author, 10.88; letter from Project Cure to author, (with HBO ratings data), 9.21.89; "Twenty-Five Best Censored Stories," *Project Censored*, 1990.

[48] Kennedy Center, Terrace Theater, 5.11.88.

[49] National Public Radio, 5.11.88.

[50] "'Hoxsey' Goes to Washington," *Film & Video Monthly*, 7.88.

CHAPTER 18:
Patented Medicine: A Way of Business

[1] Chester A. Wilk et al. vs. American Medical Association, Joint Commission on Accreditation of Hospitals, American College of Physicians, and American Academy of Orthopaedic Surgeons, in the US District Court for the Northeastern District of Illinois, Eastern Division, Nos. 76C—3777, judgement for Permanent Injunction Order against AMA, 8.27.87.

[2] Ibid; also see "The American Medical Association Found Guilty of Conspiracy," pamphlet published by Motion Palpation Institute (Huntington Beach, CA, 1987)

with highly detailed analysis of all issues including data and studies on chiropractic therapy presented in trial; Gary Null, "The War on Chiropractic," *Penthouse*, 10.85; Null, "Painful Treatment," *Penthouse*, 11.85.

[3] Wolinsky and Brune, op. cit., pp. 124–41.

[4] Getzendanner, Memorandum Opinion and Order, Permanent Injunction Order against AMA, op. cit.; "US Judge Find Medical Group Conspired Against Chiropractors," *New York Times*, 8.29.87; Ellen Rupert Shell, "The Getting of Respect," *Atlantic Monthly*, 2.88, pp. 78–80.

[5] Personal interview.

[6] American Cancer Society, "Cancer Facts and Figures—1995" (Atlanta: ACS, 1995); According to the American Cancer Society, cancer accounts for about 10 percent of the total $1 trillion annual cost of disease in the U.S.

[7] Robbins, op. cit., p. 229; Moss, *Questioning Chemotherapy*, pp. 77–78; M.L. Brown, "Special Report: The National Economic Burden of Cancer: An Update," *Journal of the National Cancer Institute*, Vol. 82, 1990, pp. 1811–14 (cites $100 billion as of 1990).

[8] E. Marshall, "Reader to Join Exodus from NCI," *Science*, Vol. 267, 1995, p. 21, (cited in Moss, *The Cancer Industry*).

[9] Robbins, op. cit., p. 229.

[10] Epstein, op. cit., p. 367.

[11] Personal interview.

[12] Personal interview; Moss, *Questioning Chemotherapy*, pp. 75–77.

[13] Personal interview.

[14] Epstein, op. cit., pp. 368–69 (charts); Moss, *The Cancer Industry*, "Appendix A: Structure and Affiliation of the Memorial Sloan-Kettering Cancer Center Leadership," pp. 441–50; Moss, *Questioning Chemotherapy*, pp. 79–80.

[15] Peter Montague, "Corporate Science," *YES! A Journal of Positive Futures*, Summer 1998, p. 19, citing Robert N. Proctor, *Cancer Wars: What We Know and Don't Know about Cancer*; Epstein, op. cit., p. 469.

[16] Moss, *Questioning Chemotherapy*, p. 75; Frost & Sullivan Market Intelligence, "World Cancer Therapeutics Markets" [Executive Summary], (Mountain View, CA: 1993), citing 13.1 percent compound annual growth rate from 1992-1999.

[17] Moss, Ibid, p. 74.

[18] Ibid, p. 76.

[19] Personal interview.

[20] Moss, *The Cancer Industry*, p. 86; "Dependence of Medicine on Industrial Invention and Research," (press release), Memorial Hospital, 3.8.40.

[21] Moss, *The Cancer Industry*, pp. 66–67.

[22] Ibid, p. 67.

[23] Ibid, p. 67, citing *Memorial Sloan-Kettering Annual Report*, New York, 1987.

[24] "Chemical Corporations Profit Off Breast Cancer," *Censored 1999: The News That Didn't Make the News* (New York, Toronto, London: Seven Stories Press, 1999), p. 35.

[25] Epstein, op. cit., p. 539; Epstein, "Awareness Month Keeps Women Perilously Unaware," *Chicago Tribune*, 10.27.97.

[26] "Too Much Unnecessary Surgery: Interview with Dr. Paul Hawley," *US News and World Report*, 2.20.53, pp. 48–55.

[27] Moss, *The Cancer Industry*, p. 389.

[28] Epstein, op. cit., p. 495; J. Bleifuss, "Cancer Politics," *In These Times*, 5.1.95; L. Fellers, "Taxol is One of the Best Cancer Drugs Ever Discovered by the Federal Government: Why Is It Beyond Some Patients' Reach?" *The Washington Post Magazine*, 5.31.98; Russell Mokhiber and Robert Weissman, *Corporate Predators* (Monroe, Maine: *Common Courage Press*, 1999), p. 103.

[29] Epstein, op. cit., p. 496; J.P. Love, "Comments on the Need for Better Government Oversight of Taxpayer-supported Research and Development," Center for Study of Responsive Law, Washington DC, testimony before the Subcommittee on Business Opportunities, and Technology of the Committee on Small Business, US House of Representatives, 7.11.94.

[30] Moss, *The Cancer Industry*, p. 87; Alan Klass, *There's Gold in Them Thar Pills* (Baltimore: Penguin Books, 1975).

[31] "Four Big Drug Makers' Nets Are Higher on Strong Sales," *New York Times*, 4.22.98; Frost & Sullivan Market Intelligence, op. cit.

[32] "Four Big Drug Makers' Nets Are Higher on Strong Sales," *New York Times*, 4.22.98.

[33] Epstein, op. cit., p. 495; J. Bleifuss, "Cancer Politics," *In These Times*, 5.1.95; L. Fellers, "Taxol is One of the Best Cancer Drugs Ever Discovered by the Federal Government: Why Is It Beyond Some Patients' Reach?" *The Washington Post Magazine*, 5.31.98.

[34] Jennifer Steinhauer, "Hospitals in New York Escalate Competition for Cancer Patients," *New York Times*, 1.4.99.

[35] "The Biggest Deals," (chart), *New York Times*, 6.2.98.

[36] Ken Silverstein, "Millions for Viagra, Pennies for Diseases of the Poor," *The Nation*, 7.19.99, p. 14.

[37] "Two Drug Giants Expected to Announce a $70 Billion Merger," *New York Times*, 11.4.99; "Fighting for the Top Spot," chart, *New York Times*, 11.5.99, p. C19.

[38] Silverstein, op. cit., p. 15; Hess, op. cit, p. 160.

[39] Robert Teitelman, *Profits of Science: The American Marriage of Business and Technology* (New York: Basic Books, 1994).

[40] Teitelmann, op. cit., pp. 162–70.

[41] Ibid, pp. 160–61.

[42] Ibid, cited on p. 163: *Fortune*, 8.65.

[43] Ibid, p. 161.

[44] Ibid, p. 162.

[45] Ibid, p. 164.

[46] Lily Giambarba Casura, "'Twenty Questions' with Ralph Moss, Ph.D.," *Townsend Letter for Doctors & Patients*, 1.98, p. 53.

[47] Moss, *The Cancer Industry*, p. 149; see pp. 153–85 for full account.

[48] Moss, *The Cancer Industry*, p. 394.

[49] Ibid, "Appendix A: Structure and Affiliation of the Memorial Sloan-Kettering Cancer Center Leadership," pp. 441–50.

[50] Moss, *The Cancer Industry*, pp. 399–406; Epstein, op. cit., pp. 288–91, 334–41, 463–72; Moss, *Questioning Chemotherapy*, pp. 25–27; Richard Carter, *The Gentle Legions*, op. cit., pp. 152–62.

[51] Starr, op. cit., p. 343.

[52] Moss, *The Cancer Industry*, p. 98–118 [table p. 109–112]; six of those listed were diagnostic tools, not cancer treatments.

[53] American Cancer Society, *Cancer Journal for Clinicians*, 1.91; "Unproven Methods of Management: Hoxsey Method/Bio Medical Center," *CA–A Journal for Clinicians*, Vol. 40, No. 1, Jan/Feb 1990, p. 54.

[54] Moss, *The Cancer Industry*, p. 198–218; Ward, "History of BCG," OTA contract report, 6.88.

[55] Robbins, op. cit., p. 248, citing S. Batt, op. cit, p. 226.

[56] E.S. Mahoney Jr., "Dr. Frank Rauscher Jr.: An Appreciation," *Journal of the National Cancer Institute*, Vol. 85, 1993, pp. 174–75; Epstein, op. cit., pp. 209–10, 495.

[57] Sharon Blatt and Liza Gross, "Cancer, Inc.," *Sierra*, September/October 1999, p. 38.

[58] Epstein, op. cit., pp. 463–72.

[59] Epstein, op. cit., p. 463.

[60] Moss, *The Cancer Industry*, p. 91.

[61] H. Hall and G. Williams, "Professor vs. Cancer Society," *The Chronicle of Philanthropy*, 1.28.92, p. 26.

[62] Epstein, op. cit., p. 465.

[63] T.J. DiLorenzo, "One Charity's Uneconomical War on Cancer," *Wall Street Journal*, 3.15.92, p. A10.

[64] Epstein, op. cit., p. 464.

[65] J.D. Salant, "Cancer Society Gives to Governors," A.P. Release, 3.30.98.

[66] "CPC Call for an Economic Boycott of the American Cancer Society," Cancer Prevention Coalition, 8.99.

[67] National Cancer Institute Act, S. 2067, 75th Congress, 8.5.37; Epstein, op. cit., p. 483; for detailed discussions, see: Moss, *The Cancer Industry*, pp. 406–11, and Epstein, op. cit., pp. 473–500.

[68] Epstein, op. cit., p. 495; M. Eliott, "Broder to Join Exodus from the NCI," *Science*, Vol. 267, 1995, p. 24.

[69] Houston, op. cit., p. 29.

[70] Wallace Janssen, "The Food and Drug Administration: How Those Regulations Came To Be," *Medical News*, 10.18.85; Janssen, "Cancer Quackery—The Past in the Present," FDA, 1979.

[71] Ibid.

[72] For detailed descriptions, see: Moss, *The Cancer Industry*, pp. 411–17, and Epstein, op. cit., references throughout too numerous to cite.

[73] Moss, *The Cancer Industry*, p. 411, citing *Science*, 6.11.76.

[74] Ibid, p. 412; *New York Times*, 1.20.76.

[75] "Bad Medicine: Drug Firm's Probe of the FDA Threatens Major Agency Scandal," *Wall Street Journal*, 6.9.89.

[76] Epstein, op. cit., "Ralph W. Moss: Congressional Testimony," 2.4.98, p. 556.

[77] Teitelman, op. cit., p. 156.

[78] Ibid, p. 167.

[79] Jane E. Brody, "Cancer Gene Tests Turn Out to Be Far From Simple," *New York Times*, 8.17.99.

[80] Nicholas Wade, "With a Death, Advocates of Gene Therapy Express Concerns for the Future of the Field," *New York Times*, 9.30.99; Sheryl Gay Stolberg, "A Death puts Gene Therapy Under Increasing Scrutiny," *New York Times*, 11.4.99.

[81] Andrew Kimbrell, *The Human Body Shop* (New York: HarperCollins, 1993), pp. 176–77.

[82] "Short Telomeres in Cloned Sheep," *Genetic Engineering News*, 6.15.99, p. 6; Gina Kolata, "With Cloning of a Sheep, the Ethical Ground Shifts," *New York Times*, 2.24.97.

[83] Jeremy Rifkin, "The Biotech Century: Human Life as Intellectual Property," *The Nation*, 4.13.98, p. 16.

[84] Mae-Wan Ho, *Genetic Engineering – Dream or Nightmare: The Brave New World of Bad Science and Big Business*, (Bath, UK: Gatrway Books, 1998).

[85] Sheryl Gay Stolberg, "Drug Review Is Effective, Agency Says," *New York Times*, 5.11.99.

[86] L. Fellers, op. cit.; also cited by Epstein, op. cit., back cover.

CHAPTER 19
Two Centuries of Trade Wars—The Allopaths Against the Empirics

[1] Griggs, op. cit., p. 26.

[2] For in-depth discussion of this area, see: Barbara Ehrenreich and Deirdre English, *Witches, Midwives and Nurses: A History of Women Healers*, (Old Westbury, NY: The Feminist Press, 1973); *The Burning Times*, part two of *Women and Spirituality* series, directed by Donna Read, Produced by Mary Armstrong and Margaret Pettigrew, National Film Board of Canada, distributed by Direct Cinema (310-396-4774); Robbins, op. cit., pp. 60–65; Starhawk, *Dreaming the Dark*, (Boston: Beacon Press, 1982, 1988) Appendix A, pp. 183–219.

[3] Griggs, op. cit., pp. 51–62.

[4] Cited in Moss, *Herbs Against Cancer*, p. 63; Julie Stone and Joan Matthews, *Complementary Medicine and the Law* (Oxford: Oxford University Press, 1996).

[5] Griggs, op. cit., p. 58, citing Statutes of the Realm, Henry VIII, c. 1547, pp. 34–35.

[6] Coulter, op. cit., p. 94; for scholarly, highly detailed accounts of this period, see Coulter, op. cit., Starr, op. cit., and Griggs, op. cit.

[7] Coulter, op. cit., pp. 112–19.

[8] Coulter, op. cit, pp. 91–100; Starr, op. cit., pp. 51–54.

[9] Starr, op. cit., p. 52.

[10] Coulter, p. 93, citing Scudder, *A Brief History of Eclectic Medicine*, c. 1888, (no publisher), p. 7; Starr, op. cit., p. 99.

[11] Coulter, op. cit., pp. 143, 152, 179–90; Starr, op. cit., pp. 116–18, 198–232.

[12] Coulter, op. cit., p. 194, 206.

[13] Coulter, op. cit., p. 119, citing Leondias M. Lawson, *A Review of Homeopathy, Allopathy, and 'Young Physic'* (Lexington, KY: Scrugham and Dunlop, 1846), p. 33.

[14] Starr, op. cit., p. 23.

[15] Coulter, op. cit., pp. 258–76.

[16] Coulter, op. cit., p. 245, citing *Boston Post*, 1864, quoted in Massachussetts Medical Society, *Medical Comm.* Vol. X, 1866, p. 386; and *Buffalo Medical and Surgical Journal*, Vol. X, 1870–1871, p. 133.

[17] Starr, op. cit., pp. 27, 103, 109–10.

[18] Coulter, op. cit., p. 215, citing *JAMA*, Vol. II, 1884, p. 35.

[19] Coulter, op. cit, p. 216, citing *An Ethical Symposium*, published by New York physicians, p. 53.

[20] Coulter, op. cit., citing *Transactions of the Medical Society of the State of New York*, 1883, p. 60.

[21] Coulter, op. cit., p. 314, citing quotation in *Transactions of the Homeopathic Medical Society of the State of New York*, Vol. XVIII, 1883, p. 79.

[22] Coulter, op. cit., p. 315, citing *New York Times*, 3.21.90, quoted in *Transactions of the Homeopathic Medical Society of the State of New York*, Vol. XXV, 1890, p. 551.

[23] Coulter, op. cit., p. 216.

[24] Coulter, op. cit., pp. 402–19; Starr, op. cit., pp. 130–44.

[25] Coulter, op. cit., pp. 403–04.

[26] Coulter, op. cit., pp. 404–09.

[27] Coulter, op. cit., p. 416; Starr, op. cit., pp. 113–14.

[28] Coulter, op. cit., p. 415, citing *JAMA*, Vol. XXXIV, 1900, p. 1041, and *Ohio State Medical Journal*, Vol. I, 1905, p. 84.

[29] F.H. Todd, "Organization," *JAMA*, Vol. 39, 10.25.02, p. 1061.

[30] Starr, op. cit., p. 134.

[31] Griggs, op. cit., p. 238.

[32] Coulter, op. cit., p. 71; Starr, op. cit., pp. 128–29.

[33] Coulter, op. cit., p. 424, citing *JAMA*, Vol. XLI, 1903, p. 263, and Vol. XXXIX, 1902, p. 1061; also, pp. 119–24.

[34] Dr. J.N. McCormack, "Admission of Former Sectarians," *JAMA*, Vol. XLI, 1903, p. 736.

[35] Coulter, op. cit., pp. 428–36; Starr, op. cit., pp. 107–12.

[36] Coulter, op. cit., p. 435, citing *Journal of the American Institute of Homeopathy*, Vol. IV, 1911, p. 1363.

[37] Coulter, op. cit., pp. 442–54; Starr, op. cit., pp. 112–27.

[38] Abraham Flexner, *Medical Education in the United States and Canada*, Bulletin Number 4 of the Carnegie Endowment (New York: Carnegie Endowment, 1910).

[39] Starr, op. cit., p. 121.

[40] Ibid, p. 127, p. 142.

[41] Ibid, p. 121.

[42] Coulter, op. cit., 449–450; Starr, op. cit., 118–123; Moss, *The Cancer Industry*, pp. 390–93; Bealle, *The Drug Story*, pp. 5–12.

[43] Starr, op. cit., p. 73.

[44] Moss, *The Cancer Industry*, pp. 65–67, 123, 390–92.

[45] Robert N. Proctor, *The Nazi War on Cancer*, (Princeton: Princeton University Press, 1999); a fascinating and deeply disturbing account of the widespread public health campaign conducted by the Nazis.

[46] Ibid, pp. 392–94; Moss, *The Cancer Industry*, pp. 392–93, 423; Hess, op. cit., pp. 64–67; Edmund L. Andrews, "I.G. Farben: A Lingering Relic of the Nazi Years," *New York Times*, 5.2.99. I. G. Farben went on to become notorious as "the Devil's chemist" for its central role in Nazi Germany's industry, which included manu-

facturing poison gas for World War I and Zyklon B nerve poison for the Nazi gas chambers of World War II. The concentration camp at Auschwitz was actually built to service Farben's synthetic rubber factory. The giant drug companies Bayer and BASF took over its manufacturing plants when the Nazi-era conglomerate went into "liquidation" after World War II, a process still not complete today.

[47] Moss, op. cit., pp. 391–92; Bealle, *The Drug Story*, pp. 1–2.

[48] Coulter, op. cit., pp. 463–65 in footnote #200, citing Allan Nevins, *John D. Rockefeller: The Heroic Age of American Enterprise*, Vol II (New York: Charles Scribner's Sons, 1940) p. 263, and Rockefeller Family Archives.

[49] Ibid, p. 449–450; Starr, op. cit., pp. 116–27; John K. Scudder, "Defunct Medical Colleges," *Eclectic Medical Journal*, Vol. 83, 1923, pp. 95–96; John S. Haller Jr., *Medical Protestants: The Eclectics in American Medicine, 1825-1939* (Carbondale and Edwardsville, IL: Southern Illinois Press, 1994).

[50] Starr, op. cit., pp. 118–20; Hess, op. cit., p. 62.

[51] Coulter, p. 500, footnote "h".

[52] Bealle, *Medical Mussolini*, pp. 202–09, citing study made by the Chicago Medical Society published in the *Illinois Medical Journal*, as well as a study by Dr. Alice Cutler, medical examiner of the Young Women's Christian Association which found less than 10 percent going to allopaths.

[53] "Small Business Innovative Research" grant application for Phase I CA 41953 submitted by Emprise, Inc., Solicitation # PHS 86-1, to NCI, 4.15.85; Grant # 2 R44 CA41953-02, "Evaluative Database on Questionable Cancer Remedies," 1987, p. 2B–1.

[54] Letter from Ward to Gibbons, 12.2.88, p. 5; personal interview.

[55] Eisenberg et al., "Unconventional Medicine in the United States," *New England Journal of Medicine*, Vol. 328, No. 4, 1993, pp. 246–52.

[56] Personal interview.

CHAPTER 20
A Truce in the Medical Civil War—The Office of Alternative Medicine Looks at Hoxsey

[1] Personal interview, 1998, including all following.

[2] Ibid; also see Moss, *The Cancer Industry*, pp. XXIII–XXXV.

[3] Cited in Moss, op. cit., p. XXVII, Natalie Angier, *New York Times*, 12.10.92.

[4] "Interview with Ralph Moss," *Townsend Letter for Doctors & Patients*, op. cit.

[5] Personal interview, 1998, as following.

[6] Personal interview, 1998, as following.

[7] For press and articles on Chad Green and parallel cases, see *Cancer Control Journal*, op. cit., pp. 2–60.

[8] Barasch and Hirshberg, op. cit., p. 126.

[9] "Twenty Questions with Ralph Moss," op. cit., p. 121.

[10] Gar Hildenbrand et al., "Five-year survival rates of melanoma patients treated by diet therapy after the manner of Gerson: A retrospective review," *Alternative Therapies*, 9.95, p. 29; also see: Hildenbrand et al., "The role of follow-up and retrospective data analysis in alternative cancer management: the Gerson experience." *Journal of Naturopathic Medicine*, Vol. 6, No.1, 1996, pp. 49–56.

[11] Michael M. Weinstein, "Checking Medicine's Vital Signs," *New York Times Sunday Magazine*, 4.19.98.

[12] Dr. Larry Dossey, "On Double Blinds and Double Standards: A Response to the Recent *New England Journal of Medicine* Editorial," *Alternative Therapies*, Vol. 4, No. 6, pp. 18–20; Richard Smith, "Where Is the Wisdom!" *British Medical Journal*, No. 303, 1991, pp. 798–99.

[13] James Dalen, Editor, "'Conventional' and 'Unconventional' Medicine: Can They Be Integrated?" *Archives of Internal Medicine*, Vol. 158, 11.9.98.

[14] Robert Pear, "Report Says Clinical Tests Put Patients' Rights at Risk," *New York Times*, 5.30.98.

[15] Ibid; Robert Sherrill, "A Year in Corporate Crime," *The Nation*, pp. 14–16 (includes further egregious examples of research manipulated to hide deadly side-effects and skew data).

[16] Lawrence K. Altman, "Treating Elderly's Cancers Is Frustrating Many Experts," *New York Times*, 5.20.98.

[17] Kurt Eichenwald and Gina Kolata, "Drug Trials Hide Conflicts for Doctors," *New York Times*, 5.16.99; Eichenwald and Kolata, "A Doctor's Drug Studies Turn Into Fraud," *New York Times*, 5.17.99.

[18] Kurt Eichenwald, "US Officials Are Examining Clinical Trials," *New York Times*, 7.14.99.

[19] Denise Grady, "Breast Cancer Studies Stir Doubts On a Drugs-Transplant Therapy," *New York Times*, 4.16.99; David M. Eddy and Craig Henderson, "A Cancer Treatment Under a Cloud," *New York Times*, 4.17.99.

[20] Gina Kolata and Kurt Eichenwald, "Business Thrives on Unproven Care, Leaving Science Behind," *New York Times*, 10.3.99.

[21] Sheryl Gay Stolberg, "Gifts to Science Researchers Have Strings, Study Finds," *New York Times*, 4.1.98.

[22] Peter Montague, "Corporate Science," *YES! A Journal of Positive Futures*, Summer 1998, p. 19; Montague, Tracy Baxter et al., *Censored 1999*, pp. 34–36.

[23] David Shenk, "Money + Science = Ethics Problems on Campus," *The Nation*, 3.22.99, pp. 11–18.

[24] Montague, op. cit. (both).

[25] Steve Wilson, "Fox in the Cow Barn," *The Nation*, 6.8.98; Jim Boothroyd, *Adbusters*, Winter 1998, pp. 22–23.

[26] Personal interview, Learning Center, 1998.

[27] S. Holt, "Chemoprevention of Cancer with Green Tea," *Alternative and Complementary Therapies*, 2.98, pp. 48–52; M. Muir, "(Green) Tea Time: Does It Help Prevent Cancer?" *Alternative and Complementary Therapies*, 2.98, pp. 43–47.

[28] Previous citation as well as: M. Luo et al., ""Inhibition of LDL oxidation by grewn tea extract," *The Lancet*, Vol. 349, 2.1.97, pp. 360–61; B.T. Ji et al., "Green tea consumption and the risk of pancreatic and colorectal cancers," *International Journal of Cancer*, Vol. 70, 1997, pp. 255–58; J. Erickson, "UA Researcher is Studying Green Tea Effects on Cancer," *Arizona Daily Star*, Vol. 156, No. 174, 6.23.97.

[29] Michael Muscat, "National Cancer Institute's OCCAM Partners with NCCAM to Expand Research on Unconventional Cancer Treatments," *Alternative Therapies*, Vol. 5, No. 4, July 1999, pp. 26–28; APMA Director's Report, *Townsend Letter for Doctors & Patients*, Aug/Sept. 1999, p. 158.

[30] For an extensive discussion of misteltoe: Moss, *Herbs Against Cancer*, pp. 142–58.

[31] "Burzynski Clinic Accepts Cancer Patients for Clinical Trials," *Townsend Letter for Doctors & Patients*, February/March 1999, p. 35; "Burzynski Wins Big in Houston, *Options: Revolutionary Ideas in the War on Cancer*, Vol. 3, No. 2, 8.97.

[32] "Deadly Cancer Slowed," *Dr. Andrew Weil's Self Healing* newsletter, 10.99, p. 3.

[33] "Twenty Questions with Ralph Moss," op. cit.; for a discussion of Gonzalez' work, see: Moss, *Cancer Therapy*, pp. 485–89, and Robbins, op. cit. pp. 251–53.

[34] "Moss Appointed to NCI PDQ Editorial Board," *Townsend Letter for Doctors & Patients*, 4.99.

[35] Moss, *Cancer Therapy: The Independent Consumer's Guide to Non-Toxic Treatment & Prevention* (Brooklyn, NY: Equinox Press, 1992 & 1997); *The Moss Reports*, 144 St. John's Place, Brooklyn, NY 11217: (718) 636-4433 (ph); (718) 636-0186 (fax).

[36] "OAM Elevated to Center Status," *Alternative Therapies*, Vol. 5, No. 1, 1.99, pp. 24–25; "Acting NCCAM Director Harlan Addresses House Subcommittee," *Alternative Therapies*, Vol. 5, No. 3, p. 28; Sheryl Gay Stolberg, "Alternative Care Gains a Foothold," *New York Times*, 1.31.00.

[37] Michael Muscat, op. cit., pp. 26–30.

CHAPTER 21
Look Out America! Here Come Alternative Cancer Therapies

[1] Epstein, "Winning the War Against Cancer?...Are They Even Fighting It?" *The Ecologist*, Vol. 28, No. 2, 3.4.98 (UK), p. 69, citing report by American Hospital Association. Among the most astute analyses of policy cures are: Moss, *Questioning Chemotherapy*, pp. 164–70; Houston, *Repression and Reform in the Evaluation of Alternative Cancer Therapies*, pp. 40–57; Epstein, op. cit., pp. 264–320, 501–10, 560–84; Hess, *Can Bacteria Cause Cancer?* pp. 156–73.

[2] Epstein, *The Politics of Cancer Revisited*, p. 19.

[3] Epstein, speech at Comprehensive Cancer Care Conference, 6.98.

[4] "Cancer-War Skeptic Confirms Drop in Death Rate," *New York Times*, 5.29.97.

[5] Epstein, "Winning the War Against Cancer?..." pp. 73–74.

[6] "Excerpts fom the EPA 'hit' list," *Chicago Tribune*, 3.3.83; "At EPA, They've Got a Little List," *Chicago Tribune*, 3.3.83.

[7] "Prize for US Expert Who Says Curing Cancer is Wrong Strategy," Right Livelihood Award Foundation press release, 10.7.98.

[8] Epstein, *The Politics of Cancer Revisited*, p. 483, for an extensive discussion of budgetary numbers.

[9] Epstein, "Winning the War Against Cancer?..," p. 75; also discussed extensively in *The Politics of Cancer Revisited*.

[10] "Breast Cancer and Diet Fat: No Link Found," *New York Times*, 3.10.99.

[11] Epstein, "Winning the War Against Cancer?..,"p. 74.

[12] Ibid, p. 73, citing *Cancer Prevention News*.

[13] Montague, Baxter et al., op. cit., p. 36; "Breast Cancer: Industrial Byproduct?" *Green Guide*, No. 62/63, 1.99; Theo Colborn, Diane Dumanoski, John Peterson Meyers, *Our Stolen Future* (New York: Dutton, 1996); Blatt and Gross, op. cit., p. 38.

[14] Montague, Baxter et al., op. cit., p. 36.

[15] Marian Burros, "High Pesticide Levels Seen in US Food," *New York Times*, 2.19.99.

[16] Alix Fano, "Environmental Factors in the Rise of Children's Cancer," *Green Guide*, No. 54–55, 6.1.98, p. 2.

[17] Ibid, p. 1.

[18] Blatt and Gross, op. cit., p. 40.

[19] Ibid, p. 40.

[20] Epstein, *The Politics of Cancer Revisited*, p. 202.

[21] Proctor, *The Nazi War On Cancer*, pp. 13–34; also Proctor, *Cancer Wars*, pp. 36–48.

[22] Epstein, "Winning the War Against Cancer?..,"p. 73.

[23] Epstein, *The Politics of Cancer Revisited*, p. 501–512; Epstein and D. Steinman, *SafeShopper's Bible* (New York: MacMillan Publishing Company, 1995).

[24] Robert Weissman,"Focus on the Corporation," listserve: corp-focus@essential.org, 1.22.99.

[25] Rose Marie Williams, "Municipalities Phase Out Chemical Use," *Townsend Letter for Doctors & Patients*, 6.99, p. 120.

[26] Epstein, *The Politics of Cancer*, p. 481.

[27] Gina Kolata, "Vast Advance Is Reported in Preventing Heart Illnesses," *New York Times*, 8.6.99.

[28] Proctor, *Cancer Wars*, p. 3.

[29] Lawrence K. Altman, "Researchers Find the First Drug Known to Prevent Breast Cancer," *New York Times*, 4.7.88; Altman, "Drug is Found to Fight Return of Breast Cancer," *New York Times*, 5.15.98; Epstein, *The Politics of Cancer Revisited*, pp. 484–90.

[30] K.I. Pritchard, "Is Tamoxifen Effective in Breast Cancer Prevention?" *The Lancet*, Vol. 352, No. 9122, 1998, pp. 80–81.

[31] Epstein, op. cit., pp. 485–89; Epstein, "Winning the War Against Cancer?...", p. 76; J. Raloff, "Tamoxifen Quandary: Promising Cancer Drug May Hide a Troubling Dark Side," *Science News*, Vol. 141, 1992, pp. 264–66.

[32] Dr. Susan Love, "Wondering about a Wonder Drug," *New York Times*, 8.3.99; "Study Suggests Why A Cancer Fighter Fails," *New York Times*, 7.30.99.

[33] Epstein, *The Politics of Cancer Revisited*, p. 486.

[34] Robert Pear, "Preventive Use of Tamoxifen Is Allowed," *New York Times*, 10.30.90.

[35] Blatt and Gross, op. cit., p. 37.

[36] Montague, op. cit.; Montague, Baxter et al., op. cit.; Epstein, op. cit. pp. 469, 487–89, 537–44; extensive discussion of this area by Proctor, *Cancer Wars*.

[37] Moss, *The Cancer Industry*, p. 358.

[38] Proctor, *Cancer Wars*, p. 257.

[39] Ibid, p. 9.

[40] Ibid, p. 10.

[41] Ibid, p. 269.

[42] Sally Deneen with Tracy C. Rembert, "Uprooted: The Worldwide Plant Crisis Is Accelerating," *E: The Environmental Magazine*, Vol. X, No. 4, July/August 1999, pp. 36–41.

[43] Linda Thornton, "The Ethics of Wildcrafting," *The Herb Quarterly*, Fall, 1998, pp. 41–46.

[44] Francis Brinker, "The Role of Botanical Medicine in 100 Years of American Naturopathy," *HerbalGram*, No. 42, spring, 1998, pp. 49–59.

[45] Abigail Zuger, "Scorned No More, Osteopathy is on the Rise," *New York Times*, 2.17.98.

[46] Personal communication with author.

[47] American Cancer Society, National Cancer Institute, and Centers For Disease Control and Prevention, facts and figures; Sheryl Gay Stolberg, "New Cancer Cases Decreasing in US as Deaths Do, Too," *New York Times*, 3.13.98; Lawrence

K. Altman, "Good News From the Front in the War Against Cancer," *New York Times*, 5.26.98.

[48] Epstein, "Winning the War Against Cancer?..," p. 71; Alix Fano, "Environmental Factors in the Rise of Children's Cancer," *The Green Guide*, No. 54–55, 6.1.98, p. 2; "Liver Cancer Rises Sharply; Control of Hepatitis Is Seen as Vital to Lower Rate," *New York Times*, 3.11.99.

[49] Epstein, *The Politics of Cancer Revisited*, various references.

[50] Ibid, p. 474; "Cancer 'Report Card' Gets a Failing Grade, Warns Professor of Environmental Medicine, University of Illinois, Chicago, School of Public Health," *Today's News*, Cancer Prevention Coalition, 4.2.98.

[51] "Cancer-War Skeptic Confirms Drop in Death Rate," *New York Times*, 5.29.97.

[52] Lawrence K. Altman, "Diagnoses and the Autopsies Are Found to Differ Greatly," *New York Times*, 10.14.98.

[53] Epstein, "The Experts' Press Conference," reprinted in *The Politics of Cancer Revisited*, p. 343.

[54] E. Ernst and B.R. Cassileth, "The prevalence of complementary/alternative medicine in cancer: A systematic review," *Cancer*, Vol. 83, No. 4, 1998, pp. 777–82. Other estimates vary: A 1993 survey by the ACS estimated 9 percent of cancer patients used alternative therapies, rising to 14 percent among higher-income people (B.J. Kennedy, *Journal of Cancer Education*, Vol. 8, 1993, pp. 129–31). Others put the figure at 50 or 60 percent (L.S. McGinnis, "Alternative Therapies, 1990: An Overview," *Cancer*, Vol. 67, 1991, pp. 1788–92, and S.P. Hauser, *Current Opinions in Oncology*, Vol. 5, 1993, pp. 646–54).

[55] Following are all from personal interviews either for the *Hoxsey* film or this book.

[56] Personal interview.

[57] "Well-to-Do Patients Most Likely to Seek Unproven Ca Therapies," *Internal Medicine News*, Vol. 23, No. 15, 8.1-14.90 (citing McGinnis study presented at ACS meeting); Moss, *The Cancer Industry*, p. XXXVIII.

[58] Barrie R. Cassileth et al., "Contemporary unorthodox treatments in cancer medicine," *Annals of Internal Medicine*, Vol. 101, 1984, pp. 105–12.

[59] Personal interview.

[60] Presentation at Comprehensive Cancer Care conference, 6.98.

[61] Associated Press, "Med Schools Teach Alternative Therapy," 9.1.98.

[62] *Nutrition Business Journal*, Vol. III, No. 2, 2.98, p. 18.

[63] *JAMA*, Vol. 280, No. 18, 11.11.98, pp. 1549–1640.

CHAPTER 22
"Pay Your Money and Take Your Choice"—The Corporatization of Alternative Medicine

[1] Jane E. Brody, "Alternative Medicine Makes Inroads, but Watch Out for Curves," *New York Times*, 4.28.98.

[2] D. M. Eisenberg et al., "Trends in Alternative Medicine Use in the United States, 1990-1997: Results of Follow-Up National Survey," *JAMA*, Vol. 280, No. 18, 11.11.98, pp. 1569–75.

[3] "The Herbal Medicine Boom, *Time*, 11.23.98, pp. 58–69.

[4] Dana Canedy, "Real Medicine or Medicine Show?" *New York Times*, 7.23.98; Sue MacDonald, "Herbal Alternatives," *The Cinicinnati Enquirer*, 1.11.98; M. Dodson, "Coming into their Own," *Los Angeles Times*, 12.22.97; *Nutracon '98*, conference brochure on "Nutraceutical, Dietary Supplements, Functional and Medical Foods," 7.98; Jane E. Brody, "Americans Gamble on Herbs as Medicine," *New York Times*, 2.9.99; W. Tanaka, "Brewing Competition: Pharmaceutical Companies Move In on a Booming Herbal Remedies Market," *San Francisco Examiner*, 11.23.97.

[5] Joerg Gruenwald, "Herbal Tradition and Phamaceutical Savvy: One View of the 21st Century Herbal Products Industry," *American Herbal Products Association Report*, Sept./Oct. 1998, pp. 14–15.

[6] *The Complete German Commision E Monographs: Therapeutic Guide to Herbal Medicines*, edited by Mark Blumenthal (Boston: Integrative Medicine Publications, 1998); "Acting NCCAM Director Harlan Addresses House Subcommittee," *Alternative Therapies*, Vol. 5, No. 3, 5.99; "NCCAM Awards Clinical Research Grants to Three Centers," *HerbalGram*, No. 45, Winter, 1999, p. 45; P.L. Le Bars et al., "A placebo-controlled, double-blind randomized trial of an extract of Gingko biloba for dementia," *JAMA*, Vol. 278, No. 16, pp. 1327–32.

[7] K. Linde et al., "St. John's Wort for depression — An overview and meta-analysis of randomized clinical trials " *British Medical Journal*, Vol. 313, 1996, pp. 253–58.

[8] *Nutrition Business Journal*, op. cit., p. 12.

[9] "NIH Studies St. John's Wort," *HerbalGram*, #41, fall 1997, p. 13.

[10] Mark Blumenthal, introduction to *The Complete German Commission E Monographs*, pp. 5–70.

[11] Steven Foster, "Black Cohosh: A Literature Review," *HerbalGram*, #45, Winter 1999, p. 35.

[12] *The Complete German Commission E Monographs*, introduction by Blumenthal; personal interview with Blumenthal, 1998; Nancy W. E'Piro, "Herbal Medicine: What Works, What's Safe," *Patient Care*, 10.15.97, pp. 49–68, 77.

[13] Moss, *Herbs Against Cancer*, p. 153.

[14] Personal interview, 1998, including the following; E'Piro, op. cit.

[15] Wolinsky and Brune, op. cit., p. 4.

[16] Ibid, p. 68.

[17] Ibid, pp. xii, 68.

[18] Ibid, pp. 68, 92–93, 68–93.

[19] Ellen Rupert Shell, "The Hippocratic Wars," *New York Times Sunday Magazine*, 6.28.98, pp. 34–38.

[20] Wolinsky and Brune, op. cit., p. xii.

[21] Shell, op. cit., pp. 34–38.

[22] Ibid.

[23] Health Policy Report: "AMA Retains Chief Despite Sunbeam Furor," *New York Times*, 6.18.98.

[24] Wolinsky and Brune, op. cit., p. xii.

[25] "The American Health Care System," *New England Journal of Medicine*, Vol. 340, No. 1, 1.7.99, pp. 70–76 for in-depth discussion, also see: Starr, op. cit.

[26] Starr, op. cit., p. 449.

[27] Ibid, p. 204.

[28] Ibid, p. 216.

[29] Ibid, p. 379.

[30] Ibid, p. 335.

[31] Ibid, p. 448.

[32] Peter J. Kilborn, "Reality of the HMO System Doesn't Live Up to the Dream," *New York Times*, 10.5.98.

[33] Robert Sherrill, "Medicine and the Madness of the Market," *The Nation*, 1.9-16.95, p. 46 (entire issue devoted to this subject, pp. 45–72).

[34] Health Policy Report: "The American Health Care System," op. cit.

[35] Robert Pear, "American Lacking Health Insurance Put At 16 Percent," *New York Times*, 9.26.98.

[36] "Insurers Tighten Rules and Lower Payments for Doctors," *New York Times*, 6.28.98; Peter T. Kilborn, "400 Doctors in Dallas Break Contracts With Aetna's HMO," *New York Times*, 10.20.98.

[37] Emily Yellin, "Some Doctors See Relief In Plan for AMA Union," *New York Times*, 6.25.99.

[38] Milt Freudenheim, "Medical Insurers Revise Cost-Control Efforts," *New York Times*, 12.3.99.

[39] Postman, op. cit., p. 105; Inlander et al., op. cit.

[40] Postman, op. cit., p. 105.

[41] Michael M. Weinstein, "Checking Medicine's Vital Signs," *New York Times Sunday Magazine*, 4.19.98, p. 36.

[42] Ibid, p. 36; Health Policy Report: "The American Health Care System," op. cit.

[43] Denise Grady, "Reactions to Prescribed Drugs Kill Thousands Annually, Study Says," *New York Times*, 4.15.98; J. Lazarou et al., "Incidence of Adverse Drug Reactions in Hospitalized Patients: A Meta-Analysis of Prospective Studies," *JAMA*, Vol. 279, No. 15, 4.15.98, pp. 1216–17; Lawrence K. Altman, "Experts See Need to Control Anitbiotics and Hospital Infections," *New York Times*, 3.12.98.

[44] Alisa Tang, "Staying on Guard for Medical Errors, *New York Times*, 12.5.99; Peter T. Kilborn, "All-Out Attack to Cut Mistakes in U.S. Hospitals," *New York Times*, 12.26.99.

[45] Robert Pear, "Federal Inspections of Hospitals Are Badly Flawed," *New York Times*, 7.21.99.

[46] Dr. Sandeep Jauhar, "First, Do No Harm: When Patients Suffer," *New York Times*, 8.10.99.

[47] Stephen Fried, "FDA Approval Is Just the First Step," *New York Times*, 4.25.98.

[48] Abigail Zuger, "Fever Pitch: Getting Doctors to Prescribe Is Big Business," *New York Times*, 1.11.99.

[49] Laurie McGinley, "US Health Care Costs Are Expected to Double by 2007," *Wall Street Journal*, 9.15.98; "Drug Review Is Effective, Agency Says," *New York Times*, 1.11.99.

[50] "Worldwide Drug Sales Up 7% in '98," *New York Times*, 3.23.99.

[51] David Pilling, "The Facts of Life," *Financial Times*, 12.9.98.

[52] Sherrill, op. cit., p. 60.

[53] Ibid, p. 61.

[54] Ibid, p. 60; Epstein, *The Politics of Cancer Revisited*, p. 496.

[55] Epstein, *The Politics of Cancer Revisited*, pp. 495–96.

[56] Silverstein, op. cit., p. 14; "The Drug Companies," part of "Medicine and the Madness of the Market," *The Nation*, p. 61.

[57] Montague, Baxter et al., op. cit., p. 37; Silverstein, op. cit., p. 14.

[58] "Insurers Tighten Rules and Reduce Fees for Doctors," *New York Times*, 6.28.98; "The Biggest Deals," (chart) *New York Times*, 6.2.98; Milton Freudenheim, "Concern Rising About Mergers in Health Plans, *New York Times*, 1.13.99.

[59] David C. Korten, *When Corporations Rule the World*, (West Hartford, CT: Kumarian Press, 1995) p. 221.

[60] Laurie McGinley, op. cit., 9.15.98; Robert Pear, "Sharp Rise Predicted in Health-Care Spending In Next Decade," *New York Times*, 9.15.98.

[61] Roy Porter, "Medical Waste," *New York Times*, book review section, pp. 12–13.

[62] *Alternative Therapies*, Vol. 5, No. 4, July 1999, p. 32.

[63] Dr. Larry Kincheloe, "Herbal Medicines Can Reduce Costs in HMO," *HerbalGram*, #41, fall, 1997, p. 49.

[64] "Oxford Will Cover Alternative Medical Care," *New York Times*, 10.9.96; "Now in the HMO: Yoga Teachers and Naturopaths," *New York Times*, 11.24.96.

[65] Teresa Riordan, "Patents: A Radical Policy Shift Opens the Door to a Variety of Herbal Preparations with Medicinal Purposes," *New York Times*, 11.23.98; "Herbiceutical Fingerprinting," *Genetic Engineering News*, 5.18.98 ["Our platform technology delivers a new consistency to developing herbal remedies," he [Dr. Pang] observes. "Patented herbiceuticals will limit market entry."]

[66] Speech at Social Venture Network, Mohonk, NY, 4.96.

[67] "Financier Pledges Millions For Medical Care Program," *New York Times*, 4.15.99.

[68] Personal interview.

[69] Speech at Comprehensive Cancer Care Conference, 6.98; also, Institute for Alternative Futures, *The Future of Complementary and Alternative Approaches (CAAs) in US Health Care* (Alexandria, VA: NCMIC Insurance Company, 1998); also see: Institute for Alternative Futures, *Healthy People in a Healthy World: The Belmont Vision for Health Care in America* (Alexandria, VA: Inst. for Alternative Futures, 1992); *Horizons 2013: Longer, Better Life Without Cancer*, Helene G. Brown, John R. Seffrin, Clement Bezold, editors, (Atlanta, GA: American Cancer Society, 1996).

[70] Speech at Comprehensive Cancer Care Conference, 6.98.

[71] Hess, op. cit., p. 78; "Well-to-Do Patients Most Likely to Seek Unproven Ca Therapies," *Internal Medicine News*, Vol. 23, No. 15, 8.1-14.90.

[72] Personal interview.

[73] Hoxsey vs. Fishbein et al., No. 3203, verdict 3.18.49; Federal Supplement, Vol. 83, p. 282–84.

CHAPTER 23
The Other Heroic Medicine

[1] This meeting took place in January, 1997 in Tijuana.

[2] Personal interviews, 1984-1998, *Hoxsey* film and other interviews.

[3] Certificate of Registration #2,100,998, US Patent and Trademark Office, 9.30.97.

[4] For a thorough discussion of Essiac, see: Moss, *Herbs Against Cancer*, pp. 108–35.

[5] Personal interview.

[6] Personal interview.

[7] Personal interview, 1998.

[8] Dr. Abigail Zuger, "Take Some Strychnine and Call Me in the Morning," *New York Times*, 4.20.99.

[9] Personal interview.

EPILOGUE

[1] US vs. Hoxsey Cancer Clinic, Civ. No. 4144, Judgement, 12.21.50; Federal Supplement, Vol. 94, pp. 464–68.

[2] Mary Ann Richardson et al., "Assessment of Outcomes of Alternative Medicine Cancer Clinics: A Feasibility Study," op. cit.

AFTERWORD

[1] "Herbal Cancer Treatment Pioneer Mildred Nelson Dies," *Alternative Therapies*, Vol. 5, No. 3, 5.99, p. 31; Kenny Ausubel, "In Memoriam: Mildred Nelson, 1919-1999," *HerbalGram*, #46, Spring 1999, p. 70.

Appendix:
Sources of Information
on Botanical Medicine

NAPRALERT
(Natural Products Alert botanical
   database)
Mary Lou Quinn-Beattie, Director
University of Illinois College of
   Pharmacy
833 South Wood Street (m/c 877)
Chicago, IL 60612
(312) 996-2246 (ph)
(312) 996-7107 (fax)
quinnml@uic.edu

Father Nature's Farmacy (USDA
   database)
Founded by James Duke, Ph.D.
www.ars-grin.gov/duke

James A. Duke, Ph.D.
Botanical Consultant
Herbal Vineyard
8210 Murphy Road
Fulton, MD 20759
(301) 498-1175 (ph)
(301) 498-5738 (fax)
jimduke@cpucg.org

Also from Dr. Duke:

Medical Botany Syllabus (herbal desk
   reference):
www.ars-grin.gov/duke/syllabus
Daily Herb A Day Column:
www.allherb.com/consumer

MEDLINE
Medline on the World Wide Web is a
   public site.
www.ncbi.nlm.nih.gov/PubMed

American Botanical Council
Mark Blumenthal, Executive Director
P.O. Box 144345
Austin, TX 78714-4345
(512) 926-4900 (ph)
(512) 926-2345 (fax)
Order toll-free 800-373-7105
Web site: www.herbalgram.org
The leading nonprofit research and
education organization on herbal
medicine in North America. Publisher of HerbalGram, the highly
acclaimed peer-reviewed quarterly
journal that takes no industry
advertising. ABC's Herbal Education
Catalog has over 500 books, monographs, CD-ROMs, videos, and
audiotapes for health professionals
and laypeople. Web site has lots of
highly credible information, and a
wide variety of resources and links.

Francis Brinker, N.D.
Botanical Consultant
6417 E. Hayne Street
Tucson, AZ 86710
(520) 747-1898
wacondaseeds@gci-net.com

Dennis J. McKenna, Ph.D.
Botanical Consultant and
    Pharmacognosist
Executive Director
Institute for Natural Products
    Research
P.O. Box 292
Marine on St. Croix, MN 55047
(651) 433-4440 (ph)
(651) 433-5104 (fax)
djmckenna@naturalproducts.org
www.naturalproducts.org
The Web site offers educational
monographs on botanicals for doctors,
pharmacists, medical professionals,
and others by subscription.

Gar and Christeene Hildenbrand
Epidemiology and Field
    Investigations
7807 Artesian Road
San Diego, CA 92127-2117
(858) 759-2966 (ph)
(858) 759-2967 (fax)
ghildenbrand@hotmail.com

Edward M. Croom Jr., Ph.D.
Botanical Consultant
National Center for the Develop-
    ment of Natural Products
School of Pharmacy
University of Mississippi
University, MS 38677
(601) 232-5941 (ph)
(601) 232-7062 (fax)
emcroom@olemiss.edu

National Foundation for Alternative
    Medicine
1629 K Street, NW
Suite 402
Washington, DC 20006
(202) 463-4900 (ph)
(202) 463-4947 (fax)
Founded by Berkley Bedell

United Plant Savers (UpS)
P.O. Box 98
East Barre, VT 05649
(802) 479-9825 (ph)
(802) 476-3722 (fax)
info@plantsavers.org
www.plantsavers.org
United Plant Savers is a nonprofit
grassroots membership organization
whose mission is to conserve and
restore native medicinal plants of the
United States and Canada and their
native habitats while ensuring an
abundant renewable supply of
medicinal plants for generations to
come. Their book, *Planting the
Future*, is available from Healing Arts
Press.

ALSO OF INTEREST

Eclectic Medical Publications
Eclectic Institute
36350 Industrial Way
Sandy, OR 97055
(800) 865-1487

Lloydiana
Lloyd Library and Museum
917 Plum Street
Cincinnati, OH 45202
A publication of the Eclectic Lloyd
Library in Cincinnati. Also a source
of books.

Dr. Andrew Weil's Self-Healing
    Newsletter
Thorne Communications
42 Pleasant Street
Watertown, MA 02472
(800) 523-3296
www.drweil.com

SCIENTIFIC ARTICLES RELATING TO HOXSEY REMEDIES

(These do not include nutritional, dietary, and psychoneuroimmunology citations from chapter 14).

Abe N., Ebina T., and Ishida N., "Interferon induction by glycyrrhizin and glycyrrhetinic acid in mice," *Microbiology and Immunology*, Vol. 26, No. 6, 1982, pp. 535–39.

Adolf W., and Hecker E., "New irritant diterpene-esters from roots of *Stillingia sylvatica* L. (Euphorbiaceae)," *Tetrahedron Letters*, Vol. 21, 1980, pp. 2887–90.

American Cancer Society, "Cancer Statistics, 1990," chapter: "Unproven Methods of Cancer Management: HoxseyMethod/Bio Medical Center," *CA: A Cancer Journal for Clinicians*, Vol. 40, No. 1, Jan/Feb 1990, pp. 51–55.

Amin A.H., Subbaiah T.V., and Abrasi K.M., "Berberine sulfate: antimicrobial activity, bioassay, and mode of action," *Cancer Journal of Microbiology*, Vol. 15, 1969, pp. 1067–76.

Arase Y.K., Ikeda N., et al., "The long-term efficacy of Glycyrrhizin in chronic hepatitis C patients," *Cancer*, Vol. 79, 1997, pp. 1494–1500.

Austin S., Baumgartner E., DeKadt D., and DeKadt S., "Long-term follow-up of cancer patients using Contreras, Hoxsey and Gerson therapies," *Journal of Naturopathic Medicine*, Vol. 5, No. 1, 1994, pp. 74–76.

Bannister B., Ginsburg R., and Shneerson J., "Cardiac arrest due to liquorice-induced hypokalaemia," *British Medical Journal*, 9.17.77.

Barker B.E., Farnes P.P., and Fanger H., "Mitogenic activity in *Phytolacca americana* (pokeweed)," *Lancet*, Vol. 1, 1.16.65, p. 170.

Barker B.E., Farnes P.P., and LaMarche P.H., "Peripheral blood plasmacytosis following systemic exposure to *Phytolacca americana* (pokeweed)," *Pediatrics*, Vol. 38, No. 3, 1966, pp. 490–93.

Barnes S., "Evolution of the health benefits of soy isoflavones," *Journal of the Society for Experimental Biology and Medicine*, Vol. 217, 1998, pp. 386–92.

Belkin M., Hardy W.G., Perrault A., and Sato H., "Swelling and vacuolization induced in ascites tumor cells by polysaccharides from higher plants," *Cancer Research*, Vol. 19, 1959, pp. 1050–62.

Bickoff E.M., Livingston A.L., Hendrickson A.P., and Booth A.N., "Relative potencies of several estrogen-like compounds found in forages," *Agriculture, Food and Chemistry*, Vol. 10, No. 5, 1962, pp. 410–12.

Bond E.E., "What's in the Hoxsey treatment?" National Health Federation Reprint 4H, c. 1953.

Brinker F., "The Hoxsey treatment: Cancer quackery or effective physiological adjuvant?" *Journal of Naturopathic Medicine*, Vol. 6, No. 1, 8.15.96, pp. 9–23.

Brinker F., "Periscope: Phytolacca," *The Eclectic Medical Journals*, Vol. 2, No. 5, Oct/Nov 1996, pp. 2–5.

Brinker F., "Periscope: Podophyllum and Podophyllin," *The Eclectic Medical Journals*, Vol. 2, No. 2, April/May 1996, pp. 2–5.

Brinker F., "The role of botanical medicine in 100 years of naturopathy," *HerbalGram*, No. 42, Spring 1998, pp. 49–59.

Brown D., "Herbal research review: Use of Chinese herbal combination with HIV-infected patients," *Quarterly Review of Natural Medicine*, Winter 1996, pp. 245–46.

Bryan A., "Clinical observations in treatment of chronic swellings with topical injections of potassium iodide," *The North American Veterinarian*, Vol. 7, No. 11, pp. 23–24.

Bryan A., "Therapeutic indications for potassium iodide," *Veterinary Medicine*, Vol. 25, No. 4, pp. 144–51.

Burack J.H., Cohen M.R., Hahn J.A., and Abrams D.I., "Pilot randomized controlled trial of Chinese herbal treatment for HIV-associated symptoms," *Journal of Acquired Immune Deficiency Syndrome and Human Retrovirology*, Vol. 12, No. 4, 1996, pp. 386–93.

Cheng E., Story C.D., Yoder L., Hale W.H., and Burroughs W., "Estrogenic activity of isoflavone derivatives extracted and prepared from soybean oil meal," *Science*, Vol. 118, 1953, pp. 164–65.

Cordell G.A., and Farnsworth N.R., "Experimental antitumor agents from plants, 1974–76," *Lloydia*, Vol. 40, No. 1, 1977, pp. 1–44.

Craig W.J., "Phytochemicals: Guardians of our health," *Journal of the American Dietetic Association*, Vol. 97 (suppl 2), 1997, pp. S199–S204.

Crombie L., "Amides of vegetable origin. Part III. Structure and stereochemistry of neoherculin." *Journal of the Chemical Society*, 1955, pp. 995–98.

D'Adamo P., "*Chelidonium* and *Sanguineria* alkaloids as anti-HIV therapy," *Journal of Naturopathic Medicine*, Vol. 3, No. 1, 1992, pp. 31–34.

Davis W.H., "Art. XLVIII: On the effects of *phytolacca decandra* on the glands," *Eclectic Medical Journal*, Vol. 36, 1876, pp. 259–60.

Dedio W., "Variation in estrogenic-like substances in red clover and alfalfa as related to environment, varieties and stage of growth," Diss. Abstracts, Int. B, 34, Vol. 11, 1974, pp. 5281–82.

Doll R., Hill I.D., Hutton C., and Underwood K.J., "Clinical trial of a triterpenoid liquorice compound in gastric and duodenal ulcer," *Lancet*, 10.20.62, pp. 793–96.

Dombrádi C.A., and Földeák S., "Screening report on the antitumor activity of purified *Arctium lappa* extracts," *Tumor*, Vol. 52, 1966, pp. 173–76.

Downing H.J., Kemp G.C.M., and Denborough M.A. "Plant agglutinins and mitosis," *Nature*, Vol. 2317, 1968, pp. 654–55.

Duke J., "The Herbal Shotgun Shell," *HerbalGram*, No. 18/19, Fall 1988/Winter 1989, pp. 12–13.

Durkee J.B., "Theory and application of the Hoxsey method of treating cancer," speech to National Medical Society, *Journal of the National Medical Society*, 10.17.47.

Dwivedi S.P.D., Pandey V.B., Shah A.H., and Rao Y.B., "Chemical constituents of *Rhamnus procumbens* and pharmacological actions of emodin," *Phytotherapy Research*, Vol. 2, No. 1, 1988, pp. 51–53.

Early R., "Hoxsey Therapy," unpublished, 12.12.94.

Editorial, "*Phytolacca* in carcinoma," *Eclectic Medical Journal*, Vol. 56, No. 1, January 1896, pp. 335–36.

Fackelman K., "Blocking breast cancer: Do faulty estrogen receptors make a meaner, tougher tumor?" *Science News*, Vol. 137, No. 19, 5.12.90, pp. 296–97.

Fairbairn J.W., "The active constituents of the vegetable purgatives containing anthracene derivatives," *Journal of Pharmacy and Pharmacology*, Vol. 1, 1949, pp. 683–92.

Farnes P., Barker B.E., Brownhill L.E., et al., "Mitogenic activity in *Phytolacca americana* (pokeweed), *Lancet*, Vol. 2, 11.21.64, pp. 1100–01.

Fish F., Gray A.I., Waterman P.G., and Donachie F., "Alkaloids and coumarins from North American *Zanthoxylum* species," *Lloydia*, Vol. 38, 1975, pp. 268–70.

Fish F., and Waterman P.G., "Alkaloids in the bark of *Zanthoxylum clava-herculis*," *Journal of Pharmacy and Pharmacology*, Vol. 25 (Suppl.), 1973, pp. 115P–16P.

Fishbein M., "History of cancer quackery," *Perspectives in Biology and Medicine*, Vol. 8, Winter 1965, pp. 139–66.

Földeák S., and Dombrádi G.A., "Tumor-growth inhibiting substances of plant origin. I. Isolation of the active principle of *Arctium lappa*," *Acta Univ. Szeged.*, *Acta Phys. Chem.*, Vol. 10, 1964, pp. 91–93 (*Chemical Abstracts*, Vol. 62, p. 6339c).

Gibson M.R., "*Glycyrrhiza* in old and new perspectives. *Lloydia*, Vol. 41, No. 4, 1978, pp. 349–54.

Guggolz J., Livingston A.L., and Bickoff E.M., "Detection of daidzein, forrnononetin, genistein, and biochanin A in forages," *Agriculture, Food and Chemistry*, Vol. 9, No. 4, 1961, pp. 330–32.

Hartwell J.L., "Plant remedies for cancer," *Cancer Chemotherapy Reports*, No. 6–10, May 1960, pp. 19–24.

Hartwell J.L., "Plants used against cancer: A survey," *Lloydia*, Vol. 30, 1967, pp. 379–436.

Hartwell J.L., "Plants used against cancer (index to series of installments published 1967–1971)," *Lloydia*, Vol. 34, 1971, pp. 427–28.

Hoerhammer L., Wagner H., and Hoerhammer H.P., "New methods in pharmacognostical education. XIII. Thin-layer chromatography of components of *Rhamnus* cortical drugs and their preparation," *Deut. Apoth.-Ztg.*, Vol. 107, No. 17, 1967, pp. 563–66 (*Chemical Asbtracts*, Vol. 67, p. 84920u).

Hoshi A., Ikekawa T., Ikeda Y., et al., "Antitumor activity of berberrubine derivatives," *Gann.*, Vol. 67, 1976, pp. 321–25.

Hudson T., "Escharotic treatment for cervical dysplasia and carcinoma," letter to the editor, *Journal of Naturopathic Medicine*, Vol. 4, No. 1, 1993, p. 23.

Ikram M., "A review on the chemical and pharmacological aspects of genus *Berberis*," *Planta Medicine*, Vol. 28, 1975, pp. 353–58.

Ingram D., Sanders K., Kolybaba M., and Lopez D., "Case control study of phytoestrogens and breast cancer," *Lancet*, 1997, Vol. 350, pp. 990–94.

Jacobson M., "The structure of echinacein, the insecticidal component of American coneflower roots," *Journal of Organic Chemistry*, Vol. 32, 1967, pp. 1646–47.

Kalish R.S., Wood J.A., Siegel D.M., Kaye V.N., and Brooks N.A., "Experimental rationale for treatment of high-risk human melanoma with zinc chloride fixative paste," *Dermatology and Surgery*, Vol. 24, No. 9, pp. 1021–25.

Kapuler A.M., and Gurusiddiah S., "Carrots, peas, apios and others," Vol. 4 of "The twenty protein amino acids are primary human food: a food system with nonviolent roots," *Peace Seeds Research Journal*, Vol. 7, 1994, pp. 66–74.

Kapuler A.M., and Gurusiddiah S., "More results of free amino acids in vegetables and medicinal herbs," Vol. 3, "The twenty protein amino acids are primary human food: a food system with nonviolent roots," *Peace Seeds Research Journal*, Vol. 6, 1991, pp. 9–17.

Kaufman P.B., Duke J.A., Brielman H., Boik J., and Hoyt J.E., "A comparative survey of leguminous plants as sources of the isoflavones genistein and daidzein: Implications for human nutrition and health," *Journal of Alternative and Complementary Medicine*, Vol. 3., No. 1, 1997, pp. 7–12.

Kennedy A., "The Evidence for soybean products as cancer preventive agents," *Journal of Nutrition*, 1995, pp. 125, 733.

Kitagawa K., Nishino H., and Iwashima A., "Inhibition of the specific binding of 12-O-tetradeconoylphorbol-13-acetate to mouse epidermal membrane fractions by glycyrrhetic acid," *Oncology*, Vol. 43, 1986, pp. 127–30.

Kumagai A., Nishino K., Shimomura A., Kin T., and Yamamura Y., "Effect of glycyrrhizin on estrogen action," *Endocrinologica Japonica*, Vol. 14, No. 1, 1967, pp. 344–48.

Kumazawa Y., Itagaki A., Fukumoto M., Fujisawa H., and Nishimura C., "Activation of peritoneal macrophages by berberine-type alkaloids in terms of induction of cytostatic activity," *International Journal of Immunopharmacology*, Vol. 6, No. 6, 1984, pp. 587–92.

Kupchan M.S., "Recent advances in the chemistry of tumor inhibitors of plant origin," Swain, T. (ed.), *Plants in the Development of Modern Medicine* (Cambridge, MA, and London: Harvard University Press, 1972), pp. 261–78.

Kupchan M.S., and Karim A., "Tumor inhibitors. 114. Aloe emodin: Antileukemic principle isolated from *Rhamnus frangula* L.," *Lloydia*, Vol. 39, No. 4, 1976, pp. 223–24.

Lish P.M., and Dungan K.W., "Peristaltic-stimulating and fecal-hydrating properties of dioctyl sodium sulfosuccinate, danthron, and cascara extracts in the mouse and rat," *Journal of the American Pharmaceutical Association*, Vol. 47, 1958, pp. 371–75.

Lloyd J.U., "History and names of *Rhamnus purshiana* (cascara sagrada)," *American Journal of Pharmacy*, Sept 1896, pp. 467–69.

Martin P.M., Horwitz K.B., Ryan D.S., and McGuire W.L., "Phytoestrogen interaction with estrogen receptors in human breast cancer cells," *Endocrinology*, Vol. 103, No. 5, 1978, pp. 1860–67.

Mary N.Y., Christensen B.V., and Beal J.L., "A paper chromatographic study of aloe, aloin and of cascara sagrada," *Journal of the American Pharmaceutical Association*, Vol. 45, 1956, pp. 229–32.

McKenna G.F., and Taylor A., "Screening plant extracts for anticancer activity," *Texas Reports in Biological Medicine*, Vol. 20, 1962, pp. 214–20.

Millard F.R., "Some of the uses of *Phytolacca decandra*," *Medical and Surgical Reporter*, Vol. 75, 1896, pp. 420–22.

Mitscher L.A., Park Y.H., Clark D., and Clark G.W. III, "Antimicrobial agents from higher plants: An investigation of *Hunnemannia fumariaefolia* pseudoalcoholates of sanguineriane and chelerythrine," *Lloydia*, Vol. 41, 1978, pp. 145–49.

Mohs F.E., "Chemosurgery: A microscopically controlled method of cancer excision," *Archives of Surgery*, Vol. 42, 1941, pp. 279–95.

Mohs F.E., "Chemosurgery for Facial Neoplasms," *Archives of Otolaryngitis*, Vol. 95, 1972.

Mohs F.E., "Chemosurgery: microscopically controlled surgery for skin cancer—past, present and future," *Archives of Dermatology*, Vol. 4, 1978, pp. 41–54.

Mohs F.E., "Chemosurgical treatment of cancer of the skin: A microscopically controlled method of excision," *JAMA*, Vol. 138, 11.23.48., pp. 564–69.

Morita K., Kada T., and Namiki M., "A desmutagenic factor isolated from burdock *(Arctium lappa Linne),*" *Mutation Research*, Vol. 129, 1984, pp. 25–31.

Morita K., Nishijima Y., and Kada T., "Chemical nature of a desmutagenic factor from burdock *(Arctium lappa Linne),*" *Agriculture, Biology and Chemistry*, Vol. 49, No. 4, 1985, pp. 925–32.

Nishino H., Kitagawa K., and Iwashima A., "Antitumor-promoting activity of glycyrrhetic acid in mouse skin tumor formation induced by 7,12–dimethylbenz[a]anthracene," *Carcinogenesis*, Vol. 5, No. 11, 1984, pp. 1529–30.

Owen, Tsung-Yao, Wang, et al., "A new antitumor substance—Lycobetaine," *K'o Hsueh Tung Pao*, Vol. 21, No. 6, 1976, pp. 285–87.

Phelan, Milgrom, Halina, et al., "The use of Mohs' chemosurgery technique in the management of superficial cancers," *Surgery, Gynecology and Obstetrics*, Vol. 114, 1962, pp. 25–30.

Phelan J.T., and Juardo J., "Chemosurgical management of carcinoma of the nose," *Surgery*, Vol. 53, 1963a (March), pp. 310–14.

Phelan J.T., and Juardo J., "Chemosurgical management of carcinoma of the external ear," *Surgery, Gynecology and Obstetrics*, Vol. 117, 1963b (Aug), pp. 244–46.

Rao K.V., and Davies R., "The ichthyotoxic principles of *Zanthoxylum clava-herculis*," *Journal of Natural Products*, Vol. 49, No. 2, 1986, pp. 340–42.

Reiners W., "7–Hydroxy–4'–methoxy–isoflavon (formononetin) aus sussholzwurzel. Uber inhaltsstoffe der sussholzwurzel," II. *Experientia*, Vol. 22, 1966, p. 359.

Reinherz E.L., Kung P.C., Goldstein G., and Schlossman S.F., "Further characterization of the human inducer T cell subset defined by monoclonal antibody," *Journal of Immunology*, Vol. 123, No. 6, 1979, pp. 2894–96.

Reisch J., Spitzner W., and Schulte K., "The problem of the microbiological activity of simple acetylene compounds," *Arzneimittel Forschung*, Vol. 17, 1967, pp. 816–25.

Ruggieri R., "Application of the potentiometric method in a water-free medium for the determination of anthaquinone derivatives in drugs," *Boll. chim. farm.* Vol. 96, 1957, pp. 491–94 (*Chemical Abstracts*, Vol. 55, p. 5874e).

Schmitz H., "The influence of berberine on cellular metabolism," *Z. Krebsforschung*, Vol. 57, 1950, pp. 137–41 (*Chemical Abstracts*, Vol. 46, p. 4680i).

Schulte K.E., Rucker G., and Boehme R., "Polyacetylenes as compounds of the roots of burdock," *Arzneimittel Forschung*, Vol. 17, No. 7, 1967, pp. 829–33.

Shutt D.A., "The effects of plant estrogens on animal reproduction," *Endeavor*, Vol. 35, 1976, pp. 110–13.

Shvarev I.F., and Tsetlin A.L., "Antiblastic properties of berberine and its derivatives," *Mater. Vses. Konf. Issled. Lek. Rast. Perspekt. Ikh Ispol'z. Proizvod. Lek. Prepp.*, 1972, p. 245 (*Chemical Abstracts*, Vol. 83, p. 674m).

Spaulding-Albright N., "A review of some herbal and related products commonly used in cancer patients," *Journal of the American Dietetic Association*, Vol. 97, No. 10, 1997, pp. S208–S215.

Spjut R.W., and Perdue R.E. Jr., "Plant folklore: A tool for predicting sources of antitumor activity?" *Cancer Treatment Reports*, Vol. 60, No. 8, 1976, pp. 979–85.

Stephens F., Phytoestrogens and prostate cancer: Possible preventive role," *Medical Journal of Australia*, Vol. 167, 8.4.97, pp. 138–39.

Stermitz F.R., Larson K.A., and Kim D.K., "Some structural relationships among cytotoxic and antitumor benzophenanthridine alkaloid derivatives," *Journal of Medical Chemistry*, Vol. 16, No. 8, 1973, pp. 939–40.

Stout G.H., Malofsky A., and Stout V.F. "Phytolaccagenin: a light atom x-ray structure proof using chemical information," *Journal of the American Chemistry Society*, Vol. 86, 1964, pp. 957–58.

Suess T.R., Stermitz F.R., "Alkaloids of *Mahonia repens* with a brief review of previous work in the genus *Mahonia*," *Journal of Natural Products*, Vol. 44, 1981, pp. 680–87.

Tamura Y., Nishikawa T., Yamada K., Yamamoto M., and Kumagai A., "Effects of glycyrrhetinic acid and its derivatives on D4-5a- and 5b-reductase in rat liver," *Arzneimittel Forschung*, Vol. 29, 1979, pp. 647–49.

Tangri K.K., Seth P.K., Parmar S.S., and Bhargava K.P., "Biochemical study of anti-inflammatory and anti-arthritic properties of glycyrrhetic acid," *Biochemical Pharmacology*, Vol. 14, 1965, pp. 1277–81.

Taylor A., McKenna G.F., and Burlage H.M., "Anticancer activity of plant extracts," *Texas Reports in Biological Medicine*, Vol. 14, 1956, pp. 538–56.

Tin-Wa M., Farnsworth N.R., Fong H.H.S., and Trojanek J., "Biological and phytochemical evaluation of plants. VII. Isolation of a new alkaloid from *Sanguinaria canadensis*," *Lloydia*, Vol. 33, No. 2, 1970, pp. 267–69.

Tin-Wa M., Fong H.H.S., Abraham D.J., Trojanek J., and Farnsworth N.R., "Structure of sanguidimerine, a new major alkaloid from *Sanguinaria canadensis* (Papaveraceae)," *Journal of Pharmacological Science*, Vol. 61, No. 11, 1972, pp. 1846–47.

Turova A.D., Konovalov M.N., and Leskov A.I, "Berberine, an effective cholagogue," *Med. Prom. SSSR*, Vol. 18, No. 6, 1964, pp. 59–60 (*Chemical Abstracts*, Vol. 61, p. 15242f).

Tyson R.M., Shrader E.A., and Perlman H.H., "Drugs transmitted through breast milk," *Journal of Pediatrics*, Vol. 11, 1937, pp. 824–32.

Uckun F.M., Chelstrom L.M., Tuel-Ahlgren L., et al., "Txu (Anti CD7): Pokeweed antiviral protein as a potent inhibitor of Human Immunodeficiency Virus," *Antimicrobial Agents and Chemotherapy*, Vol. 42, No. 2, 1998, pp. 383–88.

Velluda C.C., Goina T., Ticsa I., et al., "Effect of *Berberis vulgaris* extract and of the berberine, berbamine, and oxyacanthine alkaloids on liver and bile function," *Lucr. prez. conf. natl. farm.*, Bucharest, 1958, pp. 351–54 (*Chemical Abstracts*, Vol. 53, p. 15345a).

Vichkanova S.A., Rubinchik M.A., Adgina V.V., and Fedorchenko T.S., "Chemotherapeutic action of sanguinarine," *Farmakol. Toksikol.* (Moscow), Vol. 32, 1969, pp. 325–28 (*Chemical Abstracts*, Vol. 71, p. 59405e).

Vincent D., and Segonzac G., "Higher plants having antibiotic properties," *Toulouse med.*, Vol. 49, 1948, pp. 669 (*Chemical Abstracts*, Vol. 44, p. 10046i).

Wahlqvist M., and Dalais F., "Phytoestrogens: Emerging multifaceted plant compounds," *Medical Journal of Australia*, Vol. 167, 8.4.97, p. 119.

Ward P.S., "History of the Hoxsey treatment," 1987 contract report to the Office of Technology Assessment's *Unconventional Cancer Treatments*, 1990 (GPO #052-003-01203-3), pp. 75–80, 1987, republished in *Townsend Letter for Doctors and Patients*, May 1997, pp. 68–72.

Wash L.K., and Bernard J.D., "Licorice-induced pseudoaldosteronism," *American Journal of Hospital Pharmacy*, Vol. 32, No.1, 1975, pp. 73–74.

Waxdal M.J., "Isolation, characterization, and biological activities of five mitogens from pokeweed," *Biochemistry*, Vol. 13, No. 18, 1974, pp. 3671–77.

Wolf S., and Mack M., "Experimental study of the action of bitters on the stomach of a fistulous human subject," *Drug Standards*, Vol. 24, No. 3, 1956, pp. 98–101.

Yokoyama K., Yano O., Terao T., and Osawa T., "Purification and biological activities of pokeweed *(Phytolacca americana)* mitogens," *Biochem. Biophys. Acta*, Vol. 427, 1976, pp. 443–52.

Youngken H.W., and Vander Wyk R.W., "Studies of National Formulary drugs," *Journal of the American Pharmaceutical Association*, Vol. 28, 1939, pp. 17–31.

Zava D.T., Dollbaum C.M., and Blen M., "Estrogen and progestin bioactivity of foods, herbs and spices," *Proceedings of the Society for Experimental Biology and Medicine*, Vol. 217, 1998, pp. 369–78.

Some of the most promising and exciting work relating to anticancer natural products, barely mentioned in this book, is in the field of mycology—medicinal mushrooms. For an introductory overview, see:

Stamets P., and Wu Yao D., "Mycomedicinals: Information on Medicinal Mushrooms," *Townsend Letter for Doctors and Patients*, June 1998, pp. 152–69.

BOOKS

Boyle, W., *Official Herbs: Botanical Substances in the United States Pharmacopoeias 1820–1990* (East Palestine, OH: Buckeye Naturopathic Press, 1991).

Brinker, F. *Formulas for Healthful Living* (Sandy, OR: Eclectic Medical Publications, 1998).

Cancer Salves: A Botanical Approach to Treatment (Santa Fe, NM: Seventh Ray Press, and Berkeley, CA: North Atlantic Books, 1998).

Committee on National Formulary, *National Formulary*, 5th ed., (Washington, D.C.: American Pharmaceutical Association, 1926).

Committee on National Formulary, *National Formulary*, 6th ed., (Washington, D.C.: American Pharmaceutical Association, 1935).

Davis, G.S. *Organic Materia Medica*, 2nd ed. (Detroit, MI: Parke, Davis & Co., 1890).

Duke, J.A. *The Green Pharmacy* (Emmaus, PA: Rodale Press, 1997).

Duke, J.A. *CRC Handbook of Medicinal Herbs* (Boca Raton, FL: CRC Press, 1985).

Duke, J.A. *CRC Handbook of Phytochemical Constituents in GRAS Herbs and Other Economic Plants* (Boca Raton, FL: CRC Press, 1992).

Duke, J.A. *CRC Handbook of Biologically Active Phytochemicals and Their Activities* (Boca Raton, FL: CRC Press, 1992).

Felter, H.W. *The Eclectic Materia Medica, Pharmacology and Therapeutics* (Cincinnati, OH: John K. Scudder, 1922).

Felter, H.W., and Lloyd, J.U. *King's American Dispensatory*, 18th ed., 3rd rev., 1898 (Portland, OR: reprinted by Eclectic Medical Publications, 1983).

Grieve, M. *A Modern Herbal* (New York: Harcourt, Brace & Co., 1931, reprinted by Dover Publishers. Inc., New York, 1971).

Hartwell, J.L. *Plants Used against Cancer: A Survey* (Lawrence, MA: Quarterman, 1982).

Jones, E. *Cancer: Its Causes, Symptoms and Treatment* (Boston: Therapeutic Publishing Co., Inc., 1911).

Jones, E. *Cancer: Tumors and Malignant Growths Both External and Internal Permanently Cured without a Surgical Operation* (New Brunswick, 1905).

Jones, E. *Definite Medication*, 1910 (reprinted by: Jain Publishing Co., New Delhi, India, no date).

McDonald, J. *Physiologic Medication* (Chicago: Armstrong Publishing, 1900).

Mohs, F.E. *Chemosurgery: Microscopically Controlled Surgery for Skin Cancer* (Springfield, IL: Charles C. Thomas, 1978).

Mohs, F.E. *Chemotherapy in Cancer, Gangrene, and Infections* (Springfield, IL: Charles C. Thomas, 1956).

Nichols, P. *The Value of Escharotic Medicines* (Savannah, MO: Dr. Nichols Sanitorium, 1949).

Office of Technology Assessment. *Unconventional Cancer Treatments*, Chap. 4, "Herbal Treatments," pp. 69–87 (Washington, D.C.: Congress of the United States, 1990).

Taber, C.W. *Taber's Cyclopedic Medical Dictionary*, 17th ed. (F.A Davis Company, 1993).

Tyler, V. "Hazards of Herbal Medicine," in Stalker and Glymour, *Examining Holistic Medicine* (Buffalo, NY: Prometheus Books, 1985).

Tyler, V. *The New Honest Herbal: A Sensible Guide to Herbs and Related Remedies* (Philadelphia: George F. Stickley and Co., 1987).

Selected Bibliography

Ausubel, Kenny. "Cancer 'Cures'—An Outbreak of Controversy: The Silent Treatments." *New Age Journal*, September 10, 1989.

———. "The Troubling Case of Harry Hoxsey." *New Age Journal*, July/August 1998.

Bailey, Herbert. *Krebiozen: Key to Cancer?* New York: Hermitage House, 1955.

———. *A Matter of Life or Death: The Incredible Story of Krebiozen.* 2d ed. New York: Macfadden-Bartell, 1964.

Bealle, Morris A. *The Drug Story.* 2d ed. Spanish Fork, Utah: The Hornet's Nest, 1976.

Bird, Christopher. *The Galileo of the Microscope. The Life and Trials of Gaston Naessens.* Quebec: Les Presses de l'Université de la Personne, Inc., 1990.

Blumenthal, Mark, ed. *The Complete German Commission E Monographs: Therapeutic Guide to Herbal Medicines.* Boston: Integrative Medicine Publications, 1998.

Broad, William, and Nicholas Wade. *Betrayers of the Truth: Fraud and Deceit in the Halls of Science.* New York: Simon and Schuster, 1982.

Chowka, Peter Barry. "Herbal Healing: A Cancer Alternative With a Record." *New Age*, December 1980.

———. "Does Mildred Nelson Have an Herbal Cure for Cancer?" *Whole Life Times*, January/February 1984.

Coulter, Harris L. *Divided Legacy: The Conflict between Homeopathy and the American Medical Association: Science and Ethics in American Medicine: 1800–1914.* Berkeley, CA: North Atlantic Books, 1973.

Cousins, Norman. *Head First: The Biology of Hope and the Healing Power of the Human Spirit.* New York: Penguin, 1989.

———. *Human Options: An Autobiographical Notebook.* New York: W.W. Norton, 1981.

Dossey, Larry. *Healing Words: The Power of Prayer and the Practice of Medicine.* San Francisco: HarperCollins, 1993.

———. *Reinventing Medicine: Beyond Mind-Body to a New Era of Healing.* San Francisco: HarperCollins, 1999.

Duke, James A. *The Green Pharmacy.* Emmaus, PA: Rodale Press, 1997.

———. *CRC Handbook of Medicinal Herbs.* Boca Raton, FL: CRC Press, Inc., 1985.

443

————. *CRC Handbook of Phytochemical Constituents in GRAS Herbs and Other Economic Plants.* Boca Raton, FL: CRC Press, 1992.

————. *CRC Handbook of Biologically Active Phytochemicals and Their Activities.* Boca Raton, FL: CRC Press, 1992.

Gaynor, Mitchell L., and Jerry Hickey. *Dr. Gaynor's Cancer Prevention Program.* New York: Kensington Books, 1999.

Gerson, Max. *A Cancer Therapy: Results of Fifty Cases and the Cure of Advanced Cancer by Diet Therapy.* 2nd. ed. Edited by Gar Hildenbrand. Bonita, CA: Gerson Institute.

Gladstar, Rosemary, ed. *Planting the Future: Saving Our Medicinal Herbs.* Rochester, VT: Healing Arts Press, 2000.

Griffin, Edward G. *World Without Cancer: The Story of Vitamin B17.* Westlake Village, CA: American Media, 1974.

Griggs, Barbara. *Green Pharmacy: The History and Evolution of Western Herbal Medicine.* Rochester, VT: Healing Arts Press, 1981.

Hall, Stephen S. *A Commotion in the Blood: Life, Death, and the Immune System.* New York: Henry Holt and Co., 1997.

Heinerman, John. *The Treatment of Cancer With Herbs.* Orem, UT: Biworld Publishers, 1980.

Hess, David J. *Can Bacteria Cause Cancer? Alternative Medicine Confronts Big Science.* New York: New York University Press, 1997.

Hirshberg, Caryle, and Marc Barasch. *Remarkable Recovery.* New York: Riverhead Books, 1995.

Houston, Robert G. *Repression and Reform in the Evaluation of Alternative Cancer Therapies.* Washington, D.C.: Project Cure, Inc., 1987.

Hoxsey, Harry. *You Don't Have to Die.* New York: Milestone Books, 1956.

Kloss, Jethro. *Back to Eden.* 2nd. ed. Santa Barbara, CA: Woodbridge Press, 1972.

Kreig, Margaret B. *Green Medicine: The Search for Plants That Heal.* Chicago: Rand McNally & Co., 1964.

Illich, Ivan. *Medical Nemesis: The Expropriation of Health.* New York: Pantheon, 1976.

Levenson, Frederick B. *The Causes and Prevention of Cancer.* New York: Stein and Day, 1985.

Lewis, Walter H., Elvin Lewis, and P.F. Memory. *Medical Botany: Plants Affecting Man's Health.* New York: John Wiley & Sons, 1977.

Livingston-Wheeler, Virginia, and Edmond G. Addeo. *The Conquest of Cancer: Vaccines and Diet.* New York: Franklin Watts, 1984.

Lynes, Barry, with John Crane. *The Cancer Cure That Worked: Fifty Years of Suppression.* Toronto: Marcus Books, 1987.

Mendelsohn, Robert S. *Confessions of a Medical Heretic.* New York: Warner Books, 1979.

Mohkiber, Russell, and Robert Weissman. *Corporate Predators: The Hunt for Mega-Profits and the Attack on Democracy.* Monroe, Maine: Common Courage Press, 1999.

Morris, Nat. *The Cancer Blackout Amended: A History of Denied and Suppressed Remedies 1762–1976.* Los Angeles: Regent House, 1976.

Moss, Ralph W. *The Cancer Industry.* Brooklyn, NY: Equinox Press, 1996.

———. *Cancer Therapy: The Independent Consumer's Guide to Non-Toxic Treatment & Prevention.* Brooklyn, NY: Equinox Press, 1997.

———. *Questioning Chemotherapy.* Brooklyn, NY: Equinox Press, 1995.

———. *Herbs Against Cancer.* Brooklyn, NY: Equinox Press, 1998.

Naiman, Ingrid. *Cancer Salves: A Botanical Approach to Treatment.* Berkeley, CA: North Atlantic Books, 1999.

Natenberg, Maurice. *The Legacy of Doctor Wiley and the Administration of His Food and Drug Act.* Chicago: Regent House, 1957.

Proctor, Robert N. *Cancer Wars: How Politics Shapes What We Know and Don't Know About Cancer.* New York: Basic Books, 1995.

——— *The Nazi War on Cancer.* Princeton, NJ: Princeton University Press, 1999.

Robbins, John. *Reclaiming Our Health: Exploding the Medical Myth and Embracing the Source of True Healing.* Tiburon, CA: H. J. Kramer, 1996.

Sasuly, Richard. *I.G. Farben.* New York: Boni & Gaer, 1947.

Siegel, Bernie. *Love, Medicine and Miracles.* New York: HarperCollins, 1990.

Starr, Paul. *The Social Transformation of American Medicine, the Rise of a Sovereign Profession and the Making of a Vast Industry.* New York: Basic Books, 1982.

Teitelman, Robert. *Profits of Science: The American Marriage of Business and Technology.* New York: Basic Books, 1994.

Tyler, Varro E. "Some Potentially Useful Drugs Identified in a Study of Indiana Folk Medicine." In *Folklore and Folk Medicines*, edited by John Scarborough. Madison, WI: American Institute of the History of Pharmacy, 1987.

Weil, Andrew. *Spontaneous Healing.* New York: Ballantine, 1995.

Wiley, Harvey W. *The History of a Crime Against the Food Law.* Milwaukee, WI: Lee Foundation for Nutritional Research, 1955.

Wolinsky, Howard, and Tom Brune. *The Serpent on the Staff: The Unhealthy Politics of the American Medical Association.* New York: G.P. Putnam's Sons, 1994.

Young, James Harvey. *The Medical Messiahs: A Social History of Health Quackery in Twentieth-Century America.* Princeton, NJ: Princeton University Press, 1967.

Resources

The following resources in no way indicate a recommendation or endorsement. Any person facing cancer should consult with his or her doctor and other qualified medical practitioners. Because comprehensive resources in this field are amply offered elsewhere, this book mainly refers the reader to consult those for further information.

VIDEO

Hoxsey: How Healing Becomes a Crime

The award-winning feature documentary film produced by Kenny Ausubel and Catherine Salveson. "First-rate reportage whose true subject is greed and money as they have shaped medical politics." Vincent Canby, *New York Times*; 83 min.

available from:

Winstar TV & Video
(800) 283-6374
www.wellmedia.com
$24.98, plus shipping and handling
Item #E7359

Hope and a Prayer: Attitudinal Healing with Dr. Bernie Siegel

30-minute video

This rousing half-hour with Dr. Bernie Siegel provides an excellent resource for patients facing serious illness, with tips on how survivors do it and perspectives on the vital healing role of hope and a positive attitude.

available from:

Placebo Productions
c/o CHI
901 W. San Mateo Road
Suite L
Santa Fe, NM 87505
$19.95

ALSO BY KENNY AUSUBEL

Restoring the Earth: Visionary Solutions from the Bioneers (Tiburon, CA: HJ Kramer, 1997).

Kenny Ausubel's book on "biological pioneers" who use nature to heal nature. The book recounts the compelling stories of visionary innovators who, operating by a biological model of interconnectedness, have achieved significant environmental and social restoration. Also includes stories of botanical bioneers engaged in Green Medicine.

The Bioneers Conference

A highly acclaimed annual gathering of environmental visionaries, the Bioneers Conference was founded by Kenny Ausubel in 1990 to bring both practical and visionary environmental solutions to wider awareness. The conference has a very strong program each year on Green Medicine and herbs, among many other topics. For information contact:

Bioneers Conference
901 W. San Mateo Road
Suite L
Santa Fe, NM 87505
1-877-BIONEER (1-877-246-6337)
www.bioneers.org
kenny@bioneers.org

ALTERNATIVE CANCER CLINIC GUIDEBOOKS

For a comprehensive overview of treatment centers offering alternative and unconventional cancer therapies, there are three excellent books that provide detailed listings of numerous clinics worldwide:

Ralph W. Moss, *Cancer Therapy: The Independent Consumer's Guide to Non-Toxic Treatment and Prevention*. Brooklyn, NY: Equinox Press, 1992, 1997.

Michael Lerner, *Choices in Healing: Integrating the Best of Conventional and Complementary Approaches to Cancer*. Cambridge, MA: MIT Press, 1994, 1997.

John Fink, *Third Opinion: An International Directory to Alternative Cancer Therapy Centers for the Treatment and Prevention of Cancer*. Garden City Park, NY: Avery Publishing Group, Inc., 1988.

For an extensive list covering activist resources about the politics of cancer, see:

Samuel Epstein, *The Politics of Cancer Revisited*. Fremont Center, NY: East Ridge Press, 1998.

Cancer Prevention Coalition
School of Public Health
University of Illinois Medical Center, Chicago
2121 West Taylor
Chicago, IL 60612
(312) 996-2297
www.preventcancer.com

REFERRAL SERVICES

The following services offer customized referrals for cancer patients seeking information on alternative as well as conventional treatments. Reports are individualized for type of cancer, diagnosis, stage, and other factors. At times they may also provide additional perspectives of assistance to patients and their physicians seeking to make difficult choices.

The Moss Reports
144 St. John's Place
Brooklyn, NY 11217
(718) 636-4433 (ph)
(718) 636-0186 (fax)
mail@ralphmoss.com
www.cancerdecisions.com
Principal contact: Anne Beattie
Founder: Ralph Moss

CanHelp
3111 Paradise Bay Road
Port Ludlow, WA 98365-9771
(206) 437-2291 (ph)
(206) 437-2272 (fax)
www.canhelp.com
Principal contact: Pat McGrady

Alternative Therapy Program
People Against Cancer
P.O. Box 10
Otho, IA 50569
(515) 972-4444 (ph)
(515) 972-4415 (fax)
Principal contact: Frank Wiewel

TREATMENT CENTERS

Bio Medical Center (Tijuana Hoxsey clinic)
P.O. Box 727
3170 Avenida General Ferreira
Col. Juarez
Tijuana, Baja California 22150
Mexico
(011 52 66) 84 90 11 (ph)
(011 52 66) 84 97 44 (fax)
www.hoxsey.com
Mailing address:
P.O. Box 433654
San Ysidro, CA 92143

Motel:
International Motor Inn & RV Park
190 E. Calle Primavera
San Ysidro, CA 92173-2901
(619) 427-4486 (ph)
(619) 428-3618 (fax)
With convenient transportation to
the Bio Medical Center and Mexican
clinics

Burzynski Research Institute
12000 Richmond Avenue, Suite 260
Houston, Texas 77082
(281) 597-0111 (ph)
(281) 597-1166 (fax)

Gerson Therapy
P.O. Box 430
Bonita, CA 91908
(619)585-7600 (ph)
(619) 585-7610 (fax)

Nicholas Gonzalez, M.D.
36 East 36th Street, Suite 204
New York, NY 10016
(212) 213-3337 (ph)
(212) 213-3414 (fax)

Immuno-Augmentative Therapy
   Center
(242) 352-7455 (ph)
(242) 352-3201 (fax)
Write c/o People Against Cancer (see
   address at right)

Livingston Foundation Medical
   Center
3232 Duke Street
San Diego, CA 92110
(619) 224-3515 (ph)
(619) 224-6253 (fax)

EDUCATIONAL GROUPS

Project CURE
Michael S. Evers, Esq., Executive
   Director
16801 Addison Road, Suite 207
Dallas, TX 75248
(972) 732-7960 (ph)
(972) 732-7961 (fax)

People Against Cancer
Frank Wiewel, Director
604 East Street
P.O. Box 10
Otho, IA 50569
(515) 972-4444 (ph)
(515) 972-4415 (fax)
info@PeopleAgainstCancer.com
www.PeopleAgainstCancer.com

Cancer Control Society and Cancer
   Book House
2043 North Berendo Street
Los Angeles, CA 90027
(213) 663-7801

National Foundation for Alternative
   Medicine
1629 K Street, NW
Suite 402
Washington, DC 20006
(202) 463-4900 (ph)
(202) 463-4947 (fax)

SUPPORT GROUPS

Exceptional Cancer Patient Program
Bernie Siegel, M.D., Founder
522 Jackson Park Drive
Meadville, PA 16335
(814) 337-8192 (ph)
(814) 337-0699 (fax)
keb@touchstarpro.com
www.ecap-online.org

Commonweal Cancer Help Program
Michael Lerner, Founder
P.O. Box 316
Bolinas, CA 94924
(415) 868-0970

ALTERNATIVE MEDICINE WEB SITES

University of Texas Center for
  Alternative Medicine Research
www.sph.uth.tmc.edu/utcam/
default.htm

Center for Complementary and
  Alternative Medicine
www.camra.ucdavis.edu

Phytochemical and Ethnobotanical
  Databases
http://ars-grin.gov/duke

U.S. National Institutes of Health
  Office of Alternative Medicine
http://altmed.od.nih.gov

Fact Sheets on Alternative Medicine
http://cpmcnet.columbia.edu/dept/
rosenthal/factsheets.html

National Cancer Institute Office of
  Cancer Survivorship
http://dccps.nci.nih.gov

The Eclectic Physician
www.eclecticphysician.com

HealthWorld Online
www.healthy.net

Dr. Andrew Weil
www.drweil.com

Ingrid Naiman's escharotic salves
www.cancersalves.com

JOURNALS

*Alternative Therapies in Health and
  Medicine*
Larry Dossey, M.D., Executive
  Editor
101 Columbia
Aliso Viejo, CA 92656
(800) 899-1712
alttherapy@aol.com
http://alternative-therapies.com

Integrative Medicine
Andrew Weil, M.D., Editor in Chief
University of Arizona College of
  Medicine
Tucson, AZ
Publisher: Elsevier Science, Inc.
655 Avenue of the Americas
New York, NY 10010-5107
(888) 437-4636
usinfo-f@elsevier.com

The Journal of Naturopathic Medicine
American Association of Naturo-
  pathic Physicians
601 Valley Street
Suite 105
Seattle, WA 98109-4229

Townsend Letter for Doctors and Patients
Jonathan Collin, M.D., Editor in
  Chief
911 Tyler Street
Port Townsend, WA 98368-6541
(360) 385-6021 (ph)
(360) 385-0699 (fax)
www.tldp.com

Index

BOOKS OF RELATED INTEREST

Fighting Cancer with Vitamins and Antioxidants
by Kedar N. Prasad, Ph.D. and K. Che Prasad, M.S., M.D.

The Acid-Alkaline Diet for Optimum Health
Restore Your Health by Creating pH Balance in Your Diet
by Christopher Vasey, N.D.

The New Oxygen Prescription
The Miracle of Oxidative Therapies
by Nathaniel Altman

Natural Therapies for Emphysema and COPD
Relief and Healing for Chronic Pulmonary Disorders
by Robert J. Green Jr., ND, RRT

Nutrition and Mental Illness
An Orthomolecular Approach to Balancing Body Chemistry
by Carl C. Pfeiffer Ph.D., M.D.

Gesundheit!
Bringing Good Health to You, the Medical System, and Society through
Physician Service, Complementary Therapies, Humor, and Joy
by Patch Adams, M.D.
With Maureen Mylander

The High Blood Pressure Solution
A Scientifically Proven Program for Preventing Strokes and Heart Disease
by Richard D. Moore, M.D., Ph.D.

Primal Body, Primal Mind
Beyond the Paleo Diet for Total Health and a Longer Life
by Nora Gedgaudas, CNS, NTP, BCHN

Inner Traditions • Bear & Company
P.O. Box 388
Rochester, VT 05767
1-800-246-8648
www.InnerTraditions.com

Or contact your local bookseller